# THE *NEW* ATKINS

## FOR A NEW YOU

The **ULTIMATE DIET** for **SHEDDING WEIGHT** and **FEELING GREAT**

Dr. Eric C. Westman,
Dr. Stephen D. Phinney,
and Dr. Jeff S. Volek

A TOUCHSTONE BOOK
Published by Simon & Schuster
New York   London   Toronto   Sydney   New Delhi

★ Touchstone
A Division of Simon & Schuster, Inc.
1230 Avenue of the Americas
New York, NY 10020

This publication contains the opinions and ideas of its authors. It is intended to provide helpful and informative material on the subjects addressed in the publication. It is sold with the understanding that the authors and publisher are not engaged in rendering medical, health, or any other kind of personal professional services in the book. The reader should consult his or her medical, health or other competent professional before adopting any of the suggestions in this book or drawing inferences from it.

The authors and publisher specifically disclaim all responsibility for any liability, loss or risk, personal or otherwise, which is incurred as a consequence, directly or indirectly, of the use and application of any of the contents of this book.

First Touchstone trade paperback edition March 2010

For information about special discounts for bulk purchases, please contact Simon & Schuster Special Sales at 1-866-506-1949 or business@simonandschuster.com.

The Simon & Schuster Speakers Bureau can bring authors to your live event. For more information or to book an event contact the Simon & Schuster Speakers Bureau at 1-866-248-3049 or visit our website at www.simonspeakers.com.

Designed by Ruth Lee-Mui

Manufactured in the United States of America

20   19

Library of Congress Cataloging-in-Publication Data
Phinney, Stephen D.
    The new Atkins for a new you : the ultimate diet for shedding weight and feeling great forever / by Stephen D. Phinney, Jeff S. Volek, and Eric C. Westman.
        p.   cm.
    "A Touchstone Book."
    Includes bibliographical references and index.
    1. Reducing diets.   2. Low-carbohydrate diet—Recipes.   I. Volek, Jeff.
II. Westman, Eric C.   III. Title.
    RM222.2.P4952   2010
    612.2'5—dc22                          2010002849
ISBN 978-1-4391-9027-2
ISBN 978-1-4391-9028-9 (ebook)

The late Dr. Robert C. Atkins established the nutritional principles that remain the core of the Atkins Diet. This innovative thinker worked tirelessly to help people understand how to improve their health by implementing these principles. With every passing year, independent research continues to confirm the wisdom of his ideas. We are proud to carry on Dr. Atkins's legacy as we explore new frontiers in the low-carbohydrate dietary approach.

# Contents

# Foreword

That which seems the height of absurdity in one generation often
becomes the height of wisdom in another.

—*John Stuart Mill*

When does a treatment once considered alternative become mainstream?
Is it when thousands of overweight people shrink themselves and improve their diabetes control with a low-carbohydrate way of eating? Does it
require years of an obesity epidemic in the setting of a lifestyle increasingly
reliant on high-carbohydrate and processed foods? Possibly, but for physicians deciding whether to recommend a low-carbohydrate diet instead of a
low-fat diet to their patients, it comes down to one thing: *science*.

Books, newspaper articles, and Web sites are wonderful ways to share
new information; however, the ultimate way to change minds on a large
scale is to do research. When study after study shows the same startling
proof, physicians start to realize that what they previously regarded as un-
justified is now scientifically verified.

In my work as a pediatric neurologist at Johns Hopkins Hospital car-
ing for children with uncontrolled seizures, I have had the pleasure of wit-
nessing a similar revolution in thinking over the past fifteen years. The
ketogenic diet, similar to a low-carbohydrate diet, was created in 1921 as a
treatment for epilepsy. Before the 1990s, even at major teaching hospitals
in the United States, this dietary approach was often discarded as "voodoo,"
unpalatable, and less effective than medications. Today, it is a widely used
and universally accepted treatment worldwide. Skepticism is now rare,
and almost all doctors acknowledge the effectiveness of the ketogenic diet.
How did the perception of this treatment undergo such a radical change in
just a decade and a half? Was it lectures at national meetings, parent support groups, or television coverage? They all certainly helped, but again,

and even more important, research and hard scientific proof transformed disbelievers into advocates.

In *The New Atkins for a New You*, you will discover how in the same time frame science has similarly transformed the Atkins Diet from what was once considered a "fad" into an established, medically validated, safe, and effective treatment. This book also offers a wealth of new advice and insights into doing the Atkins Diet correctly, including numerous simplifications, making it easier for people everywhere to achieve the benefits of a low-carbohydrate lifestyle than ever before. As you will soon see, the volume you hold in your hands is far more than a typical diet how-to book. Not only have Dr. Eric C. Westman, Dr. Jeff S. Volek, and Dr. Stephen D. Phinney summarized the hundreds of research studies published in top medical journals, they have also authored many of them. In more than 150 articles, these three international experts on the use of low-carbohydrate diets to combat obesity, high cholesterol, and type 2 diabetes have led the way in repeatedly proving how a low-carbohydrate approach is superior to a low-fat one.

As a member of the Atkins Science Advisory Board, I have admired the work of these three clinician-scientists. It has been helpful to be able to call on each of them for their willing advice, and in a way now you can too, through this book. Their commonsense approach to starting and maintaining a low-carbohydrate diet is evident throughout the book, and their vast knowledge is especially evident in part IV, "A Diet for Life: The Science of Good Health." I know that I will often refer my patients to this section.

I find it sad that Dr. Robert C. Atkins did not live to see his diet so strongly validated both in scientific research and in this new book, which so heavily bases its recommendations on that research. Many of his ideas, personal observations based on thousands of patients, and philosophy, which appear in *Dr. Atkins' Diet Revolution* and his other books, have been validated in this book, with science to back them up. When the first edition of *Diet Revolution* was published in 1972, the low-carbohydrate concept was not one that physicians embraced, nor did they think that it would prevail. In Dr. Atkins's lifetime, his dietary approach was subject to skepticism and disbelief by much of the nutritional community. Perhaps there is no greater tribute to his memory than that this is typically no longer the case today.

I foresee exciting times ahead for the Atkins Diet. Already in my field of neurology, researchers are studying the application of low-carbohydrate diets for epilepsy in adults, as well as for Alzheimer's disease, autism, brain tumors, and Lou Gehrig's disease (ALS). There is published evidence from Dr. Westman and others that these diets help not only obesity and type 2 diabetes, but possibly even schizophrenia, polycystic ovarian disease, irritable bowel disease, narcolepsy, and gastroesophageal reflux. Obviously, there is growing evidence that low-carbohydrate diets are good for more than just your waistline! I am also personally hopeful that the Atkins Diet will become an accepted tool to combat the growing worldwide epidemic of childhood obesity. With its new content and firm underpinning of research, *The New Atkins for a New You* will also enable researchers to use it as a "bible" to develop correct protocols in low-carbohydrate studies.

I urge you to use this book not only as a guide to a healthier lifestyle but also as a scientific reference for your bookshelf. Friends and family may question why you are following the Atkins Diet, and even some physicians who have not read the latest research could discourage you from trying this approach. Although your personal results in your appearance and laboratory tests may change their minds within a few weeks, even before that, please let this book help you to enlighten them. Drs. Phinney, Volek, and Westman suggest at the beginning of chapter 13 that "you may want to share these chapters with your health care professional." I could not agree more. Be sure to also point out the more than one hundred references at the end.

So I ask again, when does a treatment believed to be "fad" science turn into an accepted fact? When does one man's "diet revolution" become the status quo for people committed to leading a healthier lifestyle? The answer is . . . *now*. Enjoy all the advice, meal plans, recipes, success stories—and most important—science this book has to offer our generation and our children's generation.

Eric H. Kossoff, M.D.
Medical Director, Ketogenic Diet Center
Departments of Neurology and Pediatrics
Johns Hopkins Hospital
Baltimore, Maryland

# Introduction

Welcome to the new Atkins.

You have a lot on your plate. Between holding down a job and/or raising a family and other activities, you're probably long on responsibilities and commitments and short on time. No doubt your to-do list grows with every passing day. So the last thing you need is a dietary approach that's complicated or time-consuming. Instead, you want an easy-to-follow way of eating that allows you to slim down quickly and stay there, address certain health problems, and boost your energy.

Atkins is the program you've been looking for.

Maybe you've heard about Atkins before. Maybe you've even tried it before. If so, this book will show you a whole new way to live the Atkins lifestyle that's easier and more effective than any previous book has offered. Welcome back. You'll love the updated Atkins.

Or perhaps you're new to the Atkins program. Read on and find out why the Atkins lifestyle is the key to not just a slimmer body but also a healthier life. Not only is doing Atkins easier than ever, a growing number of researchers have recently conducted experiments aimed at better understanding how carbohydrate restriction impacts health. In the last few years more than fifty basic and applied studies have been published which, in addition to validating the safety and effectiveness of the Atkins Diet, also provide new insights into ways to optimize the Atkins lifestyle.

We'll tell you how the right foods will help you take charge of your weight, boost your energy, and generally make you feel better. You'll learn everything that you need to know now and for a lifetime of weight control. You'll also come to understand that:

- Excess weight and poor health are two sides of the same coin.
- The quality of the food you eat affects your quality of life.

- Atkins is a way of eating for life, not a quickie weight loss diet.
- Activity is the natural partner of a healthy diet.

Before telling you more about *The New Atkins for a New You*, let's establish the logic of a low-carbohydrate lifestyle.

## BEAT THE EPIDEMIC OF OBESITY

Here's a pop quiz for you. When eaten in large amounts, which macronutrient raises your blood levels of saturated fats and triglycerides: protein, fat, or carbohydrate? You're probably tempted to answer *fat*. But the correct answer is *carbohydrate*. Second question: Which of the three *lowers* your HDL ("good") cholesterol? Again, the answer is carbohydrate.

In the last four decades, the percentage of overweight American adults and children has ballooned. As Albert Einstein once remarked, "Insanity is doing the same thing over and over, but expecting different results." In this time frame, the medical and nutritional establishment has told us to follow the U.S. Department of Agriculture (USDA) Food Guide Pyramid, skimp on calories, avoid fat, and focus on eating carbohydrate foods. Americans now consume less saturated fat than they did forty years ago but have replaced those calories—and added another 200 a day—with carbohydrates. Clearly, something is seriously wrong with the way we eat.

So has our population become thinner? Quite the contrary! Today, more than 65 percent of American adults are overweight. Likewise, the prevalence of type 2 diabetes has skyrocketed. Are you a part of this statistical nightmare? Or are you at risk of becoming part of it? If so, this book provides the tools to escape that fate. But it's not just enough to read the words, you must also truly take responsibility for your health. Remodeling your eating habits—like making any major life change—takes commitment. But if you're truly ready to exchange your old habits for new ones, your reward will be the emergence of a slimmer, healthier, sexier, more energetic person—the new you!

*The New Atkins for a New You* will make clear that doing Atkins isn't about eating only beef, bacon, and butter. Rather, it's about finding how many carbohydrates you can tolerate and making good choices among carbohydrate, protein, and fat foods. In terms of carbohydrates, that means a wide array of vegetables and other whole foods. And if you choose not to eat meat or fish or any animal protein—whether for personal or other reasons—or to minimize their intake, you can still do Atkins.

## CHANGE IS GOOD

In its almost forty-year evolution, the Atkins Diet has seen a number of modifications reflecting emerging nutritional science. This book reflects the latest thinking on the diet and nutrition and introduces several significant changes, including:

- A daily requirement of a substantial amount of high-fiber "foundation vegetables."
- An easy way to reduce or eliminate symptoms that sometimes accompany the initial conversion to a low-carb approach.
- Ways to smooth the transition from one phase to the next, ensuring the gradual and natural adoption of healthy, permanent eating habits.
- Detailed advice on how to maintain weight loss, including a choice of two paths in Phase 4, Lifetime Maintenance.
- The ability to customize the program to individual needs, including variations for vegetarians and vegans.
- An understanding that we eat many of our meals outside the home with detailed suggestions on how to strategize and what to eat on the road, in fast-food places, or in different kinds of restaurants.

The book is full of other small but significant updates, again based on recent research. For example, we now know that consuming caffeine in moderation actually modestly assists fat burning. So your eight daily cups of fluid can include some coffee and other beverages in addition to water.

Simplicity, versatility, and sustainability are essential for any dietary program to succeed—long term. Atkins meets all three challenges.

1. **Simplicity.** Above all, the goal of this book is to make Atkins simple to do. In a nutshell, here it is: The key to slimming down and enhancing your health is to train your body to burn more fat. And the way to do that, quickly and effectively, is by cutting back on sugars and other refined carbohydrates and allowing fat—including your own body fat—to become your primary source of energy. (Before you know it, you'll understand why

fat is your friend.) This book will give you all the tools you'll need to make this metabolic shift.

2. **Versatility.** Atkins now allows you to personalize the program to your lifestyle and food preferences. If you've tried Atkins before and found it too difficult, too restrictive, you'll be very pleasantly surprised with the updated approach. For example:

   - You determine which phase to start in and when to move to the next phase.
   - You can eat lean cuts of meat and poultry—or none at all—if you prefer.
   - You can do Atkins and still honor your own culinary heritage.
   - You choose when to begin a fitness program and what activities to pursue.
   - You select one of the two approaches to Lifetime Maintenance that better suits your needs.

3. **Sustainability.** Atkins doesn't just help you shed pounds and leave you there. We know—as you do—that the problem with every weight loss program is keeping the weight off for the long term. Understanding the power of fat burning is equally essential to lifetime weight maintenance. Importantly, the four-phase program trains you to gauge your personal tolerance for carbohydrates, so that you can tailor a program that not only fits you to a T but also enables you to permanently banish excess pounds and maintain improved health indicators. And once you find a way of eating that you can live with, yo-yo dieting will be a thing of the past.

## HOW TO USE THIS BOOK

Four sections allow you to get going on the program quickly, complete with lists of acceptable foods and meal plans, plus provide a grounding in nutrition and the scientific foundations of the Atkins approach.

- Part I covers the basics of nutrition, looking at carbohydrates, protein, and fats, and explains how and why Atkins works. We'll introduce the four phases that form the continuum of the Atkins Diet:

- – Phase 1, Induction
- – Phase 2, Ongoing Weight Loss (OWL)
- – Phase 3, Pre-Maintenance
- – Phase 4, Lifetime Maintenance

You'll also learn all about "Net Carbs" and how to count them. (For brevity, we'll often refer to carbohydrates as carbs.) Once you understand these basics and commit yourself to concentrating on whole foods, you'll find it easier than ever to slim down and shape up. You'll also learn how the wrong foods—think of those made with sugar and refined grains— keep you overweight, tired, and sluggish and increase your risk for health problems.

- Part II tells you how to do Atkins on a day-to-day basis and transition easily from one phase to the next. We'll guide you through the process of exploring the amounts and types of food that are right for you, with extensive lists of acceptable foods for each phase, as you customize the program to your needs. You'll find a wide variety of choices in the types of foods you can eat, whether dining in or eating out.
- Part III includes detailed meal plans, recipes for all phases of the diet, and guides to eating out.
- Part IV is for those of you who want to learn how Atkins can improve cardiovascular risk factors, reverse metabolic syndrome (prediabetes), and manage diabetes. We'll give you the short course and provide lots of reference material in case you happen to love reading scientific journals or want to share these chapters with your physician.

Just as you can tailor Atkins to your needs, you can read this book as you wish. If you're eager to get going immediately, simply start with part II, but please circle back later to learn how and why Atkins works. At the very least, read the review sections at the end of the chapters in part I. As the Success Stories sprinkled throughout the book make clear, until you understand the nutritional grounding of the Atkins Diet, it's all too easy to regard it merely as a tool for quick weight loss—instead of a healthy and permanent lifestyle.

In part I, you'll also make the acquaintance of the metabolic bully, which threatens your resolve to stay on the weight loss path, and its enemy—and your ally—the Atkins Edge. This powerful tool helps you slim down, without experiencing the hunger or cravings usually associated with weight loss.

Other diets may come and go, but Atkins endures because it has always worked. As physicians, nutritionists, and researchers, we're committed to making Atkins simpler than ever. After all, the easier it is, the more likely you are to stick with it, and—bottom line—achieve success. We can assure you that Dr. Robert C. Atkins, who was a pioneer in low-carb nutrition, would approve of the science-based changes introduced in this book, particularly any that make the program easier for you and enable you to keep excess weight off long term. The growing worldwide epidemics of obesity and diabetes mean that it's not a moment too soon.

Stephen D. Phinney, M.D., Ph.D.
Jeff S. Volek, Ph.D., R.D.
Eric C. Westman, M.D., M.H.S.

# WHY IT WORKS:

It's All About Nutrition

# Chapter 1

# KNOW THYSELF

Any diet that skimps on natural fats is inherently unsatisfying, making it extremely difficult to sustain long term and almost certainly doomed to failure.

Did you once delight in eating whatever you wanted without gaining an ounce? Were you athletic in high school or college? Was your weight never a problem until after you got your first high-stress job, started your family, or approached menopause? Have you been diagnosed with high cholesterol, or are you at risk for type 2 diabetes? If you're reading this book and the answer to any of these questions is yes, it's a safe assumption that your days of carefree eating are long gone.

Or maybe you've spent a good part of your adult life on the diet merry-go-round. You hop on to lose some weight, then dismount as soon as you've lost it. When you regain the pounds—as most of us inevitably do—you jump back on, and so forth. You might have even done Atkins several years ago and banished that extra padding. But when you reverted to your habitual way of eating, the lost pounds returned with a vengeance. Maybe you felt under the weather in the first week or two of Atkins, found the program too restrictive, or had some concerns about its healthfulness. Perhaps you simply got bored.

Since you're reading this book, we trust that you're giving Atkins a second chance. Thanks to some significant changes, you'll find that the program is now far easier to do. And new research makes it clear that Atkins is a healthy way to eat. It's one of the few low-carb diets subjected to extensive independent research. In studies that compared people following a low-calorie program to those controlling their carbohydrates, the groups that reduced their carbs showed greater weight and fat loss, better compliance, the ability to keep weight off long term, and higher satisfaction with food choices.[1] We'll circle back to some of the research later in this chapter.

Another possibility is that you're a veteran of the low-fat approach that left you unsatisfied, hungry, testy, and fantasizing about forbidden feasts, before ultimately bagging it. Or you've spent the last decade or so sampling every diet craze that came down the pike only to regain the weight—and perhaps a few extra pounds—for all your efforts.

Whether you're new to Atkins, have returned after wandering in the dietary wilderness, or are a confirmed Atkins follower interested in recent modifications, you've come to the right place. Atkins has never been just about weight, so there's also a seat at the table for already slim folks who want to improve their physique, increase their energy, overcome health problems, or simply feel better. Whatever your story, it's time to get off of the diet merry-go-round and onto a permanent path to lifetime slimness, vitality, and good health.

## TIME TO TAKE CONTROL

Does this sound familiar? Each time you've tried a new weight loss approach or renewed your commitment to stick with a program, you experience euphoria and a sense of empowerment. And you probably enjoyed some initial good results. But then you didn't follow through, and soon you'd find yourself in a downward spiral. You blamed yourself for your weakness, lack of control, and inability to defer the momentary pleasure of a piece of chocolate or a bag of chips for the long-term goal of a trimmer, more attractive you. And as all too many of you may have already learned, the challenges of losing weight pale compared to the real work of keeping it permanently at bay. The humorist Erma Bombeck was onto something when she quipped, "In two decades I've lost a total of 789 pounds. I should be hanging from a charm bracelet." But when it comes to your health and your psyche, the cycle of losing, regaining, losing, and so forth is no laughing matter. Nor are the guilt, shame, and sense of failure that accompany it.

By the end of this chapter, you'll have met the metabolic bully that stands in the way of your losing weight and achieving optimal health. We'll also introduce you to the Atkins Edge, the powerful tool that distinguishes Atkins from other diets and lets you outsmart the bully. The Atkins Edge converts your body to a fat-burning machine. Yes, we're talking about using your spare tire, beer belly, thunder thighs, heroic hips, jiggling butt, or wherever your fat deposits have landed as your primary energy source. Just as important, the process of literally restoring your body to its best shape will not only make you feel good about your body and proud of your resolve, you'll almost surely find that the sense of empowerment and confidence spills over into your personal and professional life. Feeling powerful is an aphrodisiac, so don't be surprised to find that your sex life also revives!

## IS ATKINS FOR YOU?

To help you decide whether Atkins can help you slim down—and stay there—and address any health issues, consider the following questions.

**ARE YOU HAPPY WITH YOUR WEIGHT?** If so, congratulations! But even if you're content with your appearance, you may find it an effort to maintain your weight, or you may have health problems that could be alleviated by changing your diet. Or perhaps you want to reconfigure your body by trading fat for muscle, as Atkins can do, especially if you also embark on a training program. *Bottom line:* Atkins is an effective and sustainable way to shed pounds—quickly and safely.

**WHAT ARE YOUR WEIGHT LOSS GOALS?** If you have just a few pesky pounds to lose, you can probably take them off in a month or so. Some people lose up to 15 pounds in the first two weeks on Atkins. Countless individuals have lost more than 100 pounds overall—and you could too. You'll meet some of them in this book and can read more of their success stories on www.atkins.com. Naturally, individual results vary considerably, depending upon age, gender, activity level, metabolic resistance, and other factors, plus—of course—how carefully you follow our instructions. *Bottom line:* You can lose a little or a lot on Atkins.

**DO YOU HAVE OTHER HEALTH ISSUES YOU WANT TO CORRECT OR HEAD OFF?** Individual results vary, but generally, if you go easy on carbs and focus on vegetables and other whole food carbs, you'll almost surely find that your triglycerides diminish, your "good" cholesterol rises, and your markers of inflammation improve.[2] If you have high blood pressure, you should see your numbers drop.[3] Those with elevated blood sugar and insulin levels will also see improvement. Most Atkins followers who once had to take medications and/or insulin for type 2 diabetes to control their blood sugar or diuretics to counteract fluid retention have been able, with their doctor's help, to reduce their dosage and even stop taking the drugs once they've adapted to the Atkins program. Atkins also addresses other health issues such as insulin resistance and metabolic syndrome.[4] Controlling carbs is also a time-tested and viable treatment for epilepsy.[5] *Bottom line:* Atkins is a healthy diet and, for those with medical problems, is also a corrective diet that can significantly reduce the risks for disease.

**WERE YOU SUCCESSFUL SHORT TERM BUT NOT LONG TERM ON OTHER DIETS?** Any diet that's not sustainable is almost certainly doomed to failure. About 95 percent of people who lose weight regain it—usually within a few years.[6] The point is that once you've slimmed down, raw willpower alone is not enough for you to succeed in the long term. You also need an ally, and this is where the Atkins Edge comes in. Numerous studies show better maintenance of weight loss after one and two years with Atkins compared to low-fat diets.[7] *Bottom line:* On Atkins, you lose the weight and can then maintain that loss, making it a diet for life.

**ARE YOU UNABLE TO LOSE WEIGHT OR MAINTAIN WEIGHT LOSS BY COUNTING CALORIES AND AVOIDING FAT?** A diet that skimps on natural fats is inherently unsatisfying, making it extremely difficult to sustain long term, as is a calorie-restricted diet that leaves you perpetually hungry. Atkins, on the other hand, allows you to eat many delicious foods that contain healthy fats. In fact, research shows that when people on Atkins eat as much as they want, most wind up naturally eating a suitable number of calories.[8] *Bottom line:* On Atkins, there's no need to skimp on fats or count calories.

**ARE YOU ALWAYS HUNGRY OR PLAGUED BY CRAVINGS ON OTHER DIETS?** A low-fat diet is almost always a high-carb diet, which quickly converts to glucose in your bloodstream, especially in the case of low-quality carbs. The result is a roller coaster of blood sugar highs and lows that zaps your energy and leave you craving another "fix" of quickly metabolized carbs a few hours after a meal. *Bottom line:* Eating the Atkins way (which includes two snacks a day) means you need never go hungry.

**ARE YOUR FAVORITE FOODS DOUGHNUTS, SWEETS, CHIPS, FRIES, AND OTHER HIGH-CARB FOODS?** The more of these foods you eat, the more you crave, setting up a vicious cycle of overeating foods that don't sustain your energy and have little nutritional value. A high-carb snack merely repeats the cycle. *Bottom line:* Eliminating sugars, refined carbs, and other high-carb foods from your diet allows you to get off the blood sugar roller coaster.

**DO YOU GAIN WEIGHT EASILY EVEN THOUGH YOU DON'T OVEREAT?** It's a sad fact that some people put on weight more easily and lose weight more slowly than others.[9] However, if you can't drop excess pounds when you're truly not overeating, this may be an indication that your body doesn't tolerate carbs well, which can be a precursor of type 2 diabetes. Controlling your carb intake nips the problem in the bud. *Bottom line:* Doing Atkins allows your body to bypass problems handling carbohydrates.

**WERE YOU INITIALLY SUCCESSFUL ON ATKINS IN THE PAST BUT REGAINED WEIGHT?** If you regained weight after losing it, you'll learn how to refine the lessons you learned about weight loss and apply them to the bigger challenge of slimming down for good. *Bottom line:* Atkins focuses on weight maintenance from Day 1.

**DID YOU GET HUNG UP ON INDUCTION AND DIDN'T MOVE THROUGH THE OTHER PHASES?** All too many people confuse Induction, the first phase that kick-starts weight loss, for the entire Atkins program. Remaining in Induction may produce quick weight loss, but it doesn't teach you how to achieve permanent weight control. You may also become bored with the food choices, which could diminish your commitment to stay with Atkins. *Bottom line:* This time you can be comfortable exploring the range of foods that will enable you to keep losing weight—and ultimately maintain your new weight.

**HAVE YOU TRIED ATKINS BEFORE BUT DROPPED OUT BEFORE LOSING MUCH WEIGHT?** If you found the program too restrictive, you'll be pleased to know that it's now far more flexible. For example, you can now enjoy a satisfying variety of vegetables from the get-go. You'll also learn how to dine out easily and safely—on any cuisine. If you felt the food was too expensive, we'll help you avoid overeating protein and provide you with a list of meat cuts that won't break your budget. *Bottom line:* Anyone can do Atkins anywhere, and that includes vegetarians and vegans.

## THIS TIME WILL BE DIFFERENT

If you're a veteran of the weight loss wars, we can promise you that you're in for a surprise: this time will be different. But first of all, you must understand that shedding pounds and getting healthy isn't just a matter of willpower. There are biological reasons why you feel hungry—or not. Earlier in this chapter, we mentioned the metabolic bully, which undermines your determination and tries to derail your efforts at weight loss. Because the glucose from carbohydrates must always be tapped first as a source of energy, there's rarely any need to access your body fat if you eat the typical carb-heavy American diet. So eating lots of carbohydrates acts as a metabolic bully: it blocks your body from burning its own fat, just like a playground bully who keeps other kids from using the swings.

But don't despair. You now have access to a valuable tool that will allow you to burn your own body fat for energy and keep hunger at bay. When you cut back on carbs sufficiently, your body transitions to a primarily fat-burning metabolism, forcing the bully to step aside. The messages your body transmits to your brain will change dramatically. Instead of hearing "I'm tired and hungry. Feed me sweet, starchy foods this minute," that nagging voice will be blissfully silent. You'll actually find that you can go for several hours without even thinking about food.

Scientists refer to it as a fat-burning metabolism, but we call this ally the Atkins Edge. It enables you to stop the metabolic bully in its tracks so you lose fat pounds without experiencing undue hunger, cravings, energy depletion, or any sense of deprivation. When you burn fat for energy all day (and all night), your blood sugar remains on a relatively even keel. Without question, the Atkins Edge makes it easier to stay the course and succeed in meeting your goals. Now that you know that eating too much sugar and other refined carbohydrates stands in the way of losing weight and restoring your energy, we ask again, is Atkins for you? Perhaps the more logical question is: Why *wouldn't* Atkins be right for you?

### NO CARBS, NOT!

The most persistent misconception about Atkins is that it's a no-carb diet. From the first printing of *Dr. Atkins' Diet Revolution* in 1972, the advice has always been to *limit*–not eliminate–carbs. In fact, this first version of the program included salads from Day 1. Over the years, the number and amount of vegetables permissible in Phase 1 has increased significantly, in large part because of a better understanding of the benign role of fiber in carbs. Atkins is actually about ultimately discovering which whole foods, including vegetables, fruits, nuts, legumes, and whole grains—all of which contain carbohydrates—you're able to eat without interfering with weight loss, weight maintenance, or metabolic health. Finding out how much fiber-rich carbohydrate you can eat while still maintaining your Atkins Edge is key to your long-term success.

## GROUNDED IN RESEARCH

Now that you realize the power of the Atkins Diet, let's take a brief look at some of the recent research that has evaluated its safety and efficacy. This newer research builds upon older information on carbohydrate-restricted diets, including the use of low-carbohydrate diets by a variety of aboriginal hunting cultures that persisted for thousands of years. In the last decade a multitude of studies on restricted carbohydrate intake has dramatically changed the research landscape. Among these are seven studies lasting from six months to two years, usually comparing the Atkins Diet to other common weight loss strategies.[10] In terms of total weight loss, in each case, individuals on Atkins did at least as well as—and usually better than—those on other diets, despite the fact that they could consume as many calories as they wanted as long as they stayed within the carb guidelines.

Moreover, risk factors such as high blood triglycerides, low HDL cholesterol levels, and elevated blood pressure consistently showed improvement with carbohydrate restriction. Whether over months or years, the various parameters were as good, and in most cases better, with the Atkins Diet. In no case did Atkins worsen any important parameter. It's worth mentioning that in each of these seven studies, the subjects received varying degrees of ongoing dietary support after the first few weeks or months. And they didn't select the diet that appealed to them; instead, they were randomly assigned to one of the various diets, which would tend to limit the degree of success in the group as a whole. Nonetheless, groups assigned to Atkins did better on average than those assigned a high-carbohydrate diet.

Another study didn't use the Atkins Diet per se, although it was initially similar to the Induction phase, nor did it compare a low-carb program to other diets. But this research, done in Kuwait, demonstrated the magnitude of beneficial change that a low-carb diet can provide when subjects receive ongoing support.[11] In this case, sixty-six obese individuals, some with elevated blood sugar and cholesterol, consumed 80 to 100 grams per day of protein from meat and fish, 20 grams of carbohydrate from salad vegetables, 5 tablespoons of olive oil for cooking and dressing vegetables, and a multivitamin/multimineral supplement. After twelve weeks, the carbohydrate intake was raised to 40 grams per day (similar to that in Ongoing Weight Loss), including some berries. The subjects were monitored and supported as outpatients for a year, at which time their average weight loss was more than 60 pounds. In addition, a subgroup with elevated blood sugar (some were diabetic) experienced a rapid reduction, bringing them within eight weeks into the normal range, where it remained for the duration of the study. This diet outperformed that of any of the randomized groups in the other seven studies, due in part to the fact that the subjects chose their diet, rather than being assigned to it. Additionally, the supportive office staff counseled them, including giving them specific advice on the kind of fat to eat, showing what's possible when a safe and effective low-carb diet is combined with an enabling support staff in a clinical setting.

In the following chapters, we'll cover the basics of the diet and talk more about the Atkins Edge and how it enables you to remain in control—and vanquish the metabolic bully that has threatened to take over your life. We'll also offer lots of practical advice on how to deal with the challenges you'll face day in and day out; but first meet Traci Marshall, who lost almost 100 pounds on Atkins.

# SHEDDING THE "BABY" WEIGHT

Two pregnancies left Traci Marshall heavier than she had ever been and with a number of serious health problems. Now that she's lost more than 90 pounds on Atkins, her health is restored, along with her figure and her zest for life.

## VITAL STATISTICS

Current phase: Ongoing Weight
   Loss
Daily Net Carb intake:
   40–45 grams
Age: 42
Height: 5 feet, 6 inches
Before weight: 267 pounds
Current weight: 172 pounds
Weight lost: 95 pounds
Goal weight: 150 pounds
Former waist/hips measurement:
   40 inches/48.5 inches

Current waist/hips measurement:
   29.5 inches/38.5 inches
Former blood pressure: 160/90
Current blood pressure: 118/74
Current triglycerides: 48
Current HDL ("good") cholesterol:
   58 mg/dL
Current LDL ("bad") cholesterol:
   110 mg/dL
Current total cholesterol level:
   178 mg/dL

**Has your weight always been an issue?**
Yes. I'd done Atkins in 1997 and lost 45 pounds in two and a half months. I kept that off without effort and felt terrific until 2003, when I got pregnant. I had morning sickness the whole time and spent three months in bed. By the time I became pregnant with our second son, I was 41 years old and it was an even more difficult pregnancy.

**What health problems did you have?**
I'd developed hypertension and had a heart murmur while I was expecting. Afterward, I also suffered from postpartum anxiety.

**What got you back on Atkins?**

I'd actually gone back to Atkins after my first son's birth and had lost 25 of the 50 extra pounds I'd gained before realizing I was having another baby. I now understand that I could have done the Lifetime Maintenance phase while pregnant. My doctor was totally supportive about my returning to Atkins after my second son's birth. By this time I'd read several of Dr. Atkins's books and knew that I was highly intolerant of carbs and that Atkins was a lifestyle change, not just a weight loss diet. I remembered how great it felt to live Atkins every day and stay slim. I wanted that back!

**What health improvements have you seen?**

My blood pressure and lipids are great. My doctor is really happy with my progress. My heart murmur has disappeared. I sleep better. I have way more energy, and exercise is something I look forward to now.

**What's your fitness routine?**

I walk with the kids three days a week and go by myself on other days. I belong to a gym, where I do some cardio, but have come to realize that staying active is not just going to the gym. Recently, I started doing modified push-ups, leg extensions, and other calisthenics. Almost immediately, weight loss picked up. I've learned to love exercise because it feels awesome!

**What was the worst thing about being overweight?**

I didn't feel like me. I felt lost in a huge body. I wanted to hide, and I was so embarrassed for my children to have a heavy mom.

**How did you handle the challenge of having a lot of weight to lose?**

I only thought about 10 pounds at a time. Now that I'm closer to my goal, I only think about 5 pounds at a time.

**How would you describe your eating style?**

I eat everything that other people eat, I just eat it differently. So today I'm baking a pumpkin pie for my husband, and I'm making low-carb pumpkin cheesecake for myself, baking it in single servings in muffin tins. For breakfast, I might have Brussels sprouts mashed with cream and butter and a pork chop cooked in olive oil with garlic. Lunch is usually a big salad with onion, tomato, avocado, a piece of chicken, and my own salad dressing. Snacks are usually berries and nuts. For dinner, we'll have a protein and a vegetable. I'll make rice or sweet potatoes for the rest of the family, and I'll have another low-carb vegetable.

**Has doing Atkins affected how you feed your family?**
Absolutely. If you teach kids how to eat, they'll eat right. I'm raising them on the Atkins lifestyle. I try not to have white potatoes in the house except at holiday times. I won't buy anything with high-fructose corn syrup. I read the labels of everything to make sure of the ingredients.

**What words of wisdom can you offer other people?**
Plan ahead. Make more than you need for a single meal so that you always have something at the ready. Satisfy sweet cravings with a cup of coffee with cream and low-carb sweetener. Motivate yourself by looking at old photos when you were at a good weight. Keep a food journal. Learn to adapt recipes, like using eggplant strips in lieu of pasta.

**What was the most difficult thing for you?**
The hardest part is just making the commitment to start. Once you get going, it just feels so good. For me, it gets easier the longer I stay on Atkins.

# Chapter 2

# THE ROAD AHEAD

As long as you consider a short-term diet as a solution, you're doomed to an on-again, off-again battle with your weight.

One of the main reasons for the failure of most efforts to slim down is that people simply can't sustain the prescribed way of eating. Boredom or dissatisfaction with the permissible foods, concern about the adequacy of the diet, or sheer hunger ultimately causes dieters to revert to their old habits. Eating is pleasurable, and any weight control approach that makes food the enemy is doomed to failure. In contrast, Atkins makes food your friend and is all about choice, rather than denial. By the time you've completed this chapter, you'll have a better understanding of the several pieces of the puzzle that come together to give you the Atkins Edge. This metabolic advantage will power you with a steady source of energy—and empower you to stay with the program.

## THE D-WORD

Most people are hung up on the secondary meaning of the word "diet": a limited period of deprivation to lose weight. That short-term thinking is what has gotten so many "dieters" into the same bind. They hop onto the diet wagon, lose a little excess baggage, then hop (or fall) off and regain the same old pounds.

As long as you consider a short-term diet as a solution, you're doomed to an on-again, off-again battle with your weight. Things are different in Atkins land. First of all, losing weight the low-carb way needn't involve deprivation. Secondly, although Atkins has all too often mistakenly been perceived as just a weight loss diet (and without question, it *does* help people lose weight swiftly and effectively), it's really a lifestyle that enriches your life in many ways. That's why the program's formal name is the Atkins Nutritional Approach. You can still call it the Atkins Diet—we do—as long as you remember that it's a much bigger tent. Atkins is a way of eating that will enhance the quality of your life. After three progressively liberal phases, the Atkins program culminates in Lifetime Maintenance.

## LET'S PREVIEW THE PHASES

Part II of this book is devoted to the four phases, but for now we'll briefly introduce them to make it crystal clear that Atkins is truly a recipe for life, rather than simply a weight loss diet.

**PHASE 1, INDUCTION,** is where most—but not all—people start. It lasts for a minimum of two weeks, but feel free to hang out there longer if you have a lot of weight to lose. In Induction, you'll train your body to burn fat, which will kick-start weight loss. To do so, you'll confine yourself to a daily intake of 20 grams of Net Carbs. (See the sidebar "What Are Net Carbs?") Of those 20 carb grams, at least 12 to 15 should be in the form of what we call "foundation vegetables," which you'll eat every day, along with protein and healthy, natural fats. Off the menu is anything made with sugar, fruit juices and concentrates, and flour or other grains.

**PHASE 2, ONGOING WEIGHT LOSS,** or OWL, is when you continue to explore foundation vegetables and begin adding back foods such as berries, nuts, and seeds—and perhaps even some legumes. You'll slowly increase your daily carb intake by 5 grams at a time until you find your personal tolerance for consuming carbs while continuing to lose weight, known as your Carbohydrate Level for Losing (CLL). You typically stay in this phase until you're about 10 pounds from your goal weight.

**PHASE 3, PRE-MAINTENANCE,** broadens the range of acceptable whole food carbs in the form of other fruits, starchy vegetables, and finally whole grains. (However, not everyone can add back all these foods or eat them on a regular basis.) As long as you continue to lose weight, you can slowly increase your daily carb intake in 10-gram increments. When you reach your goal weight, you'll test out the level of carb intake you can handle without regaining pounds or losing the precious metabolic adaptations you've achieved. This level is known as your Atkins Carbohydrate Equilibrium (ACE). Once your weight has stabilized for a month and your food cravings are under control, you're ready to move on.

**PHASE 4, LIFETIME MAINTENANCE,** is really not a phase at all but a lifestyle. You'll continue to consume the varied whole foods diet of Pre-Maintenance, adhering to your ACE and regularly monitoring your weight and measurements. Two approaches to Lifetime Maintenance address the needs of people across a range of ACEs. Some people may need to keep their intake of carbohydrates low and avoid certain foods to continue to enjoy the health benefits of carbohydrate restriction; others will have more latitude to consume more and a greater variety of carbohydrate foods.

In the next chapters, we'll get into the specifics of what you should be eating from Day 1 and what you'll add back as you slim down and your new eating habits become ingrained. We'll also discuss the few foods that you're better off steering clear of. The Atkins approach is not about banning foods lacking in nutrients and full of carbs, but it does make clear the dangers they present to weight control and overall good health. We trust that once you understand how these foods sabotage your good efforts, you'll pretty much write them off for good.

## WHAT ARE NET CARBS?

The only carbs that matter when you do Atkins are Net Carbs, aka digestible carbs or impact carbs. Fortunately, you don't have to be a food scientist or math whiz to figure out how to calculate them. Simply subtract the number of grams of dietary fiber in whole foods from the total number of carbohydrate grams. How come? The answer is that although it's considered a carbohydrate, fiber doesn't impact your blood sugar level. So unlike other carbs, it doesn't act as a metabolic bully. Let's do the math. A half cup of steamed green beans contains 4.9 grams of carbs, of which 2.0 grams are fiber, so subtract 2.0 from 4.9 and you get 2.9 grams of Net Carbs. Here's an even more dramatic example: a cup of Romaine lettuce contains 1.4 grams of carbs, but more than half the carbs (1.0 gram) are fiber, for a Net Carb count of 0.4 grams. No wonder you can eat lots and lots of salad greens on Atkins!

When it comes to low-carb foods, you subtract grams of sugar alcohols (including glycerin), as well as of fiber, from total grams of carbs to get the Net Carb count.

*Tip:* For a Carb Counter that provides total carbs, Net Carbs, and other nutritional data for hundreds of foods, go to www.atkins.com/tools.

## WHAT ARE SUGAR ALCOHOLS?

Many low-carb products are sweetened with such ingredients as glycerin, mannitol, sorbitol, xylitol, erythritol, isomalt, lactitol, and maltitol. These forms of sugar, called sugar alcohols (or polyols), provide a sweetness and mouthfeel similar to that of sugar without all the calories and unwanted metabolic effects. Because sugar alcohols are not fully absorbed by the gut, they provide roughly half the calories that sugar does, although each one varies slightly. The incomplete and slower absorption results in a minimal impact on blood sugar and insulin response. This means that sugar alcohols don't significantly interfere with fat burning, making them acceptable on Atkins. Other benefits may include promotion of colon health and prevention of cavities. However, a portion of sugar alcohols is not absorbed, which can produce a laxative effect and cause some gastrointestinal problems when they are consumed in excess. Individual tolerances vary, so it is best to test the waters slowly. Most people find that they can handle 20 to 30 grams a day without undesirable effects.

# MEASURING YOUR PROGRESS

Most people lose pounds quickly and steadily in the first few weeks of Atkins—in fact, some people lose up to 15 pounds in the first two weeks on the program. But numerous factors influence your individual weight loss pattern. If you have just a few pounds to lose, they may be more resistant to your efforts. Men tend to lose more quickly than women do. Younger people typically have an advantage over the middle-aged or older. Hormonal changes, such as menopause, can definitely slow your metabolism and make it more difficult to banish pounds. Some people naturally have a slower metabolism. Certain prescription drugs can also interfere with weight loss. Your spouse or friend may well lose at a different rate than you do. Just remember that getting slim and trim isn't a contest. Rather, it's a process of discovering how your own body works.

Those of you with a significant amount of weight to lose typically see steady progress week after week, but it's natural to experience some ups and downs, and with time almost everyone sees a slowdown in weight loss. Lost inches also indicate progress, sometimes even when pounds won't budge. That's why we encourage you to unroll the tape measure whenever you hop on the scale. As you'll come to understand, your goal is not just a smaller clothing size and a trimmer body, it's also to enjoy good health and well-being. If you start out with type 2 diabetes or hypertension, both of which tend to improve promptly on Atkins, your improved numbers will give you and your doctor evidence that the diet is working. We'll give you more detail on how diabetes and other serious conditions respond to Atkins in part IV.

## WATER POUNDS AND FAT POUNDS

As with any weight loss program, some of the initial weight loss you'll experience is water weight. After all, one-half to two-thirds of your body is composed of water. Atkins naturally has a diuretic effect that starts within the first few days, which is why drinking plenty of water and other fluids is important, as is taking a multivitamin/multimineral, to ensure that you don't deplete your stores of electrolytes (sodium, potassium, magnesium). (We'll discuss which supplements are important shortly.) So if you drop 10 to 15 pounds in the first few weeks, you'll be saying good-bye to some unnecessary water weight along with the initial fat pounds. But once that excess water is gone, you'll be losing primarily body fat. The Atkins Diet has been shown time and time again to result in significant fat loss, especially from the stomach area.[1] In head-to-head comparisons, Atkins consistently outperforms other diets in terms of fat loss.[2] The majority of studies indicate that when carbohydrate intake is reduced and protein intake is modestly increased, there's a greater percentage of fat loss and better retention of lean body mass. But after that, as long as you follow our food intake guidelines, you can be secure in the knowledge that the vast majority of your ongoing weight loss will come from fat.

## WHAT TO EXPECT

Your body makes a number of adjustments as it begins to focus on burning primarily fat, after which you will have gained the metabolic advantage we call the Atkins Edge. However, in those first few weeks, as your body makes this transition, you might encounter a few symptoms. The most common are headaches, dizziness, weakness, fatigue—sometimes referred to as Atkins flu—and constipation. Fortunately, all are pretty easy to avoid. We'll touch on them here and then give you more complete instructions on how to manage them in chapter 7.

As mentioned above, type 2 diabetes and hypertension sometimes improve dramatically when you are on a low-carb program, so the need for certain medications diminishes. Close cooperation with your doctor is essential so that you don't confuse the effects of too high a dose of a medication with doing Atkins itself. Also, it's not a good idea to begin a new or more intense exercise program at the same time you start the program. Give your body the benefit of two to three weeks to adjust before pushing the exercise envelope. On the other hand, if you are already very active or work out regularly and can continue to do so without any loss of energy, feel free to continue.

Consuming carbohydrates makes you retain water, but shifting over to fat burning has a diuretic effect, meaning you'll excrete more salt along with fluid. If you used to feel bloated and no longer do, that's a good thing. Moreover, if you have high blood pressure, the diuretic effect may mean that your numbers will come down nicely in the first few days or weeks. But for many of the rest of us, fluid loss can be too much of a good thing. To manage this problem, simply drink plenty of water and other fluids and make sure to consume a minimum of half a teaspoon of salt each day. You can do this with salt itself, a couple of cups of salty broth, or a measured amount of soy sauce. Follow this regimen from the start, and headaches, dizziness, fatigue, or constipation should not be a problem. Adding this modest sodium supplement—no, this does not make Atkins a high-salt diet—is one of many science-based changes in Atkins. We'll give you more details about this practice (and the few exceptions for those who should not follow it) in chapter 7.

## NUTRITION BASICS

You probably have a general idea that foods contain various amounts of protein, fat, and carbohydrates, which are commonly considered macronutrients. Does it matter whether you eat more or less of one or another? For that matter, what is a Calorie? And how do calories relate to carbs? Let's start with the easy stuff. Macronutrients are the three nutrient families that provide the body with needed energy—in the form of calories—to carry out all the bodily functions necessary for life. A few foods contain a single macronutrient, such as sugar (all carbohydrate) and olive oil (all fat). Most foods, however, contain two or all three macronutrients. For example, a cup of whole milk contains 8 grams of protein and about the same amount of fat, as well as more than 11 grams of carbohydrate. Four ounces of portobello mushrooms contain almost 6 grams of carbohydrate—of which nearly 2 grams are fiber—a miniscule amount of fat, and almost 3 grams of protein.

A Calorie (aka kilocalorie) is simply a unit of food energy. In this book, we use the word "Calorie" (with a capital C) to designate a kilocalorie, and the word "calorie" in reference to energy in general. Your body needs the energy in macronutrients, not just for physical activity but also for all its other functions, including breathing, staying warm, processing nutrients, and brain activity. A gram of protein or carbohydrate contains 4 Calories, while a gram of fat contains 9 Calories. So gram for gram, fat is a more concentrated source of energy. Some of the raw materials in macronutrients are turned into energy almost immediately; others are broken down into various components that are used for energy later.

## ATKINS IS DIFFERENT FROM OTHER DIETS

To succeed on Atkins, you may need to forget what you've learned on other diets. Here's why:

| | LOW-FAT DIET | LOW-CARB DIET | COMMENTS |
|---|---|---|---|
| Methodology | Count calories, restrict all fat | Count carbs, eliminate trans fats | Satiating foods eaten on Atkins minimize hunger, moderating calorie intake |
| Eat mostly | Carbs of all sorts | Healthy fats, protein, healthy carbs | Avoid sugar, pasta, bread, and other refined-carb foods that raise blood sugar levels |
| Weigh foods | Yes | No | Who takes a scale to a restaurant? |
| Count calories | Yes | No | Atkins emphasizes quality, not low-calorie food |
| Count carbs | No | Yes | All you need is a Carb Counter to track your intake |
| Eat prepared foods | Yes (on some programs) | No | You eat healthful whole foods, not expensive prepared meals |
| Snacks | Yes, but calorie restricted | Yes, twice a day | Who wouldn't prefer cheese, nuts, or guacamole to a celery stick? |

## HOW FOOD BECOMES ENERGY—AND FAT

Human metabolism is complex, but we'll make it as simple as possible. This chemical process converts food into either energy or the body's building blocks, which then become part of your organs, tissues, and cells. Eating the right foods can improve your body's metabolism, particularly how it handles fat. When you eat fewer carbohydrate foods—relying mostly on vegetables rich in fiber—your body switches to burning fat instead of carbs as its primary fuel source. The average normal-weight person carries about 100,000 Calories worth of energy in fat stores—hypothetically, that's enough to run at a steady pace for more than 200 hours—and some of us have much more than that. The Atkins Diet, more than any other diet, gives you the key to unlock that energy for fuel.

The concept of carbs as a metabolic bully should help you understand the implications of the switch from burning carbohydrates to burning fat. Here's how it works. When you eat carbohydrates, they're digested and converted to glucose (sugar), which your bloodstream transports throughout your body. This means that carbohydrate intake is largely responsible for blood sugar fluctuations. It's also important to understand that it's not only the amount of carbohydrates but also their quality that determine the extent of that impact. For example, eating a bowl of brown rice and beans raises your blood sugar level much more slowly and less dramatically than, say, consuming a doughnut, a glass of OJ, or a bowl of sweetened cereal. (Food need not taste sweet to convert rapidly to glucose. Prime examples are mashed potatoes and white bread.)

The amount of sugar circulating in your blood is actually very small—just a few teaspoons—so to keep your blood sugar level normal after a big carbohydrate dose, the absorbed glucose has to be rapidly transported out of your blood and into your cells. This is the job of the hormone insulin, which signals your cells to remove glucose from your bloodstream. Once inside a cell, three things can happen to glucose:

- It can be burned immediately for energy.
- It can be stored in limited amounts for later use as a starchlike material called glycogen.
- Or it can be converted to fat.

If a cell chooses this last option, making fat from glucose, it's a one-way street. There's no way that fat can be made back into glucose. It has to be either burned as fat or stored as fat.

In addition to its function as a traffic cop directing glucose into cells, insulin controls the release of stored fat from your fat cells. The higher your insulin level, the less fat is released back into your system to be used as fuel. So when you eat a high-carb meal, particularly one high in refined starches and sugar, your insulin shoots up to remove the glucose from your blood and tuck it away in cells, and your fat usage simultaneously goes way down. Simply put, your body always gives carbs priority treatment.

Why do carbs always get the kid-glove treatment? It's because your body has only a limited ability to store carbs: at most about half a day's energy supply. (Contrast this to body fat stores: Even a thin person tends to carry a two-month reserve supply.) So it makes sense that we burn as much carbohydrate as we can as soon as it's digested and absorbed. Otherwise we'd quickly run out of places to store it. Add to that the rapid pace at which sugar and other refined carbs are digested, and the whole process can get pretty dramatic. Now imagine this process taking place three, four, or five times a day, each time shutting off fat burning as your insulin level escalates to deal with the rising tide of blood sugar. Your body has no other options once you've eaten a carb-rich meal, because this metabolic bully always has to have its way. Because of this biologic imperative, fat calories are always pushed to the back of the line—where more than likely they are stored, and stored, and stored.

This whole process is pretty silent for most of us, as long as we're young and healthy, but some people have trouble with these wide swings in blood glucose. If your insulin response is too great or lasts too long, your blood sugar level drops—and bam! your energy level crashes. You may recognize it as a slump a few hours after lunch. You may have trouble concentrating, feel sleepy, and often crave something such as chocolate, chips, or candy. Then guess what happens a few hours later? Just rerun the tape. Keep up this pattern for years, and you may develop insulin resistance, meaning that more and more insulin is required to transport the same amount of glucose. What has happened is that your body is giving in to the bully and the stage is set for developing metabolic syndrome and even type 2 diabetes. (We'll discuss this in depth in chapter 14.)

Compared to the span of evolution, our bodies haven't had much time to learn how to deal with all these newfangled refined carbohydrates and sugars that have come to dominate our diet only in the last half century or so. And all along, you were blaming your thunder thighs on salad dressing and scrambled eggs! The ability to carry a "fanny pack" of energy in the form of fat actually helped our distant ancestors survive during prolonged intervals between meals (hunting doesn't always deliver each meal on time) and in times of famine. However, today, when most people eat three big squares full of refined carbs each day—not to mention sweetened double caffè lattes and midafternoon candy bars—they seldom get the opportunity to draw on their backup fat stores. As long as we keep making glucose into fat and let the bully blockade it there, we're doomed to being heavy.

Fortunately, finding the Atkins Edge gives you an exit pass off the blood sugar roller coaster by switching your body over to burning mostly fat for energy. When you eat foods composed primarily of protein, fat, and fiber, your body produces far less insulin. (If you eat a large amount of protein, some of it can convert to glucose, but protein doesn't provoke the secretion of nearly as much insulin as carbs do.) And when the carbs you do eat are in the form of high-fiber foods, which convert to glucose relatively slowly, you shouldn't experience extremes in your blood sugar levels. Your body needs to produce much less insulin, so your blood sugar level holds steady, along with your energy level.

By changing the balance of fats, carbohydrates, and protein in your diet, you convert your body to burning primarily fat instead of constantly making it switch back and forth between carbs and fat. There's nothing strange or risky about this perfectly normal metabolic process. You burn your own body fat for energy, and as a welcome side effect, you lose weight. Just in case you missed the point earlier, eating fats doesn't make you fat as long as you give your body permission to burn them. Place the blame where it belongs: overeating and overresponding to carbs. And herein lies the theme of this book—and the premise of the Atkins Diet.

We know that you're raring to begin Atkins, but hold your horses. We've deliberately placed the next three chapters on macronutrients before part II, where you'll get the nitty-gritty on how to do Atkins. Better to take a little bit of time reading this now than later on having to say, "Oops, I should have read that before I rushed into this and went astray!" The more you understand the importance of what you put into your mouth, the more you'll be committed to choosing a healthful way to eat for the rest of your life. Most people who failed on Atkins in the past actually were doing some misconception of Atkins. When you understand the correct way to eat (and *why*) and how slower, steady weight loss leads to lifetime weight control, your likelihood of long-term success increases greatly.

## REVIEW POINTS

- Atkins is a lifetime approach to eating, not just a weight loss diet.
- Atkins is comprised of four progressively liberal phases.
- Curb your carb intake, and you convert your body to burning primarily fat for energy.
- When you begin to tap into your body's fat stores, you foil the metabolic bully that normally blocks access to your fat stores.
- This metabolic adaptation, known as the Atkins Edge, provides a steady source of energy, helping control your appetite and eliminating or reducing carb cravings.
- You'll lose water weight first on Atkins, as you do on any weight loss diet, but fat loss will quickly follow.
- Consuming a modest amount of salt eliminates or moderates symptoms that may accompany the diet's diuretic effect and the metabolic shift to burning fat.
- The amount and quality of the carbohydrate foods you eat impact the amount of insulin in your bloodstream.
- Fat is easily stored in your body, but there is limited storage space for carbohydrate, so any excess converts to fat.

Now let's meet Janet Freedman, who is slim for the first time in her adult life.

# SUCCESS AT LONG LAST

From age 7, when she was seriously injured in an accident, the artist and author Janet Freedman had struggled with her weight. After spending months in bed being stuffed with food—including daily milk shakes to heal her bones—she emerged as a chunky little girl who grew into a chunky woman. But that's now history.

## VITAL STATISTICS

Current phase: Ongoing Weight
  Loss
Daily Net Carb intake: 30 grams
Age: 64
Height: 5 feet, 3 inches
Before weight: 157.5 pounds
Current weight: 132.5 pounds
Weight lost: 25 pounds

Current blood pressure: 110/70
Former triglycerides: 181
Current triglycerides: 83
Former HDL ("good") cholesterol:
  41 mg/dL
Current HDL ("good") cholesterol:
  54 mg/dL

**What was your first effort to slim down?**
I began the "old" Weight Watchers when I was 19. I lost the excess weight but remember lying in bed at night unable to sleep because my stomach hurt from hunger. Needless to say, I ultimately stopped the program and regained the weight I'd lost. Over many years I've tried a series of unsuccessful diets. Meanwhile, I gained additional weight during two pregnancies and even more as I aged. In 2004 I entered a study at the local hospital that focused on a low-calorie, low-fat diet (DASH) that included weekly educational meetings. I lost weight slowly but was hungry most of the time.

**Did you have related health issues?**
Yes. My cholesterol levels required increased medication, my joints ached, and I felt old and tired. I also wasn't able to fully participate in the exercise component of the DASH diet due to my "bad knees and

hips," which my doctor attributed to arthritis. Both coronary artery disease and diabetes run in my family, and I thought it was just a matter of time.

**What made you turn to Atkins?**
At the end of the study, I continued to eat the low-fat, low-calorie way, maintaining my weight through extreme diligence. I still felt deprived, and in the last year I followed that diet, I lost only 4 pounds. Meanwhile, my cholesterol numbers, which were supposed to come down, kept climbing. A friend told me how she lost weight and improved her health on Atkins. Since I still wasn't anywhere near a normal weight and I knew I couldn't continue the low-fat torture any longer, I decided to try it.

**How did you do?**
I reached my goal weight in five months and then set a goal of another 5 pounds, which I've surpassed. I've been able to reduce my cholesterol medicine dose, and my dry skin has disappeared. My joints no longer ache, so I've been able to increase my exercise. I fully expect to see further improvement as I continue this amazing lifestyle. And I fit into size 8 pants, which I've never worn in my entire life!

**What is your fitness regimen?**
I started walking at home on a treadmill for five minutes at 1.5 miles per hour. As I've lost weight and my knee and hip pain has decreased, I've doubled my speed and added an incline. I now walk for twenty to thirty minutes three or four times a week. Other days I ride a stationary bike, do a series of core exercises, and a short free-weight routine.

**What were the worst things about being overweight?**
People who are of normal weight have no idea of the agonies that young overweight people endure. I know that it left its mark on my self-esteem and confidence. All those continually unsuccessful diets only added to the pain.

**What do you like about Atkins?**
I love that it is healthy and sensible and promotes *real* food. The awful gnawing hunger disappears. Hunger has always made me abandon previous attempts to lose weight. No longer. When I went to my son's destination wedding, I was surrounded by lots of empty-calorie, high-carb foods, but I wasn't tempted, not even by the wedding cake. The excessive hunger and cravings are gone.

**What words of wisdom can you offer other people?**
Read everything you can about Atkins. Follow the guidelines, and give the plan two weeks to see what it can do for you. The Atkins Community will provide you with advice and support.

**Anything else you want to add?**
I got fat following the government's advice. Now my body is telling me that this is the right way to eat and the advice I'd been getting for years was dead wrong.

# Chapter 3

# THE RIGHT CARBS IN THE RIGHT AMOUNTS

White flour is better suited to glue for kindergarten art projects than to nutrition. Refined grains and the insidious sweet "poison" known as sugar fuel the food-processing industry, but such products damage the health and quality of life of people who are struggling with carb overload.

In addition to taking control of your weight and your health, an equally important and related goal is to discover a nutrient-rich pattern of eating that supplies you with a steady stream of energy. It's vital that you understand the basics of nutrition, but you also need to learn to read your own body's signals. Rebalancing your diet is the first step in this personalization process.

You probably know some lucky individuals who seem to be able to eat everything and never gain an ounce. (Don't hate them.) Then there are the rest of us who struggle with a metabolism that can't handle the high carbohydrate load typical of the modern, processed-food diet. Fortunately, your body will behave differently if you feed it differently. All you have to do to stop the struggle is banish the metabolic bully by activating the fat-burning switch, aka the Atkins Edge. In this chapter, we'll focus on how much and which carbohydrates you should be eating to do so. In following chapters, we'll explore the roles of protein and fat in weight management.

## WHAT ARE CARBS?

First let's clarify some terms. Carbs come in two general "flavors": sugars and starches (also called simple and complex). The most common simple carbs are glucose, fructose, and galactose, each containing a single sugar unit. These simple sugars can be partnered to make sucrose (glucose and fructose) or the milk sugar lactose (glucose and galactose). Sucrose is the main sugar in table sugar, honey, maple syrup, brown sugar, cane syrup, and molasses. Starches, on the other hand, are composed of long chains of glucose, but when they're digested they break down into their component glucose parts. Starches make up the majority of carbs in breads, pasta, cereals, rice, and potatoes. The leafy greens and other vegetables that are key to the Atkins Diet contain relatively small amounts of both sugars and starches, so they're often called "nonstarchy" vegetables.

## WHAT DO CARBS DO?

Carbohydrates provide energy, but if you're trying to lose weight, you clearly must reduce your energy intake—in the form of taking in fewer calories. Using that logic, lowering your carbohydrate intake makes sense. But there's another, more important, reason to curb carbs. By increasing your insulin levels, dietary carbohydrates control your body's use of fat for fuel. Insulin acts as an immediate roadblock, inhibiting your use of body fat. As we explained in the previous chapter, when you eat lots of carbs, they hobble your body's ability to burn fat. And that's why you can't shed those unwanted fat pounds.

## WHY EAT CARBOHYDRATES?

If carbs are such metabolic bullies, why eat them? Many foods that contain them also offer a range of beneficial minerals, vitamins, antioxidants, and other micronutrients, giving them a place in a healthy diet. The preferable carbohydrates come from foods with a modest number of grams per serving (after fiber grams have been subtracted) and are usually those that are digested and absorbed slowly, so that they don't interfere with your overall steady supply of energy. Unprocessed carbohydrates, such as those found in vegetables, some fruits, nuts, legumes, and whole grains, are also good sources of fiber and water. High fiber content is one reason why most complex carbs are absorbed more slowly than sugars and processed carbs.

Most vegetables and other whole food carbohydrates are fine in moderation, but in the typical American diet, a huge proportion of the foods consumed is not leafy greens, cooked vegetables, berries and other low-sugar fruit, and whole grains. Instead, they're foods made of ground-up grains, refined starches, and various forms of sugar. Think of bagels, pasta, and cookies. Other foods, such as potato chips and corn muffins, bear little resemblance to their origins. Even foods that appear at first glance to be healthful are often packed with sugar. Take low-fat yogurt, a favorite "diet" food. Of the 21 grams of carbohydrates in a 4-ounce container of a popular brand of strawberry yogurt, 19 grams come from sugar!

Atkins is not just about identifying and avoiding foods full of empty carbohydrates, it's also about finding the right carbs—in the right amounts—to suit your individual metabolism. You'll hold off eating some whole food carbohydrates in the initial weight loss phases of Atkins as you learn how sensitive your body is to carb intake. Instead, you'll focus initially on leafy greens and other nonstarchy vegetables. Some people have a metabolism that may eventually tolerate moderate amounts of legumes, whole grains, and even some starchy vegetables. All these foods are on the acceptable food lists for later phases of the Atkins Diet, but other individuals find that even these starchy whole food carbohydrates interfere with weight loss and/or maintenance. In that case, they should be avoided or eaten only occasionally. You'll know which camp you fall into after several weeks or months on Atkins.

## DO YOU SEEK COMFORT IN CARBS?

An inability to stay away from certain foods may not be a true addiction akin to alcoholism or dependence upon opiates, but eating these foods is still playing with fire, healthwise.

- Are your favorite foods bread, chips, and other snack foods and/or cookies, pastries, and other sweets?
- Are you unable to just have one (or two) portions?
- Do you snack on these foods throughout the day?
- When you're bored or depressed, do you turn to these comfort foods?
- Are you hungry again a couple of hours after a meal or snack?
- Do you find yourself eating such foods even when you're not hungry just because they're in front of you?
- Are you often tired, irritable, headachy, or unable to deal with stress or to focus in the afternoon or other times?

All these symptoms are evidence that you're caught in a vicious cycle of craving the very carbohydrate-rich foods that raise and then precipitously drop your blood sugar level. Unlike a true addiction, in this case, you do have a choice. If you can stay away from such foods for a week or two, which will give you the Atkins Edge, you'll soon find that you can be much more comfortable without them.

## A FRUIT IS NOT A VEGETABLE

Although fruits and vegetables are often considered interchangeable, they're more different than similar, both botanically and metabolically. Nonetheless, the USDA Food Guide Pyramid continues to group them together. Not a good idea. Most fruits are significantly higher in sugar and therefore behave very differently in your body than do lettuce, green beans, and other nonstarchy vegetables. On Atkins, you'll postpone eating almost all fruits until you're past Induction. The exceptions are olives, avocados, and tomatoes, which—believe it or not—are all botanically fruits but behave metabolically more like vegetables. The next fruits you'll reintroduce in OWL are berries, which are relatively low in carbs and packed with both antioxidants and fiber. A helpful way to think about fruit is to regard it as a condiment to enhance a meal or snack.

## WATCH OUT FOR THE BAD GUYS

In contrast to whole foods that contain carbs, refined-grain products, sugary treats, and many other packaged foods—the list is nearly endless—supply calories but are almost devoid of beneficial nutrients. To complicate matters, there's sugar and then there's sugar. The sugars in fruit are natural, which is not to say that you can consume them mindlessly even when you're in Lifetime Maintenance. Sugar also occurs naturally in dairy products, vegetables, and other carbohydrate foods. But added sugars, which, as the name suggests, boost the level in foods, are a huge problem. Added sugars can be either manufactured or natural, so the honey in honey mustard, for example, is still added sugar. According to the USDA, each person in this country consumes an average of 154 pounds of added sugar per year, up from an average of 123 pounds in the early 1970s. This translates into nearly 750 calories a day.[1]

This insidious sweet "poison" fuels the food-processing industry but damages the health and quality of life of people who are struggling with carb overload. Practically every item in the center aisles of the supermarket contains added sugar. Learn how to spot it by carefully reading both the Nutrition Facts panel and the list of ingredients on the product label. In addition to the obvious culprits such as soft drinks, baked goods, fruit drinks, desserts, candy, and cereals, added sugars lurk in sauces, salad dressings, ketchup, pickles, and even baby food. All manufactured sugars are full of empty carbs and have been implicated in a host of health problems from cavities to insulin resistance. Sounds as though nothing could be worse, right? Wrong!

## THE MOST DANGEROUS CHARACTER ON THE BLOCK

High-fructose corn syrup (HFCS) deserves a special place in the rogues' gallery of sugars. A manufacturing process that increases the fructose content of corn syrup (which starts out as pure glucose) creates HFCS, making it taste much sweeter. The end product typically contains 55 percent fructose and 45 percent glucose. In contrast, table sugar has equal parts fructose and glucose. Ah, you ask, what's a mere 5 percent difference among friends? As you'll learn below, this extra 5 percent of "sugar" as fructose is fated to turn into fat.

HFCS has infiltrated our food supply. Some public health officials link the doubling in the rate of obesity in the last four decades to the growing use of HFCS to sweeten soft drinks.[2] In 1970, on average, each year Americans consumed about half a pound of HFCS. Fast-forward to 1997, and annual consumption per person was a staggering 62.5 pounds.[3] From 1975 to 2000, annual soda consumption alone soared from an average of 25 gallons to 50 gallons per person![4]

The counterargument is that sucrose, which is half fructose and half glucose, occurs naturally in fruit, and humans have eaten it for thousands of years. That's why you'll see HFCS listed on food labels—and hawked in advertisements—as "all natural," even though factories produce it in tank-car quantities. Although chemically similar to the fructose in fruit, HFCS in processed foods is problematic because of the sheer quantity involved. Whole fruits (and vegetables) contain a relatively small amount of fructose, which is packaged with fiber and healthy antioxidants and other micronutrients. The manufactured stuff is just empty calories with none of fruit's benefits.

Though most cells in your body can metabolize glucose quickly, fructose is processed primarily in the liver, where most of it turns to fat. From there, it takes a direct route to your love handles. Though our forebears did okay with the small amount of natural fructose present in fruits, today we're taking in massively greater amounts. Frankly, our bodies weren't made to deal with it, as a recent study makes crystal clear.[5] Two groups of overweight people were told to eat their usual diet. Individuals in one group had to consume one-quarter of their daily calories as a specially made beverage sweetened with glucose. People in the other group had to consume an otherwise identical beverage sweetened with fructose. There were no other dietary requirements or limitations. As expected, everyone gained weight, but only the fructose-consuming subjects gained fat in the tummy—the most dangerous place to carry extra weight. They also showed increases in insulin resistance plus significantly higher levels of triglycerides. None of these indicators was present in the glucose group. Pass up any product that lists HFCS as an ingredient.

## THE WILLPOWER MYTH

THE MYTH: Successful weight loss is simply a matter of willpower.

THE REALITY: Like hair color, you inherit your metabolism, and metabolic characteristics vary greatly among individuals. Some of the best demonstrations that genes control metabolism involve research on identical twins. When many sets of twins were given the same reduced-calorie diet, all of them lost weight. However the amount of weight loss (and fat loss) varied widely across the whole group. And guess what? The individuals within each pair of identical twins lost very similar amounts of weight. That means that people with the same genes respond to energy restriction in the same way, but people with a different genetic makeup (in this case the different pairs of twins) have a wide range of responses, some losing easily and others very slowly.[6] The same similarity of response within each pair of twins and wide variation across the sets of twins occurred when they were put on an exercise program that burned 1,000 calories a day.[7] So don't be frustrated if someone else is losing weight faster than you. If, despite doing everything right, you're experiencing snaillike progress, you can blame some of it on your great-grandparents!

## AGAINST THE GRAIN

A little over a century ago, a Swiss invention changed forever the diet of people around the world. The steel roller transformed the milling of grain, making it possible to quickly and cheaply produce white flour and other refined grains. The good news turned out to be the bad news. White bread, once the exclusive preserve of the rich, was now available to anyone. However, by removing the oil-rich germ and fiber-rich bran, flour was stripped of virtually all of its essential nutrients. Only after millions of people worldwide died as a result of malnutrition from eating a diet based on bread made with white flour did the U.S. government act, mandating that flour be fortified with at least eight essential vitamins and minerals to replace some of the micronutrients removed in the germ and bran (with the notable exception of magnesium). This new and supposedly improved white flour was dubbed "enriched."

With or without fortification, white flour is better suited to glue for kindergarten art projects than for nutrition. White flour may still help kill people; it just takes longer, as diabetes and cardiovascular disease take their toll. Nonetheless, like sugar and its kin, refined flour and other refined grains—HFCS is a refined-corn product—have become mainstays of our diet. As a society, we are just as hooked on highly processed grains as we are on sugar. Sadly, people around the globe are following in our dietary footsteps.

Just as drinking an energy drink, aka sugar water with some taurine, guarana, fruit flavoring, or a splash of fruit juice added, is not the same as eating the fruit itself, grains that have been robbed of their essential nutrients are pale imitations of the whole food originals. For many people, there's a place for whole grain bread, steel-cut oatmeal, brown rice, quinoa, and the like in the later phases of Atkins. Refined grains are a whole different story. It may be unreasonable to expect you never again to touch foods made with them once you're in Lifetime Maintenance, but don't kid yourself that they hold much in the way of nutrition. If it turns out that you have insulin resistance that doesn't improve with weight loss—although fortunately, it usually does—even whole grains may be more than your metabolism can tolerate.

## CARBS CAN MAKE YOU FAT

We'll look at the misconception that eating fat makes you fat in detail in chapter 5. But carbohydrates and, to a lesser extent, protein can also metabolize into body fat. Guess what a farmer feeds a pig or a steer when he wants to fatten it for market? That's right: grain. An increasingly popular theory is that the chief culprit in America's expanding waistlines is not fat but sugar, HFCS, and white flour—the penultimate metabolic bullies. Consider the all-too-typical American diet: a toaster tart and OJ for breakfast; an on-the-run lunch of soup in a cup and a bag of chips; and a microwave dinner of breaded chicken and mashed potatoes; spiked with a few cans of soda and "junk food" snacks throughout the day. You could easily be looking at 300 grams of carbs. Moreover, most of these carbs are coming from refined grains and various forms of sugar. Low-calorie, low-fat diets also rely heavily on carbs, including lots of those less nutritious ones. In contrast, the carbs you eat on Atkins come primarily from whole foods, especially vegetables.

When you do Atkins, you *rebalance* your intake of the three macronutrients, removing the roadblock to burning fat for energy. That roadblock is—guess what?—a high blood insulin level resulting from a diet that includes too many carbohydrates. This change in diet, which allows you to burn mostly fat for energy—making it easy to lose weight—is the Atkins Edge.

## REVIEW POINTS

- Consuming less carbohydrate relative to fat and protein, and only as many whole food carbs as your metabolism can tolerate, will enable you to lose weight and keep it off.
- Consuming too many carbohydrates, even those in whole foods, blocks burning fat for energy.
- Significantly decreasing carb consumption causes your body to burn its built-up reserves of its preferred fuel, fat, for energy, a perfectly natural process.
- Eating sugar, refined grains, and other nutrient-deficient foods results in spikes in blood sugar; avoiding them eliminates both the spikes and slumps.
- Increased consumption of high-fructose corn syrup has been linked to the recent surge in obesity.
- Whole food carbs contain more fiber, which slows the digestive process and minimizes hunger.
- Gram for gram, whole food carbs are packed with far more micronutrients than manufactured ones.

After reading the next Success Story, that of Julian Sneed, who lost more than 100 pounds on Atkins, move on to chapter 4 to find out how eating protein plays a major role in weight control.

# THE BIG THREE-OH

Heavy since he was a teenager, 20-something Julian Sneed decided it was time to get serious about his weight—and health. He's already shed well over 100 pounds and is still going strong, proving he can be fitter in his thirties than his twenties.

## VITAL STATISTICS

Current phase: Ongoing Weight
  Loss

Daily Net Carb intake:
  50–75 grams

Age: 30

Height: 6 feet, 1 inch

Before weight: 306 pounds

Current weight: 199 pounds

Weight lost: 107 pounds

Goal weight: 185 pounds

**Has your weight always been an issue?**
As a kid I played basketball, and I was still slim as a young teen. But when I was seventeen, we moved from New York to North Carolina and I went from going everywhere on foot to driving everywhere. Plus there were lots of family barbecues, cookouts, and other gatherings with much richer food than I was used to. By the time I was eighteen, I weighed 240 pounds. Later, my job as a manager in a fast-food restaurant, where I could eat as much as I wanted, also made it difficult to control my weight.

**How did you hear of Atkins?**
My supervisor at the restaurant had lost about 100 pounds on Atkins. She gave me *New Diet Revolution* to read, but for a while it just gathered dust. When I did get around to reading it in April of 2007, I weighed more than 300 pounds and knew very little about nutrition. It seemed strange, but tell me that I can eat steak and eggs, and I'm there!

**Did you have any health problems other than your weight?**
No, but diabetes, hypertension, and heart disease all run in the family. My doctor told me that I needed to do something or it was just a matter of time.

**What happened after you started the diet?**
I lost an incredible 50 pounds in five months. At this point, I felt, "Wow, now I weigh 256 pounds." I felt great and kept the weight off for almost two years.

**What made you return to Atkins?**
I was turning 30 in July of 2009, and I decided to commit myself to getting fitter and healthier. I went back to Induction and lost 16 pounds in two weeks, before moving on to OWL. When I turned 30, I weighed 235 pounds, but I knew I was just getting started.

**When did you add an exercise component to your program?**
I began walking two miles every other day my second time in Induction. After my birthday, I joined a gym and hired a personal trainer. At first I struggled with her regimen, but now I love it and my body has changed. I regularly jog four miles five days a week without stopping, lift weights every other day, and work out on exercise machines.

**What do you eat on a typical day?**
For breakfast I might have oatmeal with sucralose and cream and three eggs. Lunch is a big salad with grilled chicken and dressing. For dinner, my favorite vegetable is green beans, which I might have with turkey and sometimes some brown rice. I eat whole grains a few times a week, but never anything white or bleached. I have an apple every other day and sometimes even half a banana. My snacks are usually almonds, but if my energy is low or I'm hungry, I'll have a piece of grilled chicken or some tuna fish.

**You're getting close to your goal weight. What's next?**
I want to see how fit I can get. My goal weight is now 185, but my larger objective is to be fit enough to join the police force within a year. You need to be able to run three miles and do 100 push-ups. I'm up to 50 now. I feel like I can do anything, and it's not just about weight. The sky's the limit!

**What advice do you have for others?**
I want anyone else who struggles with his weight to know that you can do it too. You'll learn so much about yourself. My first experience with Atkins was all about weight loss, but later I got into another place and realized that it's really about good health. I'm sort of a perfectionist, so I counted carbs faithfully, which I recommend. I wanted to get slim and fit so badly that I was able to resist certain foods in the beginning. Now you could put me down in front of a table full of unhealthy foods and they wouldn't tempt me in the least. That can happen to you if you do Atkins right.

# Chapter 4

# THE POWER OF PROTEIN

Its satiating nature means that a diet higher in protein results in better weight loss. When you replace some carbohydrate with protein in your diet, you experience fewer fluctuations in blood sugar.

Protein foods are crucial to your health and your low-carb lifestyle. Protein works hand in glove with dietary fat to allow you to cut down on carbs. We'll look first at the many important roles that protein plays, including its role in preserving lean tissue while promoting fat loss. Then we'll show you how to ensure you're getting adequate protein. Finally, you'll learn why Atkins is *not* a high-protein diet.

## PROTEIN WORKS OVERTIME

Protein is a component of every cell and organ in your body. Proteins are made from twenty different amino acids that are linked together like a strand of pearls. When you eat protein foods, the digestive process breaks the links apart so the amino acids can be absorbed into your bloodstream. There, they are transported throughout your body to provide the building blocks necessary to construct and repair cells. Without a continuous supply of amino acids, your existing cells shrink and new cells cannot be produced. When you embark on a weight loss diet, you want to shrink the cells that store body fat, but not muscle and other critical cells. Eating protein also increases blood levels of amino acids, contributing to:

- Increased satiety (a sense of fullness)
- More stable blood sugar levels
- Burning of more calories

A number of studies have shown that consuming protein is more satiating than consuming either carbohydrate or fat.[1] This may be one reason why diets with more than the minimum amount of protein have been shown to result in better weight loss. When you replace some carbohydrate with protein in your diet, you experience fewer fluctuations in blood sugar. Digesting and metabolizing protein consumes more than twice the energy (about 25 percent) as processing either carbohydrate or fat.[2] This means you burn more calories when digesting protein than when digesting the two other macronutrients. Higher-protein diets have been linked to prevention of obesity and muscle loss, as well as a reduced risk of developing metabolic syndrome, type 2 diabetes, and heart disease.[3]

A common assumption is that *a calorie is a calorie.* Advocates of this concept suggest that only the total calories consumed count and the proportions of carbohydrate, protein, and fat don't impact weight loss and body composition. Needless to say, this is a contentious issue among nutritionists. Why? Because unlike in lab animals or hospital patients, people live in the real world, making these factors hard to assess accurately week after week. Research shows that higher-protein diets are associated with greater retention of lean body mass during weight loss—independent of calorie intake—providing strong evidence that diets lower in carbs and higher in protein have beneficial effects on body composition.[4]

The proteins in your body are constantly being both torn down and built up. In adults, protein breakdown and synthesis are usually in balance, so the amount of lean body mass (muscle and organ tissue) remains pretty constant. When slimming down, you want to lose only fat. But with most diets, about one-quarter of the total lost pounds normally come from lean body mass. The key to maintaining lean mass is to keep your protein synthesis greater than or equal to your protein breakdown. Not surprisingly, up to a point, eating protein foods boosts protein synthesis, while inadequate protein intake may result in lost lean body mass—not a good thing. This is another reason that we recommend consuming some protein at every meal, including breakfast.

## BEEF ON A BUDGET

A careful look at the offerings in the meat department of your supermarket can literally pay off at the checkout aisle. In addition to making purchases when more expensive items are on sale and freezing them for future use, look for these cuts to pare your budget. The same cuts are sold under an array of names.

**For roasting:** Top sirloin roast (top butt, center-cut roast)

**For braising:** Top blade roast (chuck roast) or chuck 7-bone roast (the single bone looks like the numeral) is also known as center-cut pot roast or chuck roast center cut. It makes an excellent pot roast. Brisket is another budget-friendly cut that, like chuck cuts, benefits from long, slow cooking.

**For broiling and grilling:** Top sirloin is a relatively inexpensive steak. Sprinkle it heavily with salt for an hour or so before cooking to tenderize it. Rinse and pat dry before cooking. Skirt steak is tender when it's marinated for several hours. Cut it in strips against the grain either before or after grilling. It makes great fajitas. Flank steak is another, slightly pricier alternative.

**For pan searing:** Boneless shell sirloin (top butt, butt steak, top sirloin butt) and sirloin tips (sirloin tip steak) are relatively inexpensive cuts that can be used in skillet dishes and stir-fries.

**Ground beef:** Ground chuck is less expensive and more flavorful than ground round or ground sirloin, which can be dry. Look for about 80 to 85 percent lean for best flavor.

## PAIR EXERCISE WITH PROTEIN

The body's efficient use of dietary protein increases with exercise. Consuming enough protein combined with significant weight-bearing (resistance) activity, such as walking up and down stairs or lifting weights, can help preserve and tone your muscles during weight loss. With significant weight-bearing exercise, it may even be possible to add some lean body mass. In that case, you're basically trading fat for muscle. The more you can preserve and tone muscle while losing fat, the better you'll feel and look. You'll also be in better shape, more able to heft a couple of bags of groceries up the steps or keep pace with your kids. But that's not all. The added benefit of more muscle is that whether you're working up a sweat or flopped on the sofa, you'll still be burning more calories than someone at the same weight who has a greater percentage of body fat.

Just to be clear, you don't have to actually work out—although physical activity is important—especially for maintaining weight loss on Atkins. Nonetheless, many people discover a new interest in fitness as they shed pounds. Individuals with a lot of weight to lose may find that they need to slim down a bit before they can exercise comfortably. The choice is up to you. We'll discuss the role of physical activity in greater depth in part II.

## HOW MUCH PROTEIN?

The government's recommended dietary allowance (RDA) for protein is 0.36 gram per pound of body weight for adults a day. For a 150-pound person, that's about as much as you'd consume in a large chicken breast and a handful of nuts. It's important to understand that the RDA reflects the *minimum*, not the *optimal*, amount of protein an average healthy person needs. Many factors increase your minimum protein needs, such as your age, gender, body composition (ratio of fat to lean body mass), and whether you're still growing, are pregnant, have inflammation, or are dieting. Even the amount of stress you may be under can be a factor. Research indicates that adults benefit from protein intakes above the RDA, particularly when they're losing weight.[5]

## HOW MUCH PROTEIN DO *YOU* NEED?

The ranges below for women and men should give you an idea of the flexibility in protein intake allowed across all phases of the Atkins Diet, while the listing for typical protein intake will cover the general protein needs of most people.

**RECOMMENDED PROTEIN RANGES AND TYPICAL PROTEIN INTAKES FOR WOMEN AND MEN, BASED UPON HEIGHT**

| Height | Recommended Protein Range in Grams | Typical Protein Food Intake in Ounces | Recommended Protein Range in Grams | Typical Protein Food Intake in Ounces |
|---|---|---|---|---|
| | WOMEN | | MEN | |
| (In shoes, 1-inch heels) | Grams per day | Ounces per day | Grams per day | Ounces per day |
| 4' 10" | 63–125 | 13 | | |
| 4' 11" | 64–130 | 14 | | |
| 5' 0" | 65–135 | 14 | | |
| 5' 1" | 66–138 | 14 | | |
| 5' 2" | 68–142 | 15 | 74–154 | 16 |
| 5' 3" | 70–145 | 15 | 75–157 | 17 |
| 5' 4" | 71–149 | 16 | 76–159 | 17 |
| 5' 5" | 73–152 | 16 | 78–162 | 17 |
| 5' 6" | 75–156 | 16 | 79–165 | 17 |
| 5' 7" | 76–159 | 17 | 81–168 | 18 |

| (In shoes, 1-inch heels) | WOMEN | | MEN | |
| --- | --- | --- | --- | --- |
| | Grams per day | Ounces per day | Grams per day | Ounces per day |
| 5' 8" | 78–162 | 17 | 82–171 | 18 |
| 5' 9" | 80–166 | 18 | 84–175 | 18 |
| 5' 10" | 81–169 | 18 | 86–178 | 19 |
| 5' 11" | 83–173 | 18 | 87–182 | 19 |
| 6' 0" | 85–176 | 19 | 89–186 | 20 |
| 6' 1" | | | 91–190 | 20 |
| 6' 2" | | | 93–194 | 21 |
| 6' 3" | | | 95–199 | 21 |
| 6' 4" | | | 98–204 | 22 |

# THE RULE OF SEVENS

Who has time to weigh food or convert grams to ounces or vice versa? Not to worry. Now that you know about how many ounces of protein you should be aiming for each day, simply follow the Rule of Sevens. Each ounce of cooked chicken, meat, tofu, other protein food, nuts or hard cheese, cup of dairy, or large egg is equivalent to about 7 grams of protein. Consume 10 to 25 of these 1-ounce units daily, depending upon your height and choice within the ranges above, and you'll be satisfying your needs. These visual comparisons should help estimate the number of ounces in portions:

| FOOD | VISUAL |
| --- | --- |
| 1 ounce meat, poultry, tofu, etc. | Small matchbox/remote car key |
| 3 ounces meat, poultry, tofu, etc. | Deck of cards/cell phone |
| 8 ounces meat, poultry, tofu, etc. | Slim paperback book |
| 3 ounces fish | Check book/iPod |
| 1 ounce hard cheese | Four dice |

Spread your protein consumption out over the day, eating at least 4 to 6 ounces at each meal, including breakfast; tall men may need 8 ounces. Unless your initial portions are larger, there's usually no need to reduce your protein consumption as you move through the phases. On the other hand, if you're finding it difficult to lose weight and doing everything else by the book, you may want to decrease your protein portions if you're at the high end of our suggested intake range to see if that may be the holdup.

One way to judge if you're getting enough protein is simple: take the satiety test. After you've consumed what you consider an adequate amount of protein (which naturally comes with a modest dose of natural fat), ask yourself if you're satisfied. If you are, fine. If not, have a bit more. If you're still hungry, try adding some olive oil, cream, or one of our delicious salad dressings or sauces. You need to pay closer attention to your protein intake only if you think you might be eating too little or too much.

Don't waste time calculating the amount of protein you should be eating during weight loss as a percentage of your total macronutrient intake. Instead, as shown in the table above, base your optimal protein intake upon your height and gender. The midpoint of the range expressed in grams is provided in ounces, assuming that an ounce equals 7 grams of protein, but you can choose to have more or less within the range. Just pick your gram level and divide by 7 to get your daily goal in ounces.

## THE MORE VARIETY, THE BETTER

When most people think of protein, particularly in the context of the Atkins Diet, they envision beef and other meat, poultry, fish, shellfish, eggs, and dairy products. Animal products are all good sources of protein, but they're hardly the only ones. Nor are they the only ones you can eat on Atkins. In much of the world, people rely in large part on plant sources such as nuts and seeds, legumes, and whole grains for protein. Even vegetables contain small amounts. Animal protein is considered a complete, or whole, protein, meaning it contains all nine *essential* amino acids (those your body cannot make on its own). Many (but not all) plant sources have reduced levels of one or more of the nine essential amino acids, so they're considered incomplete proteins. It can be challenging to satisfy most or all of your protein needs from plant sources when you're on Atkins, but it's perfectly possible, as we'll discuss in chapter 6.

We can't stress strongly enough that the best diet for you is one composed of foods you love. When it comes to protein, you may be content to eat beef, chicken, dairy, and eggs and ignore most other protein sources. But if variety is the spice of *your* life, make an effort to have fish and shellfish two or three times a week, as well as sampling pork, lamb, and perhaps veal. You may also enjoy goat, turkey, duck, or even pheasant; real adventurers might branch out into venison, ostrich, rabbit, bison, or elk.

The more varied your overall diet, the more likely you are to obtain the full range of vitamins, minerals, and other micronutrients your body needs for optimal health. And the more varied your sources of protein, the more apt you are to consume a balance of amino acids and the essential fats you'll learn about in the next chapter. The point is, you can do whatever works for you in terms of taste and cost, as long as you take a food's carb content into consideration. Protein sources with relatively more fat tend to be more satiating, so you may feel full sooner after eating duck, for example, than a chicken breast. Because they're lower in fat (except for tofu and nut butters), plant proteins also tend to be less satiating, another reason to add healthy fats in cooking and to be keenly aware of the carb content of vegetable protein sources.

Our position has always been that when you control carb consumption, there's no need to avoid fatty cuts of meat or trim the fat. However, if you prefer, feel free to use leaner cuts. Just be sure to serve them with a crumbling of blue cheese or compound butter or a salad dressing or some olive oil on vegetables in the same meal. Again, it's your choice.

## ATKINS IS NOT A HIGH-PROTEIN DIET

Let us set your mind to rest about concerns that Atkins is overly high in protein and can therefore cause certain health problems. With a typical intake of 13 to 22 ounces of protein foods daily, Atkins can hardly be considered a high-protein diet. Instead, we regard it as an *optimal* protein diet. In any case, most of the concerns about eating too much protein are unfounded, in that they're based on limited or flawed research. For example, the misconception that a high protein intake can damage kidneys probably arose from the fact that individuals who *already have advanced kidney disease* cannot clear away the waste from even a moderate protein intake. There's absolutely no evidence that any healthy person has experienced kidney damage from eating the amount of protein consumed on Atkins. Far more dangerous is failure to drink enough water, as dehydration is a much greater stressor on the kidneys.

A high-protein diet has been shown to increase calcium excretion in the urine, prompting concern about a negative effect on bone health. However, recent research indicates that this loss of calcium is offset by increased absorption of calcium and the net effect is increased bone mass.[6] Concerns about an increased risk of developing osteoporosis in healthy individuals are likewise unfounded.[7]

## REVIEW POINTS

- Protein requirements should be based on your height, taking into consideration your activity level and other personal factors.
- Your protein needs will best be met by including protein in each meal.
- Eating a bit more than the RDA for protein helps preserve muscle mass, especially during weight loss.
- The satiating quality of protein helps keep you from overeating.
- Our recommended protein-intake range has been linked to a reduction in obesity and improvement in many other health problems.
- You'll be eating plenty of protein, but Atkins is not a *high*-protein diet.

In the next chapter, you'll learn about the crucial role that dietary fat plays in weight control *and* good health. But first let's visit with Loralyn Hamilton, who dispatched her excess pounds fourteen years ago—for good.

**SUCCESS STORY 4**

# DOING WHAT COMES NATURALLY

For fourteen years and counting, Loralyn Hamilton has followed Atkins to keep her weight under control and boost her energy. As she's come to know how her body works and to trust her instincts, living a low-carb lifestyle has become second nature.

## VITAL STATISTICS

Current phase: Lifetime
  Maintenance
Daily Net Carb intake:
  80–100 grams
Age: 35

Height: 5 feet, 6 inches
Before weight: 165 pounds
Current weight: 130 pounds
Weight lost: 35 pounds

**What motivated you to try Atkins?**

The first time I did Atkins was when I was a freshman in college. I needed to be careful about what I ate ever since I was 14, but it wasn't until I was 19 that I put on 30 pounds. Also, I wasn't feeling well. I was so tired that I couldn't easily walk from one class to another, and mentally, it was very difficult. Judging from my midmorning and midafternoon sugar crashes, my doctor said that I was borderline hypoglycemic. He told me to cut back on the sugar and eat more protein. After reading about the Atkins Diet, I decided to try it. I lost 35 pounds, had a lot more energy, and the sugar crashes stopped.

**Did you experience any major hurdles?**

Plateaus, of course, and getting those last 5 pounds off was difficult. As a college student, it was difficult to find food that I could eat. Every time I went somewhere and ordered a cheeseburger without a bun, everyone thought I was crazy. Of course, now it is the norm.

**Did you incorporate fitness into your lifestyle?**

I bought a little treadmill and walked on it for 5 minutes a day, slowly getting up to 15 minutes a day, 5 days a week. Now I stretch and work out for about 10 minutes a day on the glider.

**Did you fall off the wagon at any point?**

No, but I intentionally migrated off a couple of times. Once I tried Slim-Fast, but I was hungry all the time and was not a nice person on it! When I became pregnant, I was in the Lifetime Maintenance phase and although I thought I could stay there I wasn't really sure about the impact of it, so I took a moderately low-carb approach. I hope to become pregnant again soon, and this time I will stay in the maintenance phase.

**After fourteen years, is doing Atkins second nature?**

My husband eats the same way I do, which makes it easy. In fact, on our first date, we discovered we both watched our carbs. I'd never dated anyone else who did. We follow our own version of Atkins simply because we know what works for us and what doesn't. After a while, you come to know your system. Occasionally, I'll have a piece of bread or pancakes with sugar-free syrup. If they make me feel extra hungry the next day, I eat plenty of meat and butter and salad dressing to satiate myself.

**So basically you find it easy to maintain your weight?**
Yes. I weigh myself about three times a week. It's a motivational thing for me. My weight cycles between 130 and 135 pounds. When I'm at the top end of that, I can take off the extra 3 to 5 pounds quickly, but my body doesn't want to go below 130. If I realize I'm consuming too many carbs, I'll have eggs for breakfast and chicken or beef and some vegetables for lunch and dinner and the pounds come off in a week or so.

**What tips can you offer other people about maintaining their weight long term?**
Most people need to realize that they will be able to incorporate the foods they love back into their lifestyle once they know their Atkins Carbohydrate Equilibrium (ACE) and therefore how their body processes carbs. Focusing on the good things you can eat and enjoy works better than focusing on those you can't handle. You have to retrain your mind to think of the benefits. Resistance only makes you want something more. If you think of wanting an inappropriate food as something temporary, you can push through the difficult points and stay on track.

# Chapter 5

# MEET YOUR NEW FRIEND: FAT

The simplistic idea that eating fat makes you fat has no scientific basis, despite the old saw that you are what you eat. More accurately, you are what your body chooses to store from what you eat.

It's time to stop thinking of dietary fat as your enemy. One more time, loud and clear: fat is a key source of energy and essential nutrients, and you cannot live without it. Counterintuitive as it may be, replacing sugars and refined carbohydrates with natural fats also plays an important role in helping with weight control. In fact, fat can be a high-energy food that gives you a metabolic edge, what we call the Atkins Edge. When you increase your intake of fat in place of carbs, you'll experience a higher and more consistent energy level.

But first, let's get a few terms and definitions onto the table. When scientists refer to fat, they usually use the term "fatty acids," which are part of a group of substances called lipids. And because they are insoluble in water, dietary fats enable your body to absorb the fat-soluble vitamins A, D, E, and K, as well as certain other micronutrients in vegetables.

## MULTITASKING FATS

Fat-containing cells cushion many parts of your body, including bones and organs, and help insulate us from cold. Fatty acids are also vital ingredients in membranes, which are basically the wrappers that act as the cells' gatekeepers, controlling what comes in and goes out. Many of our cells, including brain cells, contain specific essential fatty acids that are necessary for healthy brain function, enabling our nerves and hormonal system to transmit signals to the rest of our body, among other important functions.

All well and good, you are probably saying, but what I really want to know is, how can fat make me thin? As you already know, along with protein, fat helps increase satiety. And because fat carries flavor, it makes food more satisfying. So what? Let's say, for the sake of argument, that 500 Calories of fat give you as much satiety as 1,000 Calories of refined carbs. Which is the better choice if you want to lose weight? Fat in the diet also slows the entry of glucose into the bloodstream, moderating the highs and lows of blood sugar that can lead to renewed hunger soon after eating carbs. Bottom line: eat fats in place of carbs, and you're less apt to overeat. These entwined properties are essential to the processes of both losing weight and then keeping it off.

Despite all these benefits, dietary fat has been demonized over the last half century. For too long, the public and even some nutrition scientists have bought into the simplistic idea that eating fat makes you fat. That's remarkable because there's no compelling research that shows that natural fat is bad for you. In fact, it's just the opposite. First, in and of itself, properly selected dietary fat isn't a threat to health. Secondly, there are now hard data to demonstrate that consuming as much as 60 percent of calories as fat in the early phases of Atkins poses no health hazard. But there is a big *but*—no pun intended! It's the *combination* of fat and a relatively high intake of carbohydrates—particularly refined ones—that can become a deadly recipe for obesity, diabetes, cardiovascular disease, and a host of other ills. We've touched on it before, but in this chapter, we'll prove to you that dietary fat is fine in the context of a low-carb lifestyle.

## CONFUSION OVER CALORIES

The higher calorie content per gram of fat compared to that of protein and carbohydrate has undoubtedly added to the phobia about eating fatty foods. (A gram of fat contains 9 Calories; a gram of protein or carbohydrate contains 4 Calories.) Gram for gram, reducing the amount of fat you eat would appear to be the best way to reduce calories, but the *weight* of food is not what counts. It's all about what foods *do* once they enter your body, and fat can do wonderful things when consumed in combination with the right ratio of carbs. Statistics reveal that fat intake by Americans hasn't changed much from 1971 to 2000.[1] The same cannot be said for carbohydrates. Their intake has increased in tandem with skyrocketing rates of obesity. In actuality, people have replaced some of their dietary fat with an even greater amount of carbohydrates. The real culprit is increased calorie intake in the form of carbs, aided and abetted by a lack of regular activity.

Absolute fat intake has stayed about the same or actually decreased slightly. So much for the "eat fat, get fat" misconception.

Moreover, there's a reason why restricting only calories may not get you the weight loss results you desire. Much as gasoline fuels a car, your body runs on energy provided by the food you eat. Just as you conserve gas by driving at a lower speed, your body conserves valuable energy when it senses that food is in short supply. This self-regulating process was a life-saver in the days when our ancestors had to endure periods of food scarcity. When fewer calories come in, your metabolism gets stingy with the calories it expends. So calories from healthy, natural fats may be the very thing you need to get your metabolism tuned to the right mix of fuels and sustain your energy level.

## WHAT HAPPENS TO DIETARY FAT?

What occurs when you eat fatty foods depends upon what else is on your plate and how your body responds to it. If you're young and active, you may be able to eat lots of fat—and carbs—and stay slim. On the other hand, if you've lost that youthful resilience, live a sedentary lifestyle, and continue certain dietary habits, you're likely to accumulate body fat. If you're already overweight and eating lots of carbs—with or without much fat—you'll rarely if ever tap into your excess body fat as an energy source. Instead, it just continues to accumulate, year after year. This is why the low-fat/high-carb approach has failed to work for so many of us. But cutting down on carbs releases you from this fat-holding pattern. When your carb intake is low, your body recovers its capacity to burn fat, so your fat intake can be relatively high without any adverse effect on your weight or health.

Some people mistakenly assume that a marriage of Atkins and a low-fat diet is the best of both worlds. Not so! As long as you're restricting carbohydrates, the dietary calories from fat are used directly for energy and are unlikely to be stored. Yummy foods such as nuts, guacamole, whipped cream, olives, pesto, butter, and chicken salad made with mayonnaise help provide satiety so you can keep your appetite under control. They also ensure an adequate calorie intake so your metabolism doesn't dial itself down to "low," slowing weight loss. Protein can't do the job on its own. The tag team of fat and protein keeps you from feeling deprived.

So what happens if you try to cut out fats in an effort to coax the pounds to come off faster? In short, problems arise, all of which can be managed but require close medical supervision. So yes, doctors do sometimes put hospital patients on a low-carb and low-fat program to resolve serious metabolic issues, but such a program must be closely supervised. Eating sufficient fats is key to making Atkins work safely. So stop worrying and start enjoying the delicious foods you can eat on Atkins.

Fat metabolism is perfectly natural for your body, and the fastest path to getting into the fat-burning mode is the Induction phase, in which you wean your body away from its carb and glucose habit. It can take several weeks to fully convert your metabolism to burning primarily fat, but after the first week of restricting carbs, you'll be most of the way there. However, even one high-carb meal will slow your conversion progress.

Another common misconception is that eating fatty foods initiates the burning of body fat. Not so. It's simply the restriction of carbohydrates that acts as the stimulus.[2] Nor is dietary fat burned before body fat. Rather, existing body fat stores intermingle with incoming dietary fat, much as the remaining fuel in your gas tank mixes with new gas when you start pumping more in. So when you're adapted to fat metabolism, some of the ingredients in the blend burn faster; the rest are recirculated, and the blend is remixed on a regular basis. This way, your body gets to pick and choose which fats it burns and which it keeps for later. As we will tell you over and over again, you're *not* what you eat. Rather, you are what your body chooses to store from what you eat. Your job is to give it good choices and let it do its job.

## THE CHOLESTEROL MYTH

THE MYTH: Eating fatty foods raises cholesterol to dangerous levels.

THE REALITY: The idea of eating less carbohydrate and more fat inevitably raises the specter of cholesterol and its relationship to cardiovascular health. But calm down. Like fats, cholesterol is a lipid. And like them, it's essential for life, in this case normal cellular function, hormone production, and infection fighting. Unlike fat, however, cholesterol has no calories, so your body doesn't burn it for energy. Though you do absorb some cholesterol from eating animal products—plants contain none—your own liver makes the vast majority of the cholesterol in your body from scratch, independently of how much cholesterol you eat. So, yes, the amount of cholesterol in your diet influences your cholesterol levels somewhat, but so does your genetic predisposition and, most important, the mix of other nutrients you eat. Give your body the right combination of nutrients, and it will figure out how to safely process cholesterol.

# THREE "FLAVORS" OF FAT

Although most foods contain a mixture of fat—the three main classes are based on chemical structure—they're typically categorized by their predominant fat.

- *Monounsaturated fatty acids* (MUFAs) are found in olive oil, canola oil, and in walnuts and most other nuts, as well as avocados. MUFAs are usually liquid at room temperature.
- *Polyunsaturated fatty acids* (PUFAs) are always liquid both at room temperature and in the refrigerator. They're found mostly in oils from vegetables, seeds, and some nuts. Sunflower, safflower, flaxseed, soybean, corn, cottonseed, grape seed, and sesame oils are all high in PUFAs. So are the oils in fatty fish such as sardines, herring, and salmon.
- *Saturated fatty acids* (SFAs) tend to remain solid at room temperature. Butter, lard, suet, and palm and coconut oils are all relatively rich in saturated fats.

Remember, most fatty foods contain more than one type of fat. For example, canola oil contains twice as much monounsaturated fat as polyunsaturated fat, so it's considered a MUFA. And although most people assume all the fat in a steak is saturated, certain cuts of beef actually contain almost as much MUFA as SFA and even a small amount of PUFA.

## THE SATURATED FAT MYTH

THE MYTH: Saturated fat is to blame for a host of health ills.

THE REALITY: Nothing could be further from the truth. Recent research actually points to the benefits of saturated fat as part of a balanced intake of natural fats. Harvard researchers found that the higher their subjects' intake of SFAs, the less plaque they had in their arteries.[3] And although some types of SFAs increase cholesterol levels, replacing dietary carbohydrate with either protein or any kind of fat lowers your blood triglyceride level and elevates HDL ("good") cholesterol levels.[4] Moreover, the number of small, dense LDL ("bad") particles actually decreases, becoming the fluffy, less risky type.[5] So where did the SFA go? When carb intake is restricted, the body makes less saturated fat and simultaneously burns more of it. And, strange but true, research shows that during the weight loss phases of Atkins, if you eat saturated fat, the less carbohydrate you eat, the more you reduce the saturated fat levels in your blood.[6] Even in the weight maintenance phases of Atkins, the increased intake of saturated fat is associated with decreased blood levels of SFAs.

All three of these classes of fats can be healthy, but getting the right balance in your diet is important to give your body the variety it needs. At present, the American diet tends to be high in polyunsaturates, which is fine for people who eat a low-fat diet. However at higher levels of fat intake, certain PUFAs lower both "good" and "bad" cholesterol. Though the latter is desirable, the former is not—it increases the risk for heart disease—so we recommend that you not add much more PUFAs. (This advice does not apply to fatty fish, discussed below.)

MUFAs, on the other hand, lower LDL ("bad") cholesterol and triglyceride levels without lowering HDL ("good") cholesterol levels. The higher the proportion of these oils you eat, the better, starting with olive oil. Dress salads and vegetables alike with extra-virgin olive oil. For cooking, your best bets are virgin olive oil, canola, and high-oleic safflower oil (which is labeled for high-heat use), all rich in MUFAs and with relatively high smoke points. Safflower imparts no taste to foods. Both canola and safflower oil are inexpensive; however, canola should be refrigerated to guard against rancidity. Canola oil also can impart an off taste when heated. Feel free to cook with butter and add a pat to vegetables, meat, or fish at the table. Coconut oil is also fine in the context of a low-carb diet. Be careful not to heat oils to their smoke point or burn them, as that causes chemical changes that can turn a good fat bad.

Interestingly, no matter which natural fats you eat, when you have the Atkins Edge, your body has its way with them. When body fat from people of all ethnic and geographic groups is analyzed, it tends to be primarily MUFA. This means that your body picks and chooses from what you give it to obtain its preferred mix for storage as body fat.

## DOUBLE-TALK ABOUT TRANS FATS

In the last decade, researchers have found that an increased intake of trans fats is associated with an increased heart attack risk.[7] More recently, trans fats have been shown to increase the body's level of inflammation.[8] (For more on trans fats and inflammation, see chapter 13.) Since 2006, the Food and Drug Administration (FDA) has mandated that the Nutrition Facts panel indicate the amount and percentage of trans fats in all packaged foods. Though the FDA did not ban trans fats outright, leaving it to the consumer to be vigilant, the result was that many manufacturers reduced the amount in their products or eliminated them altogether. Among the numerous products that recently were or may still be made with trans fats are fried foods, baked goods, cookies, crackers, candies, snack foods, icings, and vegetable shortenings. Most margarine products have been reformulated, but as long as a product contains less than 0.5 gram of trans fat per serving, a manufacturer can claim that it's free of trans fats. To be sure that there are *no* trans fats in a product, also check the list of ingredients, where trans fats are listed as "shortening" or "hydrogenated vegetable oil" or "partially hydrogenated vegetable oil." If you see any of these words in the ingredient list, just say no. Also, avoid deep-fried foods in fast-food and other restaurants.

## ESSENTIAL FATS

The essential fatty acids (EFAs) are two families of compounds among dietary fats that your body cannot produce on its own. Both omega-3 and omega-6 EFAs are polyunsaturated fats essential to your health and well-being. The former start their way up the food chain as the leaves of green plants and green algae and wind up in the fat of shellfish and cold-water fish. Omega-6 fats are found primarily in seeds and grains, as well as in chickens and pigs, which pass along to us much of these essential fats from the feed they ate. Unless you're following a very-low-fat diet, you're likely to get much more than the recommended amount of omega-6s—far in excess of what your ancestors or even your grandparents did. The latest recommendation from the American Heart Association is that 5 to 10 percent of your daily calories should be made up of omega-6s. That intake is associated with a reduced risk for cardiovascular disease.[9]

Both omega-6 and omega-3 EFAs are needed for human cell membranes to function; however, the two compete with each other to get into membranes, so keeping their intake in balance is important. In the current American diet, which relies heavily on products made from soy, corn, and their oils, omega-6s dominate. In addition, the meat of animals fattened on soy and corn is full of omega-6 fats. As a result, the ideal dietary ratio of 1 to 1 between omega-6 and omega-3 EFAs has been disrupted. For example, soybean oil has an omega-6 to omega-3 ratio of 10 to 1 and corn oil a ratio of 100 to 1! Perfect balance is difficult to achieve, so 2 to 1 or 3 to 1 omega-6 to omega-3 is a more realistic goal. To achieve a desirable ratio:

• Emphasize olive, canola, high-oleic safflower, and other high-MUFA oils for dressing foods and cooking.

- Eat foods or take supplements rich in omega-3s, such as cold-water ocean fish or fish oil. (See the sidebar "Where to Get Your Omega-3s.")
- Avoid corn, soybean, sunflower, cottonseed, and peanut oils, which are all high in omega-6s.

## WHERE TO GET YOUR OMEGA-3S

Salmon and such other cold-water fish such as tuna, sardines, herring, and anchovies are superb sources of omega-3s. Why these fish and not their tropical counterparts? The colder the water, the more omega-3 fat fish need to survive. Farmed salmon now has omega-3 levels that come close to those of wild-caught salmon. Even 2 to 3 ounces of water-packed canned tuna provide one day's requirement of omega-3s. If you don't like the taste of fish or fish oil capsules, an alternative is fish oil with lemon or orange oil to mask the fish taste. Nonfish sources—flaxseed, almonds, walnuts, and canola oil—are generally not as concentrated as fish oil and contain a form of omega-3 that your body must process extensively to convert to usable omega-3. A new product that may appeal to vegetarians or others who prefer not to use fish oil is a DHA supplement extracted from microalgae. It's about as close as you can get to what fish low on the food chain eat. The American Heart Association recently increased its dietary recommendation from two to three portions of fatty fish a week, or 1 gram of omega-3s a day.

When your body burns fat for energy, both omega-3 and omega-6 fats are metabolized along with monounsaturated and saturated fat. In fact, the omega-3 fats are actually burned off faster than the others.[10] As a result, after significant weight loss, a person tends to have reduced stores of this EFA, making it all the more important to consume omega-3s both during weight loss and for some time afterward. (See the sidebar "Where to Get Your Omega-3s.") On the other hand, one of the benefits of carbohydrate restriction is that it allows your body to make better use of the EFAs it does have in order to construct good membranes.[11] This means that the combination of cutting back on carbs and adding omega-3 fats to your diet is an excellent way to improve your cell membrane function.

If you're confused about the difference between dietary fat and essential fats, a helpful analogy is gasoline and motor oil. Both gasoline and motor oil are derived from the stuff that gushes from oil wells, but the former goes into your car's gas tank and the latter into the crankcase. Gasoline is burned for energy, while motor oil lubricates the machinery so that it runs without friction, reducing wear and tear. Dietary fats differ from each other in many ways, but most contain a mixture of nonessential fats, the saturates and monounsaturates; and essential fats, the omega-6s and omega-3s that are in the polyunsaturated group. Think of the nonessential fats as fuel and the essential fats as metabolic lubricators.

## THE REBALANCING ACT

You now understand that to effectively reboot your metabolism, you'll have to change the ratio of carbohydrate, fat, and protein in your diet. If your first reaction is "Yuck. I don't want to eat lots of fat," please take a careful look at the Phase 1, Induction, meal plans in part III. You'll see that in a typical day, you'll be eating a cornucopia of vegetables along with ample muscle-building protein. To enhance those foods, you'll add your favorite acceptable salad dressings, sauces, and oils. If you're at a loss for ideas, our recipe section, also in part III, focuses on such sauces, dressings, and condiments.

### SAVOR, DON'T SMOTHER

It's essential that you eat enough natural fats to provide satiety, the satisfying sense of fullness, keep your fat metabolism humming along, and make foods tasty. But that doesn't mean you should eat so much that you wind up with a calorie bomb. For most of us on Atkins, our natural appetite response gives us good guidance as to how much fat to eat. But here are some tips. Use enough oil when sautéing food to keep it from sticking to the pan. Use about a tablespoon of oil (plus lemon juice or vinegar) to dress a small salad. These are general guidelines. Petite women may need less, and tall men may be able to have more. Feel free to swap out one fat source for another. For example, if you don't use cream in your coffee, you can have a bit more cheese. If you have two salads a day and need more olive oil for dressing, forgo a pat of butter. You get the picture. A typical day's intake of fat might include the following:

- 2 tablespoons oil for dressing salads and cooking
- 1 tablespoon butter
- 1 ounce cream
- 2 ounces cheese
- 2–3 eggs
- 2–3 servings of meat, poultry, fish, or shellfish
- 10 olives and/or ½ Haas avocado
- 2 ounces nuts or seeds (after the first two weeks of Induction)

## REVIEW POINTS

- Dietary fat is essential to good health and plays a key role in weight control.
- In the context of a low-carb diet, natural fats pose no health risk; rather, it is the combination of fat and a high intake of carbohydrates that is linked to heart disease and other serious conditions.
- As long as you're eating a high-carb diet, you won't burn your own body fat for energy. But reduce carb intake enough, and you will burn both dietary and body fat.
- A low-fat version of Atkins is unnecessary and inadvisable.
- Your body uses three kinds of fat for fuel: monounsaturated, polyunsaturated, and saturated.
- The standard American diet is tilted toward polyunsaturated fat. To restore the proper balance, use olive and other monounsaturated oils for cooking and dressing vegetables.
- When you control your carb intake, there is no health risk in eating foods high in saturated fats.
- Eating fatty fish several times a week or taking an omega-3 supplement can remedy the imbalance between omega-6 and omega-3 essential fatty acids.
- Your cholesterol levels are primarily a factor of your genetics, not your diet.

Now let's move on to part II, where you'll learn how to personalize Atkins to meet your needs and food preferences and embark on your healthy new lifestyle. But first, meet Sara Carter, who after losing about 100 pounds quit her job and started her own business.

# NEW BODY, NEW CAREER

After Sara Carter trimmed 100 pounds from her frame, she got motivated to quit her desk job and start her own business. Eight years later, she's still slim and her business is thriving.

## VITAL STATISTICS

Current phase: Lifetime
  Maintenance

Daily Net Carb intake:
  50–60 grams

Age: 46

Height: 5 feet, 9 inches

Before weight: 235 pounds

Current weight: 135 pounds

Weight lost: 100 pounds

Former blood sugar: 163 mg/dL

Current blood sugar: 80 mg/dL

Current HDL cholesterol: 50 mg/dL

Current LDL cholesterol: 111 mg/dL

Former total cholesterol: 235 mg/dL

Current total cholesterol: 175 mg/dL

Current triglycerides: 66 mg/dL

**Has your weight always been an issue?**
I was heavyset for years. I carried most of my weight below my waist and when I was wearing stretch pants and standing with my legs together, I looked like a double scoop on a sugar cone. My weight would fluctuate, depending upon what diet my mother had me on, but I was always hungry, cranky, and sneaking food.

**What motivated you to try Atkins?**
My mother was diagnosed with diabetes about eight years ago and told to lose weight or else. Her weight just started coming off. Well, I was not about to have my mother be thinner than me! So I started Atkins too, and wow! I lost 8 pounds the first day and 70 pounds in three months. This was the only diet that felt natural to me. Every other diet was a fight, like "die" with a "t." Eating the Atkins way was how I always wanted to eat but was told was wrong.

**How long did it take you to lose the 100 pounds?**

I stayed in Induction for two weeks to get rid of my carb cravings, then moved to OWL, where I lost most of the weight. I lost weight every single day. When I got close to my goal weight, I started adding carbs until I got to between 50 and 60 grams a day. All in all, it took me six months to go from a size 24 to a size 6. Later, when I would grocery shop, I would pick up a fifty-pound bag of dog food and heft it over my shoulder just to see what it felt like; I would be amazed that I'd lugged around the equivalent of two bags for years.

**Did you see any health benefits?**

After three months, my total cholesterol went from 235—interestingly, the same number as my start weight—to 175, all the while I was eating a four-egg omelet with cheese for breakfast every day. My blood sugar went from about 163 to 80. Once I was taking many pills for depression and pain from fibromyalgia and sometimes had to walk with a cane because my knees were starting to buckle. Now that I watch my carb and gluten intake, I only need to take ibuprofen sometimes. My mother is doing well too. She lost 60 pounds and doesn't need any diabetes medications at this time. And my dad is doing Atkins too.

**How did losing weight change other things in your life?**

For twenty years I sat in a chair working as a secretary until I decided to start my own business. I clean up foreclosed properties, which means that I'm lifting things, mowing lawns, and hauling trash all day. I'm not an exercise person, but I'm so active now that I don't need to be.

**After eight years, do you watch what you eat?**

It's still a battle but I keep a tight rein on myself. I can eat pretty much what I want because I'm so active, but I weigh myself every other day. It's become a habit not to put sugar in my coffee. It shoots through me like a rocket. And eating bread makes me feel tired and sick. It's difficult to stay away from certain foods, but I know how I'll feel if I eat them and ask myself whether the price is worth paying. Usually, it isn't.

**What advice can you offer other people?**
Always have food that can quell cravings handy. I precook chicken breasts and nuke them in the microwave when I'm in a hurry. I often have to leave the house without making breakfast, so I keep sliced pepperoni and roast beef in the fridge so I can grab them and go. I'm in the car a lot, so I always keep Atkins bars and a can of mixed nuts there for snack attacks. And I know where the convenience stores are so that if I get caught without a snack on me I can pull in.

# Part II

# WHAT TO EAT:

### How to Tailor Atkins to Your Needs and Goals

# Chapter 6

# ATKINS FOR YOU: MAKE IT PERSONAL

You can customize Atkins to your own metabolism, goals, and
time frame, for example, choosing to start in OWL instead of
Induction. Just as important, you can mold the program to your
culinary preferences and dietary restrictions.

Now that you understand why and how Atkins works, let's focus on the
nitty-gritty of doing it. After covering the basics, we'll show you how to
tailor it to your needs, including deciding which path to pursue at several
forks in the road. As long as you understand and adhere to the underlying principles of the program, this approach will provide you with lots of
freedom as you give your body permission to burn primarily fat for energy,
which, as you've learned, is the essence of the Atkins Edge. But first let's
review the principles underlying Atkins.

Atkins is based upon seven concepts that ensure optimal health and
weight control. We introduced most of these principles in part I, but let's
review them quickly.

- *Focus on Net Carbs.* This means that you count only the grams of
  carbohydrate that impact your blood sugar level, not of total carbs,
  since fiber doesn't sabotage your body's use of fat.
- *Eat adequate protein.* In addition to building and fortifying all the cells
  in your body, protein helps you feel full and keeps your blood sugar and
  insulin levels on an even keel. Have a minimum of 4 to 6 ounces of protein
  with each meal. Taller guys may need closer to 8 ounces.
- *Understand the power of fat.* Fat carries flavor, making food satisfying
  and filling, working hand in glove with protein. Increase your intake of
  monounsaturated fats, while holding back on most polyunsaturated fats
  with the exception of omega-3s. Saturated fats are fine in the context of a
  low-carb diet.

- *Get adequate fiber in food.* In addition to its role in blood sugar management, fiber is filling, so it helps make you feel full, moderating your hunger.
- *Avoid added sugar and refined carbs.* Eliminating these empty carbs is essential to good health, appetite management, and weight control.
- *Supplement your diet with vitamins, minerals, and other vital nutrients.* Although Atkins is a whole foods diet, it's hard to achieve optimal levels of some micronutrients, such as omega-3 fatty acids and vitamin D, on any eating program.
- *Explore and find enjoyable forms of physical activity* to incorporate into your lifestyle, as your weight loss and improved energy level allow.

## WHAT YOU'LL EAT

You now know that your objective is to curb your carbs while eating more healthy fat, along with adequate protein. You'll be getting your carbs primarily, at least in Induction, from the leafy greens and other nonstarchy vegetables known as foundation vegetables. You'll find an extensive list of Acceptable Foods for Induction in the next chapter, along with foods to avoid in this phase. With each of the next two phases, we'll provide similar lists of acceptable foods. (Foods for Lifetime Maintenance are the same as those for Pre-Maintenance.) Some people will be able to add back most or all of these foods; others will not. We'll help you understand what works for you and what doesn't. Unless you're blessed with total recall, photocopy these lists. That way, you can have this crucial information—which will be the key to your success—with you at all times. Over time, of course, it will become second nature.

## LEARN TO COUNT

Central to doing Atkins is lowering your carbohydrate intake enough to unlock the gate that blocks fat burning. The initial amount that works for just about everyone is 20 grams of Net Carbs a day. So for at least the first two weeks of Phase 1, Induction, your objective is to stay at or very close to that number. Counting grams of Net Carbs allows precision as long as your portions match those listed in the carb gram counter. (For most packaged foods, you'll have to read the Nutrition Facts panel to find the carb count, subtracting fiber from total carbohydrate to calculate Net Carbs.) Our Induction-level meal plans in part III are designed to ensure that you eat about 20 grams of Net Carbs per day, of which 12 to 15 grams will come from foundation vegetables.

Be sensible, not obsessive, about both carbs and portions. You needn't split hairs about whether a serving contains 0.4 or 0.8 gram of Net Carbs. Round off to 0.5 gram in the first case and 1.0 gram in the second, as we've done in our meal plans. Nor will you hit 20 grams of Net Carbs on the button each day. Your intake may be a couple of grams under 20 one day and a little over the next. Don't count calories, although we do ask you to use common sense. In the past, some individuals made the mistake of thinking that they could stuff themselves with protein and fat and still lose weight. If the pounds are falling off, forget about calories. But if the scale won't budge or it seems to be taking you forever to lose, you might want to do a reality check, caloriewise. (See page 107.) You could probably guess that too many calories will slow your weight loss, but here's a surprise: too *few* will slow down your metabolism, also threatening your progress.

## THOU SHALT EAT REGULARLY...

That's right. No starving yourself! Regardless of the phase in which you start, you should be eating three regular-sized meals (with your choice of up to two snacks) every day. You may be surprised how quickly that old devil hunger diminishes when you eliminate the blood sugar roller coaster. One reason we want you to put something into your stomach at least three times a day is to provide enough protein to prevent lean-tissue loss, as well as to avoid cravings that may tempt you to hijack the office doughnut cart. Also, a low-carb late-afternoon snack, perhaps half an avocado or a couple of ounces of cheese, will make you less likely to chow down everything in sight at dinner. Are snacks mandatory? Not if your appetite is under control at meals and you're not feeling fatigued. Try cutting out one or both snacks, see what happens, and proceed accordingly. Or simply cut back a bit at meals and continue the snacks. Some people do best on four or five small meals. Do what works for you.

## ...AND DRINK REGULARLY

There are numerous health reasons for drinking adequate fluid. When you're not properly hydrated—and many people are borderline dehydrated much of the time—your body releases a hormone that makes your kidneys retain salt and water, but it does this at the expense of wasting your body's stores of potassium. This essential mineral is vital to keeping your muscles and heart happy. The key to maintaining a healthy amount of potassium is to drink plenty of water, eat your foundation vegetables, *and* consume a modest amount of salt every day (unless you're on a diuretic medication). We'll discuss how to do this in detail in chapter 7. Consuming adequate salt, particularly in Induction, keeps your circulation primed and your energy level high. People often misread the body's signal for more fluid as hunger, so staying well hydrated also helps you not overeat.

To determine if you're drinking enough fluids, simply check the color of your urine, which should be clear or pale yellow. Also make sure that you're passing urine at least every four to six hours. Thirst is clearly a sign as well, but you need to rehydrate long before you actually feel thirsty. Despite the old saw that everyone should drink eight 8-ounce glasses of water a day, individual needs vary. Larger, more active people need more than small, sedentary folks. Vigorous exercise or airplane travel (thanks to the dry air) increases your needs as well.

The bulk of your daily fluids should come from water, clear broth, and herb teas. Drinking coffee and other caffeinated beverages increases urine output, but research indicates that it doesn't contribute to creating water or electrolyte imbalances.[1] Caffeine also gently assists the body in burning fat.[2] That means that you can count coffee and caffeinated tea (in moderation) toward your fluid intake. You won't be drinking fruit juice (with the exception of small amounts of lemon and lime juice) or sodas sweetened with sugar or high-fructose corn syrup, all of which are full of carbs. The same goes for milk—and that includes skim milk, which is naturally rich in milk sugar (lactose). Spread out your fluid intake over the day, although you may want to stop a couple of hours before bedtime to avoid middle-of-the-night trips to the bathroom.

## SUPPLEMENTARY INSURANCE

Vitamins, minerals, antioxidants, and other micronutrients in food are just as vital to your health as protein, fat, and carbohydrate. Vitamins and minerals help convert calories into useful energy and perform a host of other functions that are vital for your body's optimal performance. With lots of vegetables, ample protein, and healthy fats, at the very least you'll be getting the daily minimum of micronutrients that you need. You should also take a daily multivitamin with minerals that includes magnesium and calcium but no iron (unless your doctor has diagnosed you as iron-deficient). Also, take an omega-3 supplement to ensure a proper balance of essential fatty acids. Finally, consider taking additional vitamin D if you don't spend a lot of time in the sun.

## BECOME GOAL-ORIENTED

As with any new endeavor, the first step is to set specific goals. We encourage a realistic long-term weight goal. If you're dealing with health issues, work with your health care provider to quantify both long-term and short-term goals. Blood sugar, insulin, triglyceride, and blood pressure indicators usually improve quickly on Atkins, but changes in some markers may take up to six months. As with any journey, you need to know your destination or you might get lost or distracted along the road. The more specific your goal, the more likely you'll achieve it. For example:

- I want to lose 30 pounds in six months.
- I want to be able to fit into Mom's size 10 wedding dress for my wedding in June.
- I want to get my blood sugar level down to normal in the next three months.
- I want to maintain my 30-pound weight loss for a year.

Don't make the mistake of setting yourself up for failure by trying to return to the twiggy figure you may have had thirty years ago. But don't sell yourself short either. There's usually no reason why you can't be slim again—or even for the first time. Having that goal weight firmly planted in your mind will help you confront momentary temptations. Setting short-term goals is equally important, especially if you know you have a long road ahead of you. Step-by-step goals provide an ongoing sense of accomplishment, so you don't start feeling that you'll never reach your ultimate goal. If you have a long way to go, you might set interim goals in 10-pound increments or smaller clothes sizes. If your weight loss goals are more modest, 5-pound increments may be more appropriate.

Once you've established your goal, imagine how achieving each one of your objectives will make you look and feel. These visualizations should be more than just idle daydreams. Close your eyes, clear your mind, and create a distinct image of the new you. Visualize the person you are becoming on a daily basis.

## LET'S GET PERSONAL

You can customize Atkins to your own metabolism, goals, and time frame, for example, choosing to start in Phase 2, Ongoing Weight Loss (OWL) instead of Phase 1, Induction. Just as important, you can mold the program to your culinary tastes and any dietary restrictions you may have. If you don't care to eat beef, fine. Concentrate on poultry, pork, fish, and lamb. If you're allergic to dairy products, there are plenty of alternative products that you can enjoy. You can even do Atkins while following kosher dietary rules.* One of the reasons that Atkins is so popular worldwide is that it can be adapted to almost any cuisine.

## VERSATILE ENOUGH FOR VEGETARIANS

No, that's not a typo! It's perfectly possible to be a vegetarian—or simply minimize your intake of animal protein, add variety to your meals, and trim your food budget—and still do Atkins. The typical American vegetarian often consumes far too many carbohydrates in the form of pasta and other refined grains. As long as you consume at least two varieties of plant protein each day, you can get a balance of essential amino acids. Which leads to the second challenge. Plant proteins are "packaged" with carbohydrate. Your objective is to consume enough protein without simultaneously getting so much carbohydrate that it interferes with weight loss or weight maintenance. To adapt Atkins to your needs as a vegetarian:

- Make sure to get sufficient protein in eggs, cheese, and soy products (see page 42 to gauge your needs).
- Start in Ongoing Weight Loss at 30 grams of Net Carbs and introduce nuts and seeds before berries.
- Or, if you have no more than 20 pounds to shed and are willing to swap slower weight loss for more food variety, you may start in Phase 3, Pre-Maintenance, at 50 grams of Net Carbs.
- Add extra olive, canola, high-oleic safflower, walnut, flaxseed, and other oils to salads and vegetables to make up for the smaller amount of fat in most of your protein sources, so as not to interfere with fat metabolism.

* See groups.yahoo.com/group/Kosher-Low-Carb.

You'll find vegetarian meal plans in part III. We'll go into greater detail on this variation of Atkins in the chapters on OWL and Pre-Maintenance.

## ATKINS FOR VEGANS

It's more challenging for vegans, who don't eat eggs and dairy products, to do Atkins, but not impossible. The trick is to get sufficient protein from seeds, nuts, soy products, soy and rice cheeses, seitan, legumes, and high-protein grains such as quinoa. Weight loss may proceed more slowly because of the higher carb intake than that of those following the standard Atkins program. Vegans should make the following modifications:

- Start in Ongoing Weight Loss at 50 grams of Net Carbs so that you can have nuts, seeds, and their butters, plus legumes, from the start.
- If you don't have much weight to lose, begin in Pre-Maintenance at 60 grams of Net Carbs, in order to include small amounts of whole grains and other plant protein sources from the start.
- Make sure you're getting sufficient protein in plant sources (see "How Much Protein Do *You* Need?" on page 42 to gauge your needs).
- In order not to interfere with fat metabolism, add extra flaxseed, olive, canola, walnut, and other oils to salads and vegetables to make up for the smaller amount of fat in most of your protein sources.

You'll find a 50-gram Net Carbs vegan meal plan in part III and you can modify the vegetarian plans at higher levels. We'll go into greater detail on this variation of Atkins in the chapters on OWL and Pre-Maintenance.

## ATKINS WITH A LATIN BEAT

As the number of Latinos in the United States continues to grow, so, unfortunately do their rates of obesity and diabetes, making them one of the most at-risk populations in the nation. All this argues for overweight Hispanics or those with a family history of obesity or diabetes to seriously consider Atkins, which has been shown to reduce risk factors for type 2 diabetes and even reverse its progression. Although their traditional diets include lots of corn, rice, and beans, most Latinos didn't suffer from metabolic disorders in disproportionate numbers until they migrated to this country or started eating the typical American diet full of refined grains, sugar, and other processed foods. You can honor your Hispanic culinary traditions and still do

Atkins. (We understand that from Peru to Puerto Rico, and from Mexico to Cuba, each cuisine is different, so our recommendations are general in nature.) Start in Phase 1, Induction, regardless of the amount of weight you need to lose and focus on simply prepared protein dishes flavored with traditional seasonings minus high-carb sauces. Specific recommendations appear in the chapters on Ongoing Weight Loss and Pre-Maintenance.

## RESEARCH REPORT: LOW-CARB DIETS AND EXERCISE

Two common beliefs of nutritionists and athletes are that it's necessary to consume carbohydrates to have the energy to exercise, and therefore high-carb diets optimize exercise capacity. So, the logic goes, because Atkins is a low-carb diet, it must play havoc with your ability to be physically active. Right? Wrong! The reality is that your body adapts to a low-carb diet, allowing access to your fat stores and burning more fat for fuel, which are the same desirable outcomes associated with exercise training. In fact, being able to burn fat for energy and thus spare carbohydrate stores while exercising is a major goal of endurance athletes. From a purely metabolic perspective, the Atkins Diet and exercise are highly complementary.

One researcher looked at elite cyclists who ate a diet similar to the Atkins Lifetime Maintenance phase.[3] Given their very low carbohydrate intakes, conventional wisdom would have predicted severely impaired performance. Indeed, for the first week or two, they struggled to maintain their training schedule. Four weeks later, however, when the amount of time it took for the cyclists to reach the point of exhaustion was tested, the results were virtually identical to their previous performance while on a high-carb diet. There were, however, dramatic changes in fuel selection. After the four-week period, the cyclists used almost exclusively fat during exercise, making very little use of blood sugar (which remained at the normal level) and muscle glycogen (stored glucose).

Atkins and weight training are highly compatible as well. In another study, overweight men followed a diet comparable to the Ongoing Weight Loss phase of Atkins while participating in an intense resistance training program.[4] After twelve weeks, the men showed extraordinary changes in body composition. They lost an average of 16 pounds of fat, attributable mainly to their low-carb diet. Meanwhile, their lean body mass actually increased by 2 pounds, credited mainly to the resistance training. These and other studies clearly shatter the common misconception that you need a high-carb diet to benefit from exercise.

## GET PHYSICAL—OR NOT

Numerous health benefits are associated with regular physical activity, making it a natural partner to a healthy diet. The primary benefit of exercise weightwise is to promote long-term weight maintenance. Research reveals that physical activity appears to help some people lose weight but not others, meaning that your genes make this determination.[5] But there are numerous other benefits of regular physical activity, including:

- Increasing your energy level.
- Complementing the effects of a low-carb diet to unlock your fat stores.
- Inducing calmness, thanks to the release of endorphins, which could temper stress experienced as a result of changing eating habits.
- Building muscle (in the case of some types of high-resistance exercise) so you look better in and out of clothes.
- Instilling a sense of accomplishment.

But go slowly. If physical activity is already a part of your life, you may need to reduce the duration or intensity in the first few weeks as you adapt to Atkins, before building back up again—or not. Listen to your body's signals. Sedentary folks should wait until they are at least two weeks into the program before adding activity. Build your skills and tolerance gradually so that by the time you reach your goal weight, your fitness program will help you maintain it. We also understand that some of you need to trim off a few pounds before you move on to exercise. Over time, however, there's no reason why most people can't incorporate physical activity into their routine. Begin with walking, which can be done almost anywhere and is also less likely to result in injuries. You can personalize the type and degree of activity to suit your skills, preferences, and schedule. Embarking on a vigorous fitness program at a later date is one of those possibilities that is entirely up to you.

You may find it easier to incorporate walking, hiking, and swimming into a busy schedule by combining them with family time, socializing, and even chores like walking the dog. Because it's more natural than a formal exercise program, many people are more likely to stay with such physical activities for the long term. Much like your new eating style, being active should become a habit. Just as you're more likely to eat delicious foods, you're more apt to regularly pursue activities you find enjoyable. The Department of Health and Human Services Physical Activity Guidelines for Americans recommend two and a half hours of moderate activity per week.

## TALK TO YOUR DOCTOR

See your physician before embarking on any weight loss or health improvement program, both to make sure that there is no health reason that might interfere with your success and to have baseline tests performed. He or she will check your blood pressure and blood sugar level as well as order a lipid panel (total, HDL, and LDL cholesterol and triglycerides). In three to six months, or after you've reached your goal weight (whichever comes first), these health markers will serve as bases for comparison. If you're taking any medications, discuss whether they might interfere with weight loss, as certain antidepressants, insulin, steroids, and beta-blockers can. Perhaps you can reduce the dosage or switch to another medication. If you're taking insulin, controlling your carb intake will likely reduce your blood sugar level, often necessitating a prompt reduction in your dosage. This is a good thing, but you need to discuss with your doctor how to manage it safely. People with high blood pressure also often see a quick improvement, so if you are on diuretics or other medication for this condition, take your own readings and keep in touch with your physician. *Caution: Do not stop taking or reduce the dosage of any drugs without consulting your physician.*

## GET READY, GET SET

As Henry Ford once said, "Before everything else, getting ready is the secret of success." Once you've experienced the appetite-controlling benefits of burning your own body fat, you'll find it much easier to deal with the psychological baggage associated with weight loss. The control you'll wield will enable you to accept on a profound level that you're going to succeed. You'll find that you can get past your history and perhaps a poor self-image and form new habits. With the Atkins Edge, you'll enjoy a wonderful sense of mastery as you realize that you're capable of modifying your responses to certain situations and temptations. Before you begin your Atkins journey, address these motivational and practical matters.

- *Finish reading this book.* You'll want to return to various sections as you enter each new phase, but it's important to have an overview before beginning.
- *Get a carbohydrate gram counter.* Print it out from www.atkins.com/tools or pick up *Dr. Atkins' New Carbohydrate Gram Counter,* which fits in your pocket or purse.
- *Pick the right time.* Don't embark on Atkins when you're under a lot of stress or unusually busy. You want to have as much control as you can over

external events in your first weeks on the program, to ensure getting off to a good start. Likewise, don't begin over a holiday or just before a vacation. On the other hand, don't keep coming up with excuses to delay starting the program.

- *Make maintaining your goal weight a priority* from Day 1.
- *Enlist the support of family and friends.* It's a courtesy to tell them what you're up to, but make it clear that you're not requesting approval or permission. Remember, this is all about taking control of your life, and it starts with this decision. Even those nearest and dearest to you may have some ambivalence. Their assistance can buoy you up, but their doubt, scorn, or refusal to accept your decision could torpedo your efforts. Remind them that you need all the help you can get, which includes not sabotaging your efforts.
- *In with the good and out with the bad.* Stock your kitchen with the right foods and snacks (see Acceptable Induction Foods on page 82). Equally important, remove everything that's off limits for now. If housemates or family members aren't joining you on Atkins, isolate the foods that you'll be avoiding for now. Also, be sure to have the recommended nutritional supplements on hand.
- *Make meal plans.* Advance planning puts you in the driver's seat. Review the Acceptable Foods List and the meal plans for the phase in which you're starting. Get into the habit of planning your meals *before* you go grocery shopping so you have everything on hand. Otherwise, you may find yourself grabbing the first thing you can find in the fridge or pantry.
- *Dust off your scale and find a tape measure.* These two tools are equally essential to establishing baseline figures for comparison in the weeks and months to come. Weigh yourself and take your measurements at the chest, waist, upper arms, thighs, and hips. Although the scale is not a particularly reliable tool on a day-to-day basis, it's still useful to track your progress. (See the sidebar "The Myth of the Daily Weigh-in.")
- *Change small but impactful habits.* If your morning ritual has been to stop by a bakery to get a jelly doughnut with your morning cuppa Joe, find a place where pastries don't beckon when you get your caffeine fix. If necessary, take another route so you don't wind up succumbing to the familiar sweet aroma.
- *Duplicate behavior that's been successful in other areas of your life.* By regarding being overweight or in poor health as a problem with a potential

solution rather than a personal failing, you'll be more able to come to grips with these issues.

- *Develop strategies for social situations.* To succeed on any weight loss program, you must decide how to respond to situations that threaten your control *before* you confront them.
- *Find an Atkins buddy* in the flesh or online to share the load, the successes, and the inevitable times when you're tempted to eat foods you know will undermine all your good work to date. Many people find that it's perfectly possible to team up with a friend who lives elsewhere, checking in daily by phone or online.
- *Keep a journal* to track your weight loss and health improvements, as well as your feelings, goals, challenges, and victories. First record your current weight and measurements, along with your long- and short-term goals, and include a current photo. (Go to www.atkins.com/support to use our online journal or print out the format.) Make daily entries and review them regularly to see what's working, where you may have gone off track, and what foods may be interfering with continued weight loss or causing cravings.
- *Use interactive aides.* The Atkins Web site offers a whole toolbox of them at www.atkins.com/tools. One tracks your daily carb intake and keeps a record as you proceed. Other tools include a way to track your weight and meal plans customized to your preferences for vegetables and protein sources, as well as any food allergies you may have.
- *Participate in online support networks and blogs.* The Atkins Community includes numerous chat rooms. There are also other low-carb and unofficial Atkins sites, but only www.atkins.com is monitored daily for accuracy by an Atkins nutritionist and incorporates the latest research and thinking on the diet.

One more thing: don't obsess about perfection. At this very moment, you're probably making promises to yourself about controlling your weight. If you're like most of us, you'll keep many of those promises and other times you'll fall short. As long as such failures of will occur only occasionally, regard them as an opportunity to revise your strategy and take control from that moment on. We all make mistakes, but the biggest mistake is confusing a single error with failure. When you do misstep, acknowledge it to yourself and then keep going in the right direction. Managing your weight and enhancing your health are all about taking charge.

## THE MYTH OF THE DAILY WEIGH-IN

THE MYTH: The scale doesn't lie.

THE REALITY: Unless you wisely interpret what your scale says, it will drive you crazy! Even the newest digital scales suffer from an age-old flaw: they can't tell what's in your body with enough accuracy to give you day-to-day guidance on the progress of your diet. Here's why. A typical adult's body contains about forty quarts of water, but it can safely range between thirty-nine and forty-one quarts. Since each quart weighs 2 pounds, your body weight randomly varies across a 4-pound "gray zone." Thirst and kidney function kick in only when you get to the bottom or top of this zone. Cutting your carb intake to less than 50 grams per day clears a few pounds of extra water, but that just pushes your 4-pound gray zone that much lower, without narrowing the range. Add to this the 2 to 5 pounds of water that premenstrual women typically retain, and you'll see why the scale cannot possibly be completely precise in measuring progress when you're losing, say, 3 pounds of fat per week. And forget about day to day. Instead, consider these options:

- Don't weigh yourself at all, focusing rather on how your clothes fit and how good you feel.
- Weigh yourself once a week to get a sense of your general progress, thus providing yourself fewer opportunities to hate your scale.
- Weigh yourself daily and record the number in your journal. Each day, take the last three values, average them—you can even do this on your cell phone—and write that number down in a second column. This running three-day mean smoothes out much of the random noise. Even better, keep a running average for the whole week.

Whatever method you prefer, don't let a stupid scale and a few pounds of water control your mood or sense of self-worth.

## WHERE SHOULD YOU START?

In the next chapters, we'll guide you through the four phases. But first decide whether to start in Phase 1, Induction, or a later phase. You'll find many opportunities to customize the Atkins Diet to your needs, starting with this important decision. For many people, Induction is a brief jump-start phase to get them off on the right foot before moving on. Others may remain there longer to achieve considerable weight loss before transitioning to the next phase. We advise people with more pounds to lose or certain health issues to start in Induction, but otherwise you can start in Phase 2 or beyond if you prefer. The self-test that follows should help you make the choice that's right for you. Obviously, the more grams of carbs you're consuming—progressively more in each phase—the more slowly excess weight will come off.

**Do you have less than 15 pounds to lose?**
If so, you could probably start in Phase 2, Ongoing Weight Loss (OWL), especially if you're young and active. On the other hand, if you're a bit older, you might choose to start in Induction, as weight loss will likely occur more slowly.

**Do you have from 15 to 30 pounds to lose?**
You'll probably still want to start in Induction. You can also start in Ongoing Weight Loss if you want to add more variety in food options in exchange for slower weight loss.

**Do you have more than 30 pounds to lose?**
You'll definitely want to begin in Induction.

**Do you lead a sedentary lifestyle?**
Start in Induction unless you have less than 15 pounds to lose, in which case you could start in Ongoing Weight Loss and lose more slowly.

**Have you gained and lost and regained weight for years?**
You may have become resistant to weight loss. Start in Induction to get off on the right foot.

**Are you over age 50?**
Your metabolism usually slows with the passage of years. Start in Induction and move to Ongoing Weight Loss after two weeks if the pounds come off easily and you're so inclined.

**Do you have type 2 diabetes?**
Start in Induction and remain there at least until you get your blood sugar and insulin levels under control.

**Does your waist measure more than 40 inches (if you're a guy) or is it larger than your hips (if you're a gal), and do you have high blood pressure, high triglycerides, and low HDL?**

Chances are that you have metabolic syndrome, or prediabetes (see chapter 13). Have your doctor check your blood sugar, blood pressure, and insulin levels. Then working with him or her, start in Induction, and remain there until you get your blood sugar and insulin levels under control.

**Do you have high triglycerides?**

Starting in Induction will help you improve your triglyceride level more quickly.

**Are you a vegetarian or vegan?**

See pages 70–71 for guidance on where to start.

Even if you decide to start in a later phase, be sure to read the following chapter to understand what foods you can eat and what to expect in your first few weeks on Atkins. Then take a few minutes to make the acquaintance of mom-to-five Jennifer Munoz, who gained weight with each successive pregnancy.

# KEEPING UP WITH THE FAMILY

With a family and a full-time job, Jennifer Munoz was short on time and low on energy. After struggling with her weight for years and giving birth to five children, she decided to do Atkins. More than halfway to her goal weight, she loves that she now has the energy to keep up with her kids.

## VITAL STATISTICS

Current phase: Ongoing Weight
  Loss
Daily Net Carb intake:
  30–40 grams
Age: 33

Height: 5 feet, 3 inches
Before weight: 198 pounds
Current weight: 159 pounds
Weight lost: 39 pounds

**What motivated you to do Atkins?**
Because of my weight I was tired all the time. My cholesterol was high and so was my blood pressure. There is a history of heart attacks in my family, so I knew I needed to get the extra weight off. Five months after the birth of my daughter, it was time. One of my office mates at the order management firm for car dealers where I work and I decided to do Atkins together because we'd heard that it was the best way to lose weight.

**Had you put on excess weight during your pregnancy?**
Actually, I didn't gain that much when I was pregnant, but I sure gained it afterward. I was eating everything in sight, and on the weekends, I'd eat fast food. My family is from Mexico, and I love Mexican food—rice, beans, and enchiladas—so those high-carb foods weren't helping either. I've moved away from them because I'm still afraid of them, although I have started using low-carb tortillas.

**How did the first few months go?**
The beginning was a breeze; I started in Induction and lost 25 pounds in the first two months. My blood pressure has normalized, so I no longer need medication, and I'm full of energy. Recently my weight loss has slowed down to about 3 or 4 pounds a month.

**How are you dealing with that?**
I keep myself motivated. When I started Atkins, I found a Web site that takes a photo of you and manipulates it to show how you'll look when you've reached your goal weight. When I am tempted by foods I know I shouldn't eat, I look at that photo, and it keeps me going. I also religiously write down everything I eat. My work friend and I try to incorporate exercise by taking three 10-minute walks every day, and I walk everywhere I can. I also get on the treadmill to watch a video when I get home from work. Every day I fill up a gallon jug with water and make sure to drink it all.

**What do you eat in a typical day?**
For breakfast I might have a sausage and cheese slices minus the bun. For lunch, it's usually a salad topped with chicken or steak. Or I'll have a taco meat salad without the taco shell. Dinner is similar. I'll grill chicken, a steak, hamburgers, or turkey burgers and serve it with lots of salad. I'm not big on cooked vegetables. My usual snacks are string cheese with cucumbers or pork rinds with lemon juice.

**What tips do you have for other people?**
Keep junk food out of the house, not just for you but for your kids as well. Have a diet buddy to help you out. Keep your eye on the ball.

# Chapter 7

# WELCOME TO PHASE 1, INDUCTION

Food is necessary for life. And a major component of succeeding on Atkins is enjoying what you eat. If it's blah, boring, or nutritionally inadequate, there's no way you're going to stay the course long enough to become slim and healthy.

Induction, as the name implies, is your initiation into the Atkins Diet. In Induction, also called Phase 1, you'll consume 20 grams of Net Carbs each day, which will come primarily from foundation vegetables. It's not essential to start here, but Induction is the fastest way to blast through the barrier that blocks your fat stores, transforming your cells into an army of fat-burning soldiers. Induction will also likely energize and empower you.

At the end of the last chapter, we asked a series of questions to help you ascertain where you should start Atkins. (We'll do the same at the end of this chapter and the next two chapters to help you decide whether to stay there or move on.) There are no ironclad rules about the timing. Instead, we'll give you the tools so you can make the choice that's right for you. For example, if you have a lot of weight to shed, you're more likely to see significant results sooner if you stay in Induction longer than two weeks. However, if losing more slowly is a trade-off you're willing to make for reintroducing nuts and berries into your diet and upping your carb intake slightly, that's your choice.

If you haven't already decided whether to start in Induction, a glimpse of what you get to eat in Phase 1 should also help you make up your mind.

## ACCEPTABLE INDUCTION FOODS
This is an extensive list but cannot include all foods. When in doubt, leave it out!

## MEAT, FISH, AND POULTRY

Most fish, poultry, and meat that are not breaded contain few or no carbs. We've noted those that do in the footnotes below.

**All fish, including:**

| | |
|---|---|
| Cod | Sardines |
| Flounder | Sole |
| Halibut | Trout |
| Herring* | Tuna |
| Salmon | |

**All shellfish, including:**

| | |
|---|---|
| Clams | Oysters‡ |
| Crabmeat† | Shrimp |
| Lobster | Squid |
| Mussels‡ | |

**All poultry, including:**

| | |
|---|---|
| Cornish hen | Ostrich |
| Chicken§ | Pheasant |
| Duck | Quail |
| Goose | Turkey§ |

**All meat, including:**

| | |
|---|---|
| Beef¶ | Pork, bacon, ham¶ |
| Goat | Veal |
| Lamb | Venison |

---

* Avoid pickled herring prepared with added sugar and all "batter-dipped" fish and shellfish.
† Avoid artificial crab (surimi), sold as "sea legs," and other processed shellfish products.
‡ Oysters and mussels contain carbs. Limit your consumption to about 4 ounces per day.
§ Avoid processed chicken and turkey products, such as chicken nuggets and other products with breading or fillers.
¶ Some processed meat—think pepperoni, salami, hot dogs, and the like—bacon, and ham are cured with sugar, which adds to their carb count. Also steer clear of cold cuts and other meats with added nitrates, and meat products made with bread crumbs such as meatballs, meat loaf, and Salisbury steak.

**Eggs any style, including:**

| | |
|---|---|
| Boiled | Omelets |
| Deviled | Poached |
| Fried | Scrambled |

*Note:* One egg contains 0.6 gram Net Carbs.

## SOY AND OTHER VEGETARIAN PRODUCTS

| Product | Serving Size | Grams of Net Carbs |
|---|---|---|
| Almond milk, unsweetened | 1 cup | 1.0 |
| Quorn burger | 1 | 4.0 |
| Quorn roast | 4 ounces | 4.0 |
| Quorn unbreaded cutlet | 1 | 3.0 |
| Seitan | 1 piece | 2.0 |
| Shirataki soy noodles | ½ cup cooked | 1.0 |
| Soy "cheese" | 1 slice | 1.0 |
| Soy "cheese" | 1 ounce | 2.0 |
| Soy milk, plain, unsweetened | 1 cup | 1.2 |
| Tempeh | ½ cup | 3.3 |
| Tofu, firm | 4 ounces | 2.5 |
| Tofu, silken, soft | 4 ounces | 3.1 |
| Tofu "bacon" | 2 strips | 2.0 |
| Tofu "Canadian bacon" | 3 slices | 1.5 |
| Tofu "hot dogs" | 1 | 2.0–5.0 (depending on brand) |
| Tofu bulk "sausage" | 2 ounces | 2.0 |
| Tofu link "sausage" | 2 links | 4.0 |
| Vegan "cheese," no casein | 1 slice | 5.0 |
| Vegan "cheese," no casein | 1 ounce | 6.0 |
| Veggie burger | 1 burger | 2.0 |
| Veggie crumbles | ¾ cup | 2.0 |
| Veggie "meatballs" | 4–5 balls | 4.0 |

*Note:* Check individual products for exact carb counts. Quorn products contain milk and eggs, making them unsuitable for vegans. Soy cheeses that contain casein, a milk product, are also unsuitable for vegans.

## CHEESE

Most cheese contains less than 1 gram of Net Carbs per ounce. You may have up to 4 ounces of cheese per day. An ounce is about the size of an individually wrapped slice of American cheese or a bit larger than a 1-inch cube. A tablespoon or two of any grated cheese contains a negligible amount of carbs. Avoid ricotta and cottage cheese in Induction. Also, steer clear of cheese spreads that contain other ingredients—strawberry cream cheese, for example—that may raise the carb count. Also skip "diet" cheese, "cheese products," and whey cheeses, none of which is 100 percent cheese. Soy or rice "cheese" is acceptable, but check the carb count.

Other than that, you can enjoy most cheeses, including:

| Cheese | Serving Size | Grams of Net Carbs |
|---|---|---|
| Blue cheese | 2 tablespoons | 0.4 |
| Brie | 1 ounce | 0.1 |
| Cheddar or Colby | 1 ounce | 0.4 |
| Cream cheese | 2 tablespoons | 0.8 |
| Feta | 1 ounce | 1.2 |
| Goat cheese, soft | 1 ounce | 0.3 |
| Gouda | 1 ounce | 0.6 |
| Mozzarella, whole milk | 1 ounce | 0.6 |
| Parmesan | 1 ounce | 0.9 |
| Swiss | 1 ounce | 1.0 |

*Note:* For a more extensive list of cheeses, see www.atkins.com/tools.

## FOUNDATION VEGETABLES

These include both salad vegetables and others that are usually cooked. They'll continue to be the foundation upon which you will build your carb intake as you move through the phases. The 12 to 15 grams of Net Carbs of foundation vegetables you'll eat each day are equivalent to approximately six cups of salad and up to two cups of cooked vegetables, depending upon the ones you select.

## SALAD VEGETABLES

A serving of raw vegetables is usually a cup, which is roughly the size of your fist. Measure the following salad vegetables raw (except for artichoke hearts). Note that tomatoes, onions, and bell peppers are higher in carbs than are other salad vegetables, so use them in small portions. Also included are other fruits generally thought of as vegetables, such as avocados and olives.

| Vegetable | Serving Size | Grams of Net Carbs |
|---|---|---|
| Alfalfa sprouts | ½ cup | 0.2 |
| Artichoke hearts, marinated | 4 pieces | 2.0 |
| Artichoke hearts, canned | 1 heart | 1.0 |
| Arugula | 1 cup | 0.4 |
| Avocado, Haas | ½ fruit | 1.8 |
| Beans, green, snap, string, wax | ½ cup, raw | 2.1 |
| Bok choy (pak choi) | 1 cup, raw | 0.4 |
| Boston/Bibb lettuce | 1 cup, raw | 0.8 |
| Broccoli florets | ½ cup | 0.8 |
| Cabbage, green, red, Savoy | ½ cup, shredded | 1.1 |
| Cauliflower florets | ½ cup | 1.4 |
| Celery | 1 stalk | 0.8 |
| Celery root (celeriac) | ½ cup, grated | 3.5 |
| Chicory greens | ½ cup | 0.1 |
| Chinese cabbage | ½ cup, shredded | 0.0 |
| Chives | 1 tablespoon | 0.1 |
| Cucumber | ½ cup, sliced | 1.0 |
| Daikon radish | ½ cup | 1.0 |
| Endive | ½ cup | 0.4 |
| Escarole | ½ cup | 0.1 |
| Fennel | ½ cup | 1.8 |
| Greens, mixed | 1 cup | 0.4 |
| Iceberg lettuce | 1 cup | 0.2 |
| Jicama | ½ cup | 2.5 |
| Loose-leaf lettuce | 1 cup | 1.0 |
| Mesclun | 1 cup | 0.5 |
| Mung bean sprouts | ½ cup | 2.1 |
| Mushrooms, button, fresh | ½ cup | 1.2 |
| Olives, black | 5 | 0.7 |
| Olives, green | 5 | 0.0 |
| Onion | 2 tablespoons, chopped | 1.5 |
| Parsley (and all fresh herbs) | 1 tablespoon | 0.1 |
| Peppers, green bell | ½ cup | 2.1 |
| Peppers, red bell | ½ cup | 2.9 |
| Radicchio | ½ cup | 0.7 |
| Radishes | 6 | 0.5 |

| Vegetable | Serving Size | Grams of Net Carbs |
|---|---|---|
| Romaine lettuce | 1 cup | 0.4 |
| Scallion/green onion | ¼ cup | 1.2 |
| Spinach | 1 cup | 0.2 |
| Tomato | 1 small (3–4 ounces) | 2.5 |
| Tomato | 1 medium | 3.3 |
| Tomato, cherry | 5 | 2.2 |
| Watercress | ½ cup | 0.0 |

## COOKED VEGETABLES

Because most of the following foundation vegetables are usually served cooked, we've indicated their carb counts as such, unless otherwise noted. Some also appear on the salad vegetable list, but cooking compacts them, which explains the differences in carb counts. A standard serving of a cooked vegetable is a half cup. A number of these vegetables are slightly higher in carbs than the salad vegetables listed above. Unless otherwise noted, be sure to measure them *after* you cook them. Note that some, such as Brussels sprouts, celery root, kohlrabi, leeks, mushrooms, onions, and pumpkin, are higher in carbs than most, so we have usually indicated smaller portions. You can steam, sauté, stir-fry, or braise most of these vegetables. Boiling destroys and/or removes nutrients (unless you drink the broth). *Note:* Vegetables *not* on this list should not be consumed in Induction.

| Vegetable | Serving Size | Grams of Net Carbs |
|---|---|---|
| Artichoke | ½ medium | 3.5 |
| Asparagus | 6 spears | 2.4 |
| Bamboo shoots, canned, sliced | ½ cup | 1.2 |
| Beans, green, wax, string, snap | ½ cup | 2.9 |
| Beet greens | ½ cup | 3.7 |
| Bok choy (pak choi) | ½ cup | 0.2 |
| Broccoflower | ½ cup | 2.3 |
| Broccoli | ½ cup | 1.7 |
| Broccoli rabe | ½ cup | 2.0 |
| Brussels sprouts | ¼ cup | 1.8 |
| Cabbage, green | ½ cup | 1.6 |
| Cabbage, red | ½ cup | 2.0 |
| Cabbage, Savoy | ½ cup | 1.9 |

| Vegetable | Serving Size | Grams of Net Carbs |
|---|---|---|
| Cardoon | ½ cup | 2.7 |
| Cauliflower | ½ cup | 0.9 |
| Celery | ½ cup | 1.2 |
| Chard, Swiss | ½ cup | 1.8 |
| Chayote | ½ cup | 1.8 |
| Collard greens | ½ cup | 2.0 |
| Dandelion greens | ½ cup | 1.8 |
| Eggplant | ½ cup | 2.0 |
| Escarole | ½ cup | 0.1 |
| Fennel | ½ cup | 1.5 |
| Hearts of palm | 1 heart | 0.7 |
| Kale | ½ cup | 2.4 |
| Kohlrabi | ¼ cup | 2.3 |
| Leeks | ½ cup | 3.4 |
| Mushrooms, button | ¼ cup | 2.3 |
| Mushrooms, shiitake | ¼ cup | 4.4 |
| Mustard greens | ½ cup | 0.1 |
| Nopales (cactus pads) | ½ cup | 1.0 |
| Okra | ½ cup | 2.4 |
| Onion | ¼ cup | 4.3 |
| Peppers, green bell, chopped | ¼ cup | 1.9 |
| Peppers, red bell, chopped | ¼ cup | 1.9 |
| Pumpkin | ¼ cup | 2.4 |
| Rhubarb, unsweetened | ½ cup | 1.7 |
| Sauerkraut | ½ cup, drained | 1.2 |
| Scallions | ½ cup | 2.4 |
| Shallots | 2 tablespoons | 3.1 |
| Snow peas/snap peas in the pod | ½ cup | 3.4 |
| Sorrel | ½ cup | 0.2 |
| Spaghetti squash | ¼ cup | 2.0 |
| Spinach | ½ cup | 2.2 |
| Summer squash | ½ cup | 2.6 |
| Tomatillo | ½ cup | 2.6 |
| Tomato | ¼ cup | 4.3 |
| Turnips (white), mashed | ½ cup | 3.3 |
| Water chestnuts | ¼ cup (canned) | 3.5 |
| Zucchini | ½ cup | 1.5 |

## SALAD DRESSINGS

Any prepared salad dressing with no more than 3 grams of Net Carbs per serving (1–2 tablespoons) is acceptable. A better—and lower-carb option—is to make your own. (See recipes in part III.)

| Dressing | Serving Size | Grams of Net Carbs |
|---|---|---|
| Blue cheese dressing | 2 tablespoons | 2.3 |
| Caesar salad dressing | 2 tablespoons | 0.5 |
| Italian dressing | 2 tablespoons | 3.0 |
| Lemon juice | 2 tablespoons | 2.5 |
| Lime juice | 2 tablespoons | 2.9 |
| Oil and vinegar | 2 tablespoons | 1.0 |
| Ranch dressing | 2 tablespoons | 1.4 |

## FATS AND OILS

No carbs to worry about here. A serving size is approximately 1 tablespoon. Oils labeled "cold pressed" or "expeller pressed" are preferable because they haven't been subjected to nutrient-destroying heat. Use extra-virgin olive oil only for dressing salad and vegetables and sautéing and olive oil, canola, or high-oleic safflower for other cooking. Never use specialty oils such as walnut or sesame oil for cooking; instead, use them to season a dish after removing it from the heat. Avoid products labeled "lite" or "low fat" and all margarines and shortening products, which still contain small amounts of trans fats. The term "no trans fats" actually means that a product may contain up to 0.5 gram per serving. (See chapter 5 for more on selection of oils.)

| | |
|---|---|
| Butter | Mayonnaise* |
| Canola oil | Olive oil |
| Coconut oil | Safflower oil, high-oleic |
| Flaxseed oil | Sesame oil |
| Grape-seed oil | Walnut oil |

* Most commercial mayonnaise is made with soybean oil. Find a brand made with canola or high-oleic safflower oil and without added sugar. Or make your own with our recipe in part III.

## NONCALORIC SWEETENERS

Count each packet as 1 gram of Net Carbs and consume no more than three per day.

> Splenda (sucralose)
> Truvia or SweetLeaf (natural products made from stevia)
> Sweet'N Low (saccharin)
> Xylitol (available in health food stores and some supermarkets)

## LOW-CARB CONVENIENCE FOODS

Some low-carb food products can come in handy when you're unable to find appropriate food, can't take time for a meal, or need a quick snack. More and more companies are creating healthy food products that can be eaten during the Induction phase of Atkins. Just remember two things:

- Not all low-carb bars, shakes, and other convenience products are the same. Check both the list of ingredients and the Nutrition Facts panel to ascertain the number of grams of Net Carbs. ("Sugar free" does not necessarily mean "carb free" or "low carb.") Products suitable for Induction should contain no more than 3 grams of Net Carbs per serving.
- Such foods can make doing Atkins easier, but don't overdo them. Don't substitute them for any of your 12–15 grams of Net Carbs from foundation vegetables.

## CONDIMENTS, HERBS, AND SPICES

Hidden carbs lurk in many condiments. Read labels carefully, and be on the lookout for added sugar, flour and cornstarch, and other off-limits thickeners. Most ketchups, marinades, and barbecue sauces contain added sugar (often listed as corn syrup, corn syrup solids, cane syrup, or something else). Salt, black and cayenne pepper, most spices, basil, cilantro, dill, oregano, rosemary, sage, tarragon, thyme, and other dried herbs contain practically no carbs. But make sure that any herb or spice mixture contains no added sugar. The following products are suitable. Check the list of ingredients of any products that aren't listed before consuming them.

| Condiment, Herb, or Spice | Serving Size | Grams of Net Carbs |
|---|---|---|
| Ancho chili pepper | 1 pepper | 5.1 |
| Anchovy paste | 1 tablespoon | 0.0 |
| Black bean sauce | 1 teaspoon | 3.0 |
| Capers | 1 tablespoon | 0.1 |
| Chipotle en adobe | 2 peppers | 2.0 |
| Clam juice | 1 cup | 0.0 |
| Coconut milk, unsweetened | ½ cup | 1.9 |
| Cocoa powder, unsweetened | 1 tablespoon | 1.2 |
| Enchilada sauce | ¼ cup | 2.0 |
| Fish sauce | 1 teaspoon | 0.2 |
| Garlic | 1 large clove | 0.9 |
| Ginger | 1 tablespoon grated root | 0.8 |
| Horseradish sauce | 1 teaspoon | 0.4 |
| Jalapeño chili pepper | ½ cup sliced | 1.4 |
| Miso paste | 1 tablespoon | 2.6 |
| Mustard, Dijon | 1 teaspoon | 0.5 |
| Mustard, yellow | 1 teaspoon | 0.0 |
| Pasilla chili pepper | 1 pepper | 1.7 |
| Pesto sauce | 1 tablespoon | 0.6 |
| Pickapeppa sauce | 1 teaspoon | 1.0 |
| Pickle, dill or kosher | ½ pickle | 1.0 |
| Pimento/roasted red pepper | 1 ounce | 2.0 |
| Salsa, green (no added sugar) | 1 tablespoon | 0.6 |
| Salsa, red (no added sugar) | 1 tablespoon | 1.0 |
| Serrano chili pepper | ½ cup | 1.6 |
| Soy sauce | 1 tablespoon | 0.9 |
| Tabasco or other hot sauce | 1 teaspoon | 0.0 |
| Taco sauce | 1 tablespoon | 1.0 |
| Tahini (sesame paste) | 2 tablespoons | 1.0 |
| Vinegar, balsamic | 1 tablespoon | 2.3 |
| Vinegar, cider | 1 tablespoon | 0.9 |
| Vinegar, red wine | 1 tablespoon | 1.5 |
| Vinegar, rice (unsweetened) | 1 tablespoon | 0.0 |
| Vinegar, sherry | 1 tablespoon | 0.9 |
| Vinegar, white wine | 1 tablespoon | 1.5 |
| Wasabi paste | 1 teaspoon | 0.0 |

**BEVERAGES**

- Clear broth/bouillon (*not* low sodium and without added sugars, hydrogenated oils, or MSG).
- Club soda.
- Cream, heavy or light, or half-and-half (1 to 1.5 ounces a day).
- Caffeinated or decaffeinated coffee.
- Caffeinated or decaffeinated tea.
- Diet soda sweetened with noncaloric sweeteners.
- Lemon juice or lime juice; limit to 2 to 3 tablespoons a day. Note that 2 tablespoons of lemon juice contain 2.5 grams Net Carbs; the same amount of lime juice contains 2.9 grams.
- Plain or essence-flavored seltzer (must say "no calories").
- Herb tea (without added barley or fruit sugars).
- Unsweetened, unflavored soy or almond milk. An 8-ounce portion contains 1.2 and 1 gram Net Carbs, respectively.
- Water (tap, spring, filtered, or mineral).

## WHAT'S OFF LIMITS?

For now you need to stay away from certain foods. Clearly, we cannot list every food you should avoid. Follow these guidelines, and use your common sense. Avoid the following:

- Fruits and juices (other than fruits listed with vegetables and lemon and lime juice).
- Caloric sodas.
- Foods made with flour or other grain products (exclusive of low-carb products with no more than 3 grams of Net Carbs per serving) and/or sugar, including but not limited to bread, pasta, tortillas, muffins, pastries, cookies, chips, cakes, and candy.
- Any food with added sugar, no matter what kind. Look for terms such as brown syrup, evaporated cane juice, glucose, dextrose, honey, and corn syrup.
- Alcohol of any sort.
- Nuts and seeds, nut and seed butters (in the first two weeks of Induction), except for flaxseeds, which are acceptable.
- Grains, even whole grains: rice, oats, barley, quinoa, buckwheat groats, and so on.

- Kidney beans, chickpeas, lentils, and other legumes.
- Any vegetables not on the Acceptable Induction Foods list, including starchy vegetables such as parsnips, carrots, potatoes, yams, sweet potatoes, acorn squash, and other winter squash.
- Dairy products other than hard cheese, cream, sour cream, and butter. No cow or goat milk of any sort, yogurt, cottage cheese, or ricotta for now.
- "Low-fat" foods, which are usually high in carbs.
- "Diet" products, unless they specifically state "no carbohydrates" or have no more than 3 grams of Net Carbs per serving. Such foods are mostly suitable for low-fat diets, not low-carb plans. Don't be fooled by the words "sugarless," "sugar free," "natural," or "no sugar added." Go by the carb content, which must be stated on the label.
- "Junk food" in any form.
- Products such as chewing gum, breath mints, cough syrups and drops, even liquid vitamins, which may be filled with sugar or other caloric sweeteners. (You can have breath mints and gums sweetened with sorbitol or xylitol and count 1 gram per piece, up to three a day.)
- Any foods with manufactured trans fats (hydrogenated or partially hydrogenated oils).

When in doubt, pass it up.

## TURNING LISTS INTO MEALS

Your objective is to build meals around a wide array of protein sources, natural fats, and foundation vegetables. If you love salads, eat them to your heart's content. When it comes to cooked vegetables, choose from almost fifty selections, from artichoke to zucchini. Steam, sauté, roast, or stir-fry vegetables, but don't boil them, which destroys their nutrients, unless you drink the broth or add it to soups. Likewise, meats, poultry, fish, shellfish, and tofu may be broiled, grilled, roasted, stir-fried, poached, or braised—but not breaded or floured and deep-fried. Enjoy the odd fruits that pretend to be vegetables—think avocados, olives, and tomatoes—in moderation. Refer to the Induction meal plans in part III, which you can modify according to your needs, as long as you comply with the Acceptable Induction Foods list and tally the carbs.

## INDUCTION GUIDELINES

Many people see remarkably fast weight loss results on Induction. Others find it slow going. Whatever your pace, you'll need to follow the rules precisely to achieve success. This applies equally to those of you who are working on improving your blood sugar and insulin levels or your lipids. Otherwise, you could become frustrated before you've had a chance to see what Atkins can really do for you. Read the following rules of Induction, and then read them again to ensure that they're engraved on your brain!

- Eat either three regular-size meals a day or four or five smaller meals. Don't skip meals or go more than six waking hours without eating.
- At each meal, eat at least 4 to 6 ounces of protein foods. Up to 8 ounces is fine if you're a tall guy. There's no need to trim the fat from meat or the skin from poultry, but if you prefer to do so, fine. Just add a splash of olive oil or a pat of butter to your vegetables to replace the fat.
- Enjoy butter, mayonnaise (made from olive, canola, or high-oleic safflower oils), olive oil, high-oleic safflower oil, canola oil, and seed and nut oils. Aim for 1 tablespoon of oil on a salad or other vegetables, or a pat of butter. Cook foods in enough oil to ensure they don't burn, but no more. Or spritz the pan with a mister of olive oil. See guidelines for oils on page 89.
- Eat no more than 20 grams a day of Net Carbs, 12 to 15 grams of them as foundation vegetables. This means you can eat approximately six loosely packed cups of salad and up to two cups of cooked vegetables. (See Acceptable Induction Foods on page 82.) Carb counts of vegetables vary.
- Eat only the foods on this list. This is not the time to push the envelope.
- Learn to distinguish hunger from habit and adjust the quantity you eat to suit your appetite as it decreases. When you're hungry, eat until you feel satisfied but not stuffed. If you're not sure if you're full, wait ten minutes, have a glass of water, and eat more only if you're still unsatisfied. If you're not hungry at mealtime, eat a small low-carb snack.
- Don't starve yourself, and don't restrict fats.
- Don't assume that any food is low in carbs. Read the labels on packaged foods to discover unacceptable ingredients, and check their Net Carb counts (subtract grams of fiber from total grams). Also use a carbohydrate gram counter.

- When dining out, be on guard for hidden carbs. Gravy is usually made with flour or cornstarch, both no-nos. Sugar is often found in salad dressing and may even appear in coleslaw and other deli salads. Avoid any deep-fried or breaded food.
- Use sucralose (Splenda), saccharin (Sweet'N Low), stevia (SweetLeaf or Truvia), or xylitol as a sweetener. Have no more than three packets a day, and count each one as 1 gram of carbs.
- To be safe, stick with Atkins low-carb products and only those coded for Induction. Limit them to two a day.
- Drink at least eight 8-ounce portions of approved beverages each day to prevent dehydration and electrolyte imbalances. Include two cups of broth (not low sodium), one in the morning and one in the afternoon, in this count.
- Take a daily iron-free multivitamin/multimineral combo and an omega-3 fatty acid supplement.

## WHAT TO EXPECT IN THE FIRST WEEK

If you've been eating lots of poor-quality carbohydrates, this way of eating will be a significant change for you, and it may take some time for your body to adjust. You may also be giving up many of your old high-carb comfort foods, which may leave you feeling emotionally bereft. Both reactions are normal. Record any such feelings in your diet journal, along with a list of the foods you've eaten. You can find online support and answers to specific questions on the Atkins Community forums during this transition (as well as at any other time) as well as link up with Atkins "newbies" and old hands.

Just because your best friend or spouse lost 7 pounds on Atkins in her first week of Induction, don't assume it will be the same for you. It's better to begin with no set expectations. Most people lose a couple of pounds of water weight in the first few days. Your loss may be more dramatic, or not. And don't skimp on fluids or eliminate salt to hasten water loss. Remember that lost inches are just as significant. So if your clothes seem to feel a bit looser, even if your weight is constant, you're on the right track. This is also why we recommend that you weigh yourself once a week at roughly the same time of day (or use weight averaging) and take your measurements. That way, you're more likely to see positive results and not get hung up on your body's normal day-to-day variances.

Everyone is different, and it can take some time to fully switch your metabolism over to burning primarily fat. A low-carb diet is naturally diuretic, which flushes sodium and water from your body. Fatigue, light-headedness upon standing up or with exposure to heat (in a hot shower or hot tub or while mowing the lawn on a hot day, for example), weakness, constipation, chronic headaches, and leg cramps are all signs you might not be getting enough sodium. Like fat, salt has been unjustly demonized, despite being essential to life and well-being.

The symptoms described above are not the result of the diet—too little carbohydrate, too much protein, or whatever. The real problem is the lack of just a daily pinch of sodium. Yes, individuals who are sensitive to salt may experience bloating and high blood pressure if they eat lots of salt. But interestingly, these conditions are most pronounced when people eat high-carb diets. Adapting to the low-carb state fundamentally changes how your system handles nutrients that might cause problems in a high-carb setting.

Our strategy to restore your sodium balance will stop most symptoms before they begin. In our experience, normally salting food to taste is not adequate. So don't wait until you experience symptoms; instead, have either two cups of broth, ½ teaspoon of salt, or 2 tablespoons of regular soy sauce daily from your first day on Atkins. Continue until your carb intake exceeds 50 grams of Net Carbs.

If you opt for the broth, drink one cup in the morning and another in the midafternoon. Ideally, make your own chicken, beef, or vegetable broth (see recipes in part III), but otherwise use regular (not low-sodium) canned or Tetra Pak broth or a bouillon cube dissolved in water. If you're going to be exercising vigorously, drink one portion about an hour beforehand. If you opt for salt instead, measure out the amount in the morning and sprinkle it on food throughout the day, being sure to use all of it. If you use soy sauce, make sure it is not the low-sodium kind and consume it in at least two portions as a condiment or ingredient in meals.

If you're taking a diuretic medication or have been advised to restrict your salt intake, consult your physician before adding sodium to your diet. Meanwhile, be sure to eat the recommended amount of vegetables and sufficient protein with every meal, as well as drink enough fluids and take your supplements. If symptoms do crop up or remain, you may want to temporarily increase your intake to 25 grams of Net Carbs by eating more foundation vegetables. Or have some nuts or seeds or even a half cup of tomato juice, which you would not normally have until Ongoing Weight Loss. Once you feel better, eliminate these foods for the time being and return to 20 grams of Net Carbs to speed your weight loss.

Follow this advice, and you're unlikely to experience the symptoms described above.

## YOUR ALLY, THE ATKINS EDGE

Somewhere toward the end of the first or second week, most people feel a dramatic increase in their energy level and sense of well-being. This is a clear signal that you've got the Atkins Edge and can begin to hone your low-carb skills.

Developing new habits and learning how to resist temptation are crucial to your success, but they're not enough. Another major component of succeeding on Atkins is enjoying what you eat. If it's blah, boring, or nutritionally inadequate, there's no way you're going to stay the course long enough to become slim and healthy. Having a large repertoire of enjoyable food choices and making sure that the right foods and ingredients are always in your kitchen is integral to forming habits that will result in a permanently slim you. (See the sidebar "Don't Get Caught Short.") Food is necessary for life. Once you discover which types and amounts of food are best for your metabolism, you'll set yourself up for success in terms of health and weight management as well as satisfaction, and, yes, pleasure. So let's delve deeper into what you can eat on Induction.

### DON'T GET CAUGHT SHORT

You've been following Atkins to the letter, but after a grueling day at work, the kids are clamoring for dinner and there's nothing in the house that's Atkins-compliant. So you wind up eating mac and cheese with the family. If this sounds familiar, you need to have an emergency store on hand at all times. Stock your freezer, fridge, and pantry with the following foods, and you should always be able to put together a tasty low-carb meal.

REFRIGERATOR: Eggs, tofu, cheese, herring in cream sauce (without added sugar), rotisserie chicken (not honey basted), sliced roast beef or fresh turkey, hard salami and other cold cuts with no added sugar; salad fixings.

FREEZER: Hamburger patties, lamb chops, shrimp, chicken breasts, all in individual ziplock bags for quick defrosting in a bowl of warm water.

PANTRY: Tuna or salmon in cans or vacuum bags, sardines, crabmeat, clams, Vienna sausages.

## THE VEGETABLE CHALLENGE

One of the things we hear most often from people new to Atkins is that they're having trouble getting enough vegetables into their daily carb tally. New science on the importance of fiber, minerals, and phytochemicals in vegetables has changed our recommendations about the amount of vegetables you should eat in Induction to 12 to 15 grams of Net Carbs. Have at least one, and preferably two, salads a day. To make it easier to track your carbs, we've created minirecipes for basic main course and side dish salads, which you can modify.

- *Side Dish Salad:* Start with 2 cups of salad greens (0.8 gram Net Carbs). Add 6 sliced radishes (0.5 gram), ½ medium tomato (1.6 grams), and a tablespoon of olive oil and a little vinegar, and you've spent only about 4 grams of Net Carbs. Hate radishes or tomatoes? Simply replace them with vegetables of comparable carb counts, and you're set to go. Or add a couple of slices of avocado for another gram of carbs.
- *Main Course Salad:* Start with four cups of your favorite leafy greens (1.6 grams Net Carbs). Add ¼ cup sliced scallions (1.2 grams), ½ cup sliced raw mushrooms (1.4 grams), and ½ cup cucumber slices (1.0 gram), for a total of 5.2 grams of Net Carbs. Top with a grilled chicken breast, shrimp, roast beef, tuna, tofu, hard-boiled eggs, or another protein source and dress with oil and vinegar, for roughly another gram, and you're looking at not much more than 6 grams of Net Carbs. Or pile on such low- or no-carb garnishes as crumbled bacon, diced hard-boiled egg, or grated cheese.

Making a salad is no big deal, especially if you invest in a salad spinner. To save time, wash and spin a couple of days' worth of greens, then wrap them gently in a dishtowel, seal in a ziplock bag, and pop the bag into the vegetable drawer in your fridge. Likewise, wash, trim, and cut up your other favorite salad veggies and keep in the fridge. Or, to cut out the washing and prep work, buy bagged prewashed salad greens and packaged sliced vegetables. Easier yet, stop by a salad bar and load up on acceptable vegetables. The point is, don't let anything get in the way of eating fresh greens.

## WHAT'S FOR BREAKFAST?

Most people find that it's pretty easy to eat Atkins style at lunch and dinner, and it is at breakfast too if you get "egg-cited" about the myriad ways
in which eggs can be prepared. But if eggs aren't your thing, you'll need
to get a bit more creative, as we explain below. Americans have grown up
equating the first meal of the day with sugar, in the form of sweetened cereal, jelly doughnuts, juice drinks, toaster pastries, and other foods of dubious value. But in most other countries, breakfasts are much more varied.
The Japanese often have soup for breakfast, the Scandinavians delight in
smoked fish. Time to broaden your own horizons.

Some of our Induction breakfast suggestions are variations of such
dishes, and yes, we admit, there's an egg here and there, but they're a far
cry from two over lightly. Remember, your goal is not just to control carbs
but to also get sufficient protein and fat at every meal, including the first
meal of the day. The following ideas, which all come in under 4 grams of
Net Carbs, should add some variety to your morning repertoire. Some are
portable, making them good for weekday mornings, and all serve one unless
otherwise indicated.

- *On-the-Run Roll-ups:* Wrap slices of cheese and ham around a couple of
  cucumber spears and a dab of mayonnaise mixed with mustard. Use sliced
  turkey or roast beef instead and lettuce leaves or another vegetable. Or
  wrap cream cheese in smoked salmon.
- *Chocolate-Coconut Shake:* Blend 4 ounces unsweetened soy or almond
  milk, 2 tablespoons no-sugar-added coconut milk, 1 scoop unsweetened
  whey protein powder, 2 teaspoons unsweetened cocoa powder, ½ teaspoon
  vanilla extract, 3 ice cubes, and 1 packet sucralose (optional) in a blender
  until well mixed and frothy.
- *Stuffed Peppers:* Stuff half a bell pepper with a few tablespoons of pork
  or turkey bulk sausage and microwave for 10–15 minutes on high or in
  a 350°F. oven for 45 minutes. Pour off the excess fat, and serve with
  no-added-sugar salsa or, if desired, with a poached egg and/or grated
  cheese. Make a batch ahead of time and reheat individual portions.
- *Corned Beef Hash.* Instead of the potatoes called for in most recipes, use
  white turnips or chopped cauliflower. Or replace the corned beef with
  leftover chicken or turkey.

- *Veggie Hash Browns.* Sauté cauliflower florets and cut-up white turnips and onions in bacon drippings until browned and tender. Add crumbled bacon or sausage and serve with no-added-sugar ketchup.
- *Grilled Stuffed Mushrooms:* Brush a portobello mushroom cap with oil. Broil for a minute or two on both sides. Top with browned ground beef and some grated cheese and return to the broiler for a minute or two.
- *Eggs Fu Yung:* Stir-fry a sliced scallion with ½ cup bean sprouts in a little oil until soft, then add two beaten eggs and cook, stirring, for a minute or two. Serve with soy sauce or no-added-sugar salsa. Or replace the sprouts with grated zucchini, spinach, or vegetable leftovers. Or replace the sprouts with ½ package well-rinsed and drained shirataki noodles.
- *Morning Soup:* Bring 1 cup of water to a boil. Turn down the heat and add 1 bouillon cube, 4 ounces firm tofu cut into small pieces, ½ package well-rinsed shirataki noodles, and 1 thinly sliced scallion. Simmer for a few minutes. Ladle into a soup bowl. Or replace the tofu with chunks of leftover chicken, beef, or pork and/or add watercress or baby spinach leaves.

While we're on the subject of breakfast, there's no reason to avoid caffeinated coffee. Moderate caffeine intake is actually associated with improved long-term health and regulation of body weight.[1] Coffee contains several antioxidants and has the added benefit of mildly enhancing fat burning.[2] Add cream (but not milk) and/or one of the four acceptable sweeteners, if you wish. By the way, an overwhelming desire for caffeine is not a true addiction but simply the result of consuming it regularly. You'll probably notice some withdrawal signs such as a mild headache if you miss your daily dose. This reaction is normal and isn't associated with doing Atkins. However, another common morning beverage, orange juice (along with other fruit juices), is off the table—think of it as liquid sugar, and you'll understand why.

## THE MYTH ABOUT EGGS

THE MYTH: Eggs raise cholesterol levels and increase health risks.

THE REALITY: Eggs are one of the most nutrient-dense foods you can consume. One large egg provides 6 grams of high-quality, easily digested protein and all the essential amino acids. Eggs are also a significant source of a number of vitamins and minerals. The yolk of a large egg has about 4 to 5 grams of fat, mainly the unsaturated type, and also contains choline, an important substance necessary for fat breakdown and brain function. Eggs also provide high-quality protein at a lower cost than many other animal-protein foods.

A large body of research over five decades has revealed no association between eating eggs and heart disease. Recent research involving 9,500 overweight but otherwise healthy adults showed that eating one or more eggs a day had no impact on cholesterol or triglyceride levels and didn't increase the subjects' risk of heart disease or stroke.[3] There also appears to be an association with decreased blood pressure. Subjects who ate eggs also lost more weight and felt more energetic than subjects who ate a bagel for breakfast. Both groups were on reduced-calorie diets, and the egg and the bagel breakfasts both contained the same number of calories.[4] Previous research indicated that individuals who ate eggs for breakfast felt more satisfied and were likely to consume fewer calories at lunchtime.[5] Compared to the bagel eaters, egg eaters lost 65 percent more weight and had a 51 percent greater reduction in BMI. Finally, another study that compared the results of following the Atkins Diet both with and without eggs found that eating three eggs a day is associated with a greater increase in HDL ("good") cholesterol.[6] So go ahead and enjoy your breakfast–or lunch or dinner–of eggs in all their wondrous variety, without a smidgen of guilt.

## SNACK TIME

Snacks are an important part of the Atkins Diet. A midmorning and mid-afternoon snack should help keep your energy on a level plane and head off fatigue, jitters, inability to concentrate, ravenous cravings for inappropriate food, or overeating at your next meal. But not just any snacks will do: they should be made up of fat and protein. Vegetables (and later berries and other fruit) are fine in moderation, but always eat them with some fat and/or protein to minimize the impact on your blood sugar. In addition to a low-carb shake or bar, here are ten guilt-free Induction-appropriate snacks, each with no more than 3 grams of Net Carbs.

- An ounce of string cheese
- Celery stuffed with cream cheese
- Cucumber "boats" filled with tuna salad
- 5 green or black olives, perhaps stuffed with cheese
- Half a Haas avocado
- Beef or turkey jerky (cured without sugar)
- A deviled egg
- A lettuce leaf wrapped around grated Cheddar cheese
- Sliced ham rolled around a few raw or cooked green beans

- Two slices of tomato topped with chopped fresh basil and grated mozzarella and run under the broiler for a minute

After the first two weeks you can also have one ounce of nuts or seeds.

## DESSERT ON INDUCTION

On Atkins, desserts are an option, even in Phase 1. Here's a week's worth of ideas, each with no more than 3 grams of Net Carbs—to finish off a low-carb meal. Once you're past the first two weeks and can eat nuts and seeds, your options will open up.

- *Chocolate "Pudding"*: Mix together 2 tablespoons heavy cream, 1 tablespoon unsweetened cocoa powder, and 1 packet of sucralose. Using a fork or a spatula, blend for a couple of minutes until it reaches the consistency of soft ice cream. Add a drop or two of vanilla extract if desired.
- *Mocha "Pudding"*: Add 1 teaspoon instant coffee granules to the above recipe.
- *Chocolate Coconut "Pudding"*: Add 1 teaspoon of coconut extract to the basic recipe.
- *Raspberry Mousse:* Follow the recipe on the package of raspberry sugar-free gelatin and partially set in the fridge. Whip ½ cup heavy cream. Gently blend into the gelatin. Return to the fridge until set. Makes four servings.
- *Lime Mousse:* Use sugar-free lime (or any other flavor) gelatin instead.
- *Rhubarb Compote:* Treat this vegetable like a fruit. Cut 1 stalk into 1-inch pieces and cook in a saucepan over low heat with a tablespoon of water and 1 packet of sucralose until soft. Serve warm or cold, topped with a little heavy cream. (Makes 2 servings.)
- *Vanilla Freeze:* In a large cereal bowl, dissolve 1 scoop low-carb vanilla protein powder in ½ cup unsweetened soy milk. Add a cup of cracked ice and stir until the ice turns the mixture to the consistency of soft ice cream. Add a bit more soy milk if it seems too thick. Or make in a blender after crushing the ice. Sweeten with a little acceptable sweetener, if desired.

## LET'S EAT OUT

Like many people, you may eat many of your meals outside the home. Fast food may be convenient and inexpensive, but the typical offerings are all too often full of empty carbs: in the bun, crust, breading, condiments, and, of course, the fries. Fortunately, there are other options if you take the trouble to find them. Some fried chicken chains now offer grilled, broiled, roasted, or "broasted" chicken that's not battered or breaded. Watch out for some of the sauces, however, which may be full of sugar. In a pinch, you can always peel off the battered skin of a piece of fried chicken and eat only the meat.

Many fast-food chains now offer salads with ham or chicken and even salad dressings that aren't swimming in sugar. If you ask, most will give you a cheeseburger minus the bun, or just ask for a fork and then ditch the bun. The bigger chains provide complete nutritional data for their foods on their Web sites. Burger King and Dairy Queen even allow you to add or subtract the bun and/or condiments and immediately see the nutritional impact. For example, once you remove the bun and ketchup, a Whopper goes from 51 to 3 grams of Net Carbs. For specific suggestions on what to order and what to avoid at twelve national chains, see chapter 11, "Low-Carb Fast-Food and Restaurant Meals."

What about your favorite cuisines? Again, as long as you follow certain guidelines, you can dine out on Atkins. Select simple grilled, broiled, or roasted meats and fish. Avoid deep-fried dishes, which are breaded and may contain harmful trans fats. Likewise, avoid stews, which may have potatoes or other starchy vegetables in them. Gravy is almost always thickened with flour or cornstarch, so steer clear of it. In lieu of potatoes or another starch, ask for an additional portion of (hopefully) fresh vegetables or a side salad.

Nearly every cuisine has a staple food such as potato, bread, rice, pasta, corn, or beans. Though it may seem almost impossible to eat Italian cuisine, for example, without a plate of pasta, what really gives any cuisine its identity is certain seasonings and cooking methods. Those elements can be applied to a wide variety of protein sources and vegetables. For advice on how to navigate Italian, Mexican, Indian, Chinese, Japanese, and other menus, see chapter 11, "Low-Carb Fast-Food and Restaurant Meals."

Regardless of cuisine or price point, all restaurants have some things in common.

- *They're in the service business.* And they love repeat customers. Don't hesitate to ask what's in a dish. There's no need to explain why you're interested. Specify any changes you want, such as salad dressing and any sauces on the side, and ask that the bread basket, chips, and salsa not be placed on the table.

- *Don't believe the menu.* Though many major chains and some restaurants have done their homework, just because a dish is listed in a "healthy" or "low-carb" section of the menu doesn't mean that it actually is. If carb counts aren't listed, take any claims with a large grain of salt.
- *Exercise portion control.* Most chains and many other restaurants have supersized their portions. You can always take leftovers home in a doggie bag.
- *Play it safe with a salad.* Just be sure to order dressing that has an oil-and-vinegar base, whether French, Italian, or Greek. Mayo is fine on occasion (sometimes you just can't dodge soybean oil), as is blue cheese dressing, which is either mayo- or, preferably, sour cream–based. Get it on the side for portion control, and ditch any croutons.
- *Ask your server about the dressing* and pass on it if you're not satisfied with the explanation. Many packaged dressings are full of sugar, cornstarch, or corn syrup.
- *Preview the menu.* Even smaller restaurants often post their menus online. Decide what you're going to order before you arrive so you won't be tempted to order less suitable dishes.
- *Steer clear of temptation.* If you're concerned that eating in a Mexican restaurant, for example, could tempt you with longtime high-carb favorites, go somewhere else.

## ON THE ROAD

Many of us live life on the run, commuting to work, driving kids to school and activities, rushing from one commitment to another. When hunger strikes, you're often at the mercy of a vending machine or snack bar that offers only sugary, starchy options. That's why it's essential to have a repertoire of portable low-carb foods that you can take on the road or in a plane. Some of our Induction-approved snack ideas, such as string cheese, fill the bill, as, of course, do low-carb meal replacement bars and Tetra Pak shakes. One item will do as a snack, but if you're putting together a meal, you'll need to include several items. Pack each item in a separate ziplock bag in an insulated bag. Here are some suggestions.

- Sliced vegetables with cream cheese
- Cheese slices or cubes
- Hard-boiled eggs
- Cold cuts

- Nuts and pumpkin seeds (after first two weeks on Induction)
- Vacuum-packed tuna
- Strips of cooked chicken breast, wings, or drumsticks, or sliced leftover steak

What about when you're traveling for business or pleasure? Follow our advice for eating out above. If you order from room service, specify what you *don't* want as well as what you do and have the server remove any "offending" items that make their way into your room. A pair of plump hard rolls staring you in the face as you eat dinner in front of the plasma is not a good idea. Likewise, as soon as you're done, put the tray outside the door so you don't wind up grazing hours later. Resist the impulse to check out the contents of the room's bar refrigerator. Other than bottled water, which you can get less expensively elsewhere, it's a minefield studded with sugary and starchy snacks. If you think you may give in to temptation, decline the key to the fridge or return it to the reception desk.

## HOW ARE YOU DOING?

After a week or so on Induction, you should have the basics under your belt. If you're thinking "It's a breeze!" you've obviously already lost an impressive amount of weight and are feeling energized. Do prepare yourself for a bit of a slowdown after you've lost that extra water weight you were carrying. For variety (and to avoid boredom), it's a good idea to start sampling new foods, particularly new foundation vegetables, and explore new ways of preparing old favorites.

If you've been writing in your journal each day, you'll be able to see whether you've been eating enough vegetables and drinking enough fluids. You'll also begin to recognize such patterns as an afternoon slump if you're skipping your snack. If you feel hungry on a regular basis, review your protein intake; you're almost certainly not eating enough. You may have already discovered the difference between hunger and habit. If so, bravo! Some people go through life without ever learning the distinction. If you feel weak or light-headed, check on when you had your last cup of broth. If it's been more than six or eight hours, have another.

If your first week wasn't a walk in the park or the pounds and inches aren't dropping as fast as you'd hoped, a few small adjustments may be all you need to get into first gear. If you've had trouble changing some ingrained habits, now's the time to adjust any missteps and lay the groundwork for a whole new set of habits. This is a much harder task than losing a few pounds the first week of a new diet. And we know that change doesn't happen overnight. As you move through the first three phases of Atkins, you'll have the opportunity to hone those new habits. The day will come when you can walk through the cookie, cracker, or snack food aisles or ice cream section of the supermarket without a twinge. Then you'll realize that you've banished one of your old habits. At this very moment it may be hard to believe that that day will ever come. But we promise you, it will.

Changing habits is essential, but you might simply be someone—and you are not alone—who, no matter how faithfully she—unfortunately, this is more often a problem for women—follows the program, will find it slow going. We profile such a person at the end of this chapter. Metabolic resistance simply means that your body is resistant to losing weight. This may be the case if you have lost and then regained weight in the recent past. If, after two weeks on Induction, you've lost no weight or merely the 2 pounds that typically constitute water weight, you need to confirm that you're actually doing everything right. It's the rare person who doesn't lose weight on Atkins, so the two most important pieces of advice we can give you are: first, be sure you're in full compliance with the program, and second, be patient. Occasionally, those first few pounds are maddeningly slow to disappear from your life. Even if you think you're doing everything right, this spot quiz should set you right.

### Were your expectations unrealistic?
If you've already lost more than 2 or 3 pounds (some of it water weight), you're on your way. From here on in, you'll be shedding fat. Although some people do experience more dramatic results, a loss of just a few pounds is definitely within the normal range. Stay the course, and those small increments will add up.
*Course correction:* Readjust your expectations. After the initial few weeks, your average rate of loss could be as low as 1 to 2 pounds per week.

### Are you eating too much protein?
Sometimes people new to Atkins take the freedom to eat ample amounts of protein to extremes. Protein is essential to fortify your body, but overindulging can get in the way of fat burning and stall weight loss.
*Course correction:* Cut back to a maximum of 6 ounces at each meal (unless

you're a tall man who might need a bit more) and follow the guidelines for total daily intake in chapter 4, and you should see results.

**Are you not eating enough or holding back on fat?**
Strange as it sounds, eating too little or skipping meals can slow down your metabolism. Eat three meals a day, or, if you simply aren't hungry, have a small snack that includes fat and protein. Once you're eating sufficient quantities of both, you should start shedding pounds. If your calorie intake dips too low, your metabolism slows to preserve your body's organs and muscle mass.
*Course correction:* Follow the guidelines on fat intake to ensure that you're getting enough energy to maintain your metabolic rate. Don't follow a low-carb, low-fat diet!

**Are you eating too many calories?**
Although you don't have to count calories on Atkins, if you're overdoing the protein and fat, you may be taking in too many calories. We know, we said that you don't have to count calories on Atkins, and the vast majority of people don't, but you may need a reality check.
*Course correction:* See "Savor, Don't Smother" on page 57 and refer to the recommended protein ranges on page 42. Women should shoot for a range of 1,500 to 1,800 calories a day, while men should aim for 1,800 to 2,200. Eat less if you're not losing weight. If you're accustomed to counting calories, you'll know what your range is. If not, a spot check at www.fitday.com will tell you whether you're in the ballpark. (If you're losing nicely, don't worry about calories.)

**Are you counting grams of Net Carbs?**
If you're just estimating, you may well be consuming too many carbs.
*Course correction:* Note the carb content of each item you eat in your diet journal. If you're right at about 20 grams of Net Carbs and not losing weight, make sure that you're not exceeding the recommended protein portions.

**Are you eating 12 to 15 of your carb grams in the form of foundation vegetables?**
If you're not, you may be constipated, which will obviously impact the numbers on your scale and tape measure. The fiber and moisture in vegetables also help you feel full so you'll eat less.

*Course correction:* To learn how to incorporate more foundation vegetables into your meals, see "The Vegetable Challenge" on page 98.

**Are you consuming hidden carbs?**
Unless you're reading the labels on all sauces, condiments, beverages, and packaged products, you might be unaware that you're consuming added sugars and other carbs. And do they add up fast!
*Course correction:* Eat nothing that you're not 100 percent sure contains no hidden carbs.

**Are you overdoing low-carb shakes and bars?**
The limit is two a day in Induction for products with no more than 3 grams of Net Carbs.
*Course correction:* If you're having three or more shakes and/or bars a day, cut back to two. (This almost certainly means that you're not eating enough foundation vegetables.) If you're eating two, cut back to one.

**Are you using more than three packets a day of noncaloric sweeteners?**
Sweeteners themselves contain no carbs, but they're made with a powdered agent to prevent clumping, which contains somewhat less than 1 gram of carbohydrate per packet. Those small amounts can add up all too quickly when your total is 20 grams a day.
*Course correction:* Cut back to three packets. If that doesn't work, cut out any sodas sweetened with noncaloric sweeteners.

**Are you really, truly drinking at least eight 8-ounce glasses of water and other fluids?**
Fluid helps you feel full, so you're less likely to overeat.
*Course correction:* Keep track of your fluid intake, and aim for a minimum of 64 ounces.

**Are you skipping meals and then getting ravenous before the next meal?**
One reason we recommend a morning and afternoon snack is to keep you from getting so hungry that you lose the internal gauge that alerts you when you've eaten enough.
*Course correction:* Eat three meals and two snacks to keep your appetite under control.

**Are you taking over-the-counter (OTC) drugs that could slow your weight loss?**

Nonsteroidal anti-inflammatory drugs (NSAIDs), including aspirin, ibuprofen (Motrin, Advil), naproxen (Aleve, Naprosyn), and ketoprofen (Orudis) cause water retention and may block fat burning. Other OTC drugs can also interfere with weight loss.

*Course correction:* Cut back on these drugs if possible. If you need further pain relief, use acetaminophen (Tylenol or Panadol), which is not a NSAID. Your physician may be able to suggest additional alternative anti-inflammatory remedies.

**Are you taking prescription medications that could slow weight loss?**

There are many pharmaceuticals that can interfere with weight loss. They include estrogens in hormone replacement therapies and birth control pills, many antidepressants, insulin and insulin-stimulating drugs, antiarthritis drugs (including steroids), diuretics, and beta-blockers.

*Course correction:* Speak to your doctor about whether you can use another prescription drug. Caution: *Do not go off or reduce the dosage of any drugs without medical consultation.*

**Are you under stress?**

Stress plays a profound role in weight loss efforts. When you produce a lot of the stress hormone cortisol, your body releases more insulin to buffer its effects. Insulin, as you now know, is the fat-storing hormone, and it deposits fat around the waist first. Insulin also causes sodium retention, which in turn makes you hold water. If your waist is as large as or larger than your hips, you may be particularly sensitive to cortisol, which is one reason why we recommend you take your measurements before you begin Atkins.

*Course correction:* Meditation, biofeedback, low-intensity exercise, and yoga are all known stress reducers.

## OTHER MEASURES OF SUCCESS

What if you're not losing weight—or have lost very little—but have carefully reviewed all the questions and answers above and can honestly say that none apply to you? You may have not had any extra water (bloating) to start with and therefore didn't experience the usual water weight loss. But sometimes there's no explanation for slow weight loss. Your body has its own agenda and timetable. It isn't a duplicate of anyone else's body. In the long run, it nearly always responds to sensible management, but in the short run, it may decide to go its own way, for its own inexplicable reasons. Be patient. You can outwait it. After the first few weeks, you'll have adapted to the diet by switching your metabolism to burning fat and will start to lose weight.

Remember, too, that whittling off pounds is not the only way to measure success. Look at the other markers. Are you feeling better than you used to? Do you have more energy? If so, good things are happening to your body. Have you tried on those clothes that felt a little too tight just a couple of weeks ago and found them looser? Hopefully, you've followed our advice about measuring your chest, waist, hips, thighs, and upper arms. If you're eliminating inches, the scale will eventually catch up. It's a mistake to ignore this advice. You may be losing weight but building a little muscle. If so, that's great news. Your clothes will fit better, and the scale will soon catch up with the measuring tape.

Increasing your activity may be helpful as you move through the phases. Continue to take it easy in the first two weeks of Induction, but if you stay in this phase longer, you may decide that it's time to get moving. If you've been a bona fide couch potato for years, take it slowly. Perhaps a walk around the block after dinner is all you can manage now, but even small efforts can add up. If exercise has been an asset for you in the past, it's time to switch to the "on" button for good. If you've always been active, think about ramping up your activity level a bit as your weight comes down. Many of you will find Atkins and exercise naturally complement each other.

## READY TO MOVE ON? IT'S UP TO YOU

By the end of your second week on Induction, it's decision time. Even if you got off to a rocky start, by the end of the second week you should have corrected any missteps and your results will show it. You should be losing weight and inches—although perhaps not as fast as you had hoped—and feeling energized. After the first week, low energy is very often a sign that you are not regularly consuming enough salt. Review the paragraphs about how to address sodium depletion in this chapter. Getting adequate salt also eliminates or minimizes other symptoms that may accompany switching to fat metabolism.

If you're not feeling satisfied with your meals and snacks, you're probably not eating enough protein and/or fat. Again, the combination will moderate your appetite and boost your energy level. You may also be missing the filling benefit of fiber if you're not eating the recommended amount of foundation vegetables. Skipping meals or snacks may also increase the likelihood of giving in to cravings for sugary, starchy, and other unacceptable foods. As you now know, sugars and refined carbs block fat burning.

You know what to do. So just do it. Let go of the carbs! Instead of saying that Atkins is too restrictive, explore the great foods you can eat and fill yourself up so hunger doesn't overtake your good intentions. If you can stick to the program for just two weeks, you'll experience the Atkins Edge. Among its other beneficial effects, burning fat for energy moderates hunger and cravings. Without it, it's unlikely that you'll be able to realize your dream of a healthier, slimmer body.

## DECISION TIME

Based upon your experience in the last two weeks, plus your weight goal, you've come to one of the forks in the road. It's time to decide whether to stay in Induction or move on to Phase 2, Ongoing Weight Loss, or even to Phase 3, Pre-Maintenance. Having a large amount of weight to lose is a common reason to stay longer in Induction, as you'll lose a bit more quickly and consistently in this phase than in subsequent ones. If you're content for now with the Induction food choices, you should consider staying put. But as always, the choice is yours. On the other hand, if you're close to your goal weight, losing very quickly, or being tempted to stray because of limited food choices, it's time to move to OWL.

Don't make the mistake of staying in Induction too long just because you love how the pounds are peeling off. Eventually, it's important to move through the phases to ensure that you have cured yourself of your old habits and can reintroduce foods without halting your weight loss or provoking cravings. Losing weight fast is exhilarating, but it will likely be a temporary fix if you don't find your comfort zone for eating in the "real world." Deliberately slowing your rate of weight loss as you approach your goal will make it easier to make those lost pounds history—permanently. You needn't worry about any health risks of staying in Induction, but you do need to work on moving up the ladder so you can find your tolerance for carbs, whether it's 30, 50, 60, or more grams a day.

*Move to OWL if . . .*

- You're already within 15 pounds of your goal weight. It's important for you to move on to learn a new, permanent way of eating.
- You're bored with your current food choices.
- You've been in Induction for several months and are more than halfway to your goal. Again, it's important for most people to cycle through the phases.

*You may choose to stay in Induction if . . .*

- You still have more than 30 pounds to lose.

*You should stay in Induction for now if . . .*

- You still have a large amount of weight to lose.
- You're still struggling with carb cravings.
- You have not been fully compliant with Induction.
- If you still have elevated blood sugar or blood pressure levels.
- Your weight loss is slow and you aren't physically active.

*Move on to Pre-Maintenance if . . .*

- You're within 10 pounds of your goal weight and still losing at a brisk pace.

## BEYOND TWO WEEKS

If you do choose to stay put in Induction, you'll remain at 20 grams of Net Carbs a day, but you can add nuts and seeds to your list of acceptable foods. A couple of tablespoons (1 ounce) of walnuts, almonds, pecans, pumpkin seeds, or other seeds or nuts makes a great snack. Or sprinkle them on a salad or cooked vegetables.

After two weeks, now that you're feeling more energetic, many of you should be considering incorporating physical activity into your program if you've not already done so. A regular walking program is a great way to begin. Once you get into the habit, you'll realize the benefits in terms of toning your body and improving your mood. Finally, remember to keep your diet (and fitness) journal up to date, tracking foods as you add them back to spot any problems.

As you say good-bye to Induction, move on to the next chapter to learn how to transition to Phase 2, Ongoing Weight Loss. Even if you're moving directly to Pre-Maintenance, it's important for you to review the content on OWL. But first, read about Rebecca Latham's success with Atkins after trying numerous other diets.

# HUNGRY NO MORE

After eating at "starvation level" for decades without being able to lose weight, Rebecca Latham decided to join her husband on the Atkins Diet. Unusually resistant to weight loss, she is finally seeing results and closing in on her goal weight.

## VITAL STATISTICS

Current Phase: Pre-Maintenance

Daily Net Carb intake: 25 grams

Age: 54

Height: 5 feet, 3 inches

Before weight: 150 pounds

Current weight: 140 pounds

Weight loss: 10 pounds

Goal weight: 130 pounds

Former BMI: 26.6

Current BMI: 24.8

Current blood pressure: 120/80

**What made you decide to do Atkins?**
When my husband was diagnosed with metabolic syndrome, our doctor recommended the Atkins Diet and I decided to join him. I'd started gaining weight at age 30 and over the next twenty years slowly put on 40 pounds.

**Did you have any relevant health issues?**
I have estrogen dominance and an underactive thyroid. Although there's heart disease and diabetes in my family, my lipids and other health markers were always normal.

**Have you tried other weight loss programs?**
You name it, I've tried it! I've suffered through the South Beach Diet, NutriSystem, LA Weight Loss, the Ice Cream Diet, the Hawaiian Diet, Deal-A-Meal, the Schwarzbein Principle, the Carbohydrate Addict's Diet, the GI Diet, the Nautilus Diet, the Pritikin Diet, Seattle Sutton's Healthy Eating, and Weight Watchers. My husband and I were doing The Zone just before we began Atkins. We'd both just lost a few pounds, but we were starving!

**Had you done Atkins before?**

Yes, years ago, but now I know that I was doing it incorrectly. I was eating no vegetables, and I kept cutting calories until I was down to 1,000 and then I quit.

**So what was different this time?**

I read a few Atkins books, as well as *Good Calories, Bad Calories* by Gary Taubes, which was influential in getting me to try Atkins again. I found out at www.atkins.com that severely limiting calories would make me stop losing. I know I would have failed again without the support of the Atkins Community forums. I also now know that even though weight loss may happen slowly, lost inches also indicate success. I've lost almost five inches at my navel alone!

**How did you customize Atkins to your needs?**

My hormonal imbalance and hypothyroidism made it extremely difficult to lose weight. So Atkins nutritionist Colette Heimowitz gave me a modified version of Induction to follow. I started at 11 grams of Net Carbs, with 8 of them coming from foundation vegetables. Now that I'm in Pre-Maintenance, I'm at 25 grams of Net Carbs, with at least 15 of them coming from vegetables. Occasionally, I also eat nuts, berries, yogurt, applesauce, and legumes.

**What is your fitness regimen?**

I started walking and lifting weights about three weeks after starting Atkins. When I started, my muscles were wasted and I was very weak. My doctor had told me to lose 35 pounds of fat and to gain 10 pounds of muscle. When I reached 140 pounds, the 10 pounds I'd lost actually represented the loss of almost 17 pounds of fat and the gain of almost 7 pounds of muscle!

# Chapter 8

# MOVING TO PHASE 2, ONGOING WEIGHT LOSS

Initially, the differences between Induction and Ongoing Weight Loss (OWL) are relatively minor, but the gradual additions to your diet mark the beginning of your return to a permanent way of eating. Your objective in OWL is to find how many carbs you can consume while continuing to lose weight, keep your appetite under control, and feel energized.

Welcome to Phase 2, Ongoing Weight Loss, or OWL to Atkins insiders. Initially, the differences between Phases 1 and 2 are relatively minor, but the gradual additions to your diet mark the beginning of the return to a permanent way of eating. Everything else remains the same as in Induction. You'll count Net Carbs. You'll eat the recommended amounts of protein and plenty of natural fats. You'll continue to drink about eight glasses of water and other acceptable fluids and make sure that you're getting enough salt (assuming that you don't take diuretic medications). And you'll continue with your multivitamin/multimineral and omega-3 supplements.

There is, however, one key distinction between the two phases: the slightly broader array of acceptable foods in Ongoing Weight Loss. Still, despite eating more carbs and gradually introducing a greater variety of them, it's best to regard these two changes as baby steps. Perhaps the biggest mistake you can make when you move from Induction to OWL is to regard the transition as dramatic.

Most people spend the majority of their (weight loss) time in this phase. Unless you have just a little jellyroll to lose and plan to be on your way quickly to Phase 3, Pre-Maintenance, you'll have plenty of time to get familiar with Ongoing Weight Loss. We recommend that you stay here until you're only 10 pounds from your goal weight. If you're beginning your Atkins journey in this phase, be sure to read the previous chapter on Induction, which is key to understanding much of OWL and preparing properly before beginning the program.

In this chapter, in addition to helping you transition to this phase, we'll look at how to:

- Gradually increase your carb intake in 5-gram increments without stopping weight loss and/or prompting the return of old symptoms.
- Reintroduce foods in a certain order.
- Address challenges such as plateaus and carb creep.
- Find your personal tolerance for carb consumption in this phase, known as your Carbohydrate Level for Losing (CLL).
- Integrate physical fitness into your weight control program.
- Customize OWL to suit your needs.

## LEARN THE LINGO

Newcomers to Atkins are sometimes confused by abbreviations tossed around by insiders. Here's how to translate them:

NET CARBS: Generally, grams of total carbohydrates minus grams of fiber.

OWL: Ongoing Weight Loss, Phase 2 of Atkins.

CLL: Carbohydrate Level for Losing, the maximum number of grams of Net Carbs you can eat each day and continue to lose weight.

ACE: Atkins Carbohydrate Equilibrium, the maximum number of grams of Net Carbs you can eat each day and maintain your weight.

## TRANSITION JITTERS

Before we describe exactly how to do Ongoing Weight Loss, let's address an important issue. With the freedom to choose among more carbohydrate foods comes the risk of getting out of your safety zone. After holding yourself back in Induction, you may be afraid that you'll go too far in OWL. Undoubtedly, this is one reason why some people have a hard time weaning themselves away from Induction. Furthermore, by the time you get to OWL, your initial enthusiasm may be flagging slightly and you may find it harder to focus on the work that remains. You're not alone. We'll hold your hand every step of the way. You can always back off a bit if a new food causes a problem. Let's take a moment to put your transition in perspective.

**Are you daunted by what still remains ahead?**

Of course you are. If you're on the plump side, it took a while to pad your body by eating the wrong foods. If you're struggling with health issues, they didn't occur overnight either. As the hare in Aesop's fable learned in his race with the tortoise, slow and steady wins the race. Learn to celebrate your small and incremental victories instead of focusing only on the ultimate goal.

**Are you using all the tools and help available?**

Writing in your journal and reviewing it a few days later can often offer valuable perspectives. That seeming regain of a pound or two suddenly isn't so bad a week later, when you've relost it along with a couple more pounds. Having a buddy and/or tapping into the online support network on the Atkins Web site can also prove invaluable when you need a shoulder to cry on or a platform to crow from.

**Do you have more energy than before you started Atkins?**

If you're eating enough protein, fat, vegetables, and salt, you should be bursting with energy. If not, once again, we remind you not to skip meals or skimp on protein. To maintain your energy if you're middle-aged or older, you may need to increase your protein intake within the recommended range for your height by eating a bit more meat, poultry, and fish. Cutting out sugars and other poor-quality carbohydrates should also have eliminated that all-too-common affliction, the midafternoon slump. If you've started exercising or increased your physical activity recently, you've probably also noticed that both your energy level and endurance have increased.

**How about your moods?**

Most Atkins followers report a sense of exhilaration, along with increased energy, during or shortly after the first two weeks on Atkins. That's another benefit of the Atkins Edge. Hopefully, you're also experiencing a whole complex of positive emotions about other changes you can make in your life. Physical activity is a known mood enhancer as well. That's not to say that you probably haven't battled temptation and perhaps occasionally succumbed to it. We're willing to bet that on at least one occasion you've found yourself in a situation where there was nothing you could eat. At such times, when the scale and the measuring tape just won't budge or seem headed in the wrong direction, you may have wondered whether this new lifestyle is worth it. All of this is perfectly normal. The mere fact that you're now transitioning to OWL is proof of your success to date.

## BEGINNING IN OWL

If you've decided to start in OWL rather than Induction, you presumably have one or more of these reasons:

- You're 15 or fewer pounds from your goal weight.
- Your weight loss goal is modest and you're physically very active.
- No matter what your current weight is, you want more variety in your diet than Induction offers and are willing to lose weight a bit more slowly.
- You're a vegetarian or a vegan.
- Weight isn't an issue, but you want to feel better and have more energy.

## HOW TO DO OWL

Initially, you'll increase your daily carb intake by just 5 grams to 25 grams of Net Carbs and then gradually move up in 5-gram increments, slowly building upon your Induction carbohydrate food choices. In addition to the Acceptable Induction Foods (page 82), you can now begin to select foods from the Acceptable Foods for OWL below. (Be sure to also check out the meal plans for Phase 2 in part III, which incorporate many of them.) Our recommendation is that you add nuts and seeds first, then berries and a few other fruits, then additional dairy choices, and only then legumes. Those of you who remained in Induction beyond the first two weeks are probably already enjoying the satisfying crunch of walnuts, almonds, pumpkin seeds, pine nuts, and such. But if the sweetness of a few berries (with the emphasis on *few*) matters more to you than a few nuts, rearrange the order to suit your preferences. We call these different food groups the rungs on the carb ladder. (See the sidebar "The Carb Ladder.") Later we'll address the needs of those who want to limit their intake of animal protein or omit it altogether or have a Latino culinary heritage.

Add only one new food within a certain group at a time. That way, if something reawakens food cravings, causes gastric distress, or interferes with your weight loss journey, you can easily identify it. So, for example, you might start with a small portion of blueberries one day. Assuming that they cause no problems, you could then move on to strawberries in a day or two.

## THE CARB LADDER

The carb ladder assists you in two ways. First, it provides a logical progression with which to add carbohydrate foods. Second, it prioritizes their amount and frequency. On the lower rungs are the foods you should be eating most often. On the top rungs are the foods that—even in Lifetime Maintenance—will put in an appearance only occasionally, rarely, or never, depending upon your tolerance for carbs.

*Rung 1:*  Foundation vegetables: leafy greens and other low-carb vegetables
*Rung 2:*  Dairy foods high in fat and low in carbs: cream, sour cream, and most hard cheeses
*Rung 3:*  Nuts and seeds (but not chestnuts)
*Rung 4:*  Berries, cherries, and melon (but not watermelon)
*Rung 5:*  Whole milk yogurt and fresh cheeses, such as cottage cheese and ricotta
*Rung 6:*  Legumes, including chickpeas, lentils, and the like.
*Rung 7:*  Tomato and vegetable juice "cocktail" (plus more lemon and lime juice)
*Rung 8:*  Other fruits (but not fruit juices or dried fruits)
*Rung 9:*  Higher-carb vegetables, such as winter squash, carrots, and peas
*Rung 10:*  Whole grains

## REALISTIC EXPECTATIONS

If you shed pounds quickly on Induction, know that this reliable and exhilarating pace won't continue indefinitely. Your average weekly loss will almost certainly slow as you increase your carb intake and your weight drops. This is deliberate as you gradually add more carbohydrates in greater variety and slowly adopt a new, sustainable way of eating. You may find the path ahead much like driving in heavy traffic: you'll crawl along at a snail's pace for a few miles, perhaps picking up speed for a while, and then stopping, slowing, and so forth. This bumpy progress will try your patience, no doubt, but knowing that it's not unusual should help you cope. We'll revisit how you may be able to influence your progress below.

## HOW TO REINTRODUCE CERTAIN FOODS

There are three important points to understand as you begin to reintroduce foods. First, if you've been estimating carb counts, now is the time to start counting them. Second, you're increasing your range of foods but not the *amount* of food that you're eating day to day by very much. As you continue to add small amounts of carbohydrate foods, you don't have to do anything other than make sure you're not overdoing your protein intake. Let your appetite be your guide. Stay hydrated, and the moment you feel you've had enough, stop eating. If you've always been a member of the clean-plate club, now is the time to resign. Or dish out less from the get-go. Finally, not everyone will necessarily be able to reintroduce all the acceptable foods for this phase; some of you will be able to eat them only rarely.

As you add new foods, you'll substitute some of them for other carb foods you're already eating, but not your 12 to 15 grams of Net Carbs from foundation vegetables. For example, you can now have cottage cheese in lieu of some of the hard cheese you've been eating in Induction. Instead of an afternoon snack of green olives, you might switch off with macadamias. You'll still be eating those Induction-friendly foods, but you can branch out a bit. As long as you're tracking your carb intake, eating the recommended amount of vegetables, and feeling full but not stuffed, you should do fine. Your protein portions at each meal should remain within the roughly 4-to-6-ounce range.

We can't stress enough that writing in your diet journal is particularly important as you start to add back foods. This process doesn't always happen smoothly, and you'll want to know which food is causing which response, so, if necessary, you know which to back off from. Keep on noting what you're adding, how much, and your reactions, if any.

## ACCEPTABLE FOODS FOR OWL
### NUTS AND SEEDS

Most people start by reintroducing nuts and seeds and butters made from them. Avoid honey-roasted and smoked products. An ounce or two of walnuts, pecans, or pumpkin seeds makes a perfect snack. (The following list provides portions equivalent to an ounce.) Or sprinkle them over salads or cottage cheese. Salted nuts are fine, but understand that they can be notoriously difficult to eat in moderation. Store nuts and seeds in the fridge or freezer to avoid rancidity. Peanuts, cashews, and roasted soybeans ("soy nuts") are not true nuts. The latter two are higher in carbs than true nuts, so go easy on them. (Chestnuts are very starchy and high in carbs, making them unsuitable for OWL.) Heart-healthy fiber helps moderate the carb counts of nuts and seeds, but their healthy fats make them all high in calories, so keep your intake to no more than 2 ounces (about ¼ cup) a day. Almond, macadamia, and other nut or seed butters are a great alternative to peanut butter, but avoid products such as Nutella that include sugar or other sweeteners. Nut meals and flours broaden your cooking options.

*Tip:* When you buy a large bag of nuts or seeds, divide it into 1-ounce servings; place them in small resealable bags and store in the freezer. There's no need to weigh anything; if it's a 1-pound bag, simply divide the contents into 16 equal portions. When you're ready for a nut snack, consume one—and only one—bag. Or count out the suitable number of a particular kind of nut, following the portion guidelines below, and return the rest of the bag or container to the fridge.

| Nut or Seed | Serving Size | Grams of Net Carbs |
|---|---|---|
| Almonds | 24 nuts | 2.3 |
| Almond butter | 1 tablespoon | 2.5 |
| Almond meal/flour | ¼ cup | 3.0 |
| Brazil nuts | 5 nuts | 2.0 |
| Cashews | 9 nuts | 4.4 |
| Cashew butter | 1 tablespoon | 4.1 |
| Coconut, shredded unsweetened | ¼ cup | 1.3 |
| Macadamias | 6 nuts | 2.0 |
| Macadamia butter | 1 tablespoon | 2.5 |
| Hazelnuts | 12 nuts | 0.5 |
| Peanuts | 22 nuts | 1.5 |
| Peanut butter, natural | 1 tablespoon | 2.4 |
| Peanut butter, smooth | 1 tablespoon | 2.2 |
| Pecans | 10 halves | 1.5 |
| Pine nuts (piñons) | 2 tablespoons | 1.7 |
| Pistachios | 25 nuts | 2.5 |
| Pumpkin seeds, hulled | 2 tablespoons | 2.0 |
| Sesame seeds | 2 tablespoons | 1.6 |
| Soy "nuts" | 2 tablespoons | 2.7 |
| Soy "nut" butter | 1 tablespoon | 3.0 |
| Sunflower seeds, hulled | 2 tablespoons | 1.1 |
| Sunflower seed butter | 1 tablespoon | 0.5 |
| Tahini (sesame paste) | 1 tablespoon | 0.8 |
| Walnuts | 7 halves | 1.5 |

## BERRIES AND OTHER FRUITS

There's a good reason why the first (sweet) fruits you'll add back are berries. They're relatively high in fiber—the seeds help—which lowers their Net Carb gram count. They're also packed with vitamins and antioxidants. The brighter the color of a fruit or vegetable, the higher its antioxidant level. And what could be bolder than the blue, black, and red of most berries? Melon (but not watermelon) and cherries are slightly higher in carbs than most berries. Eat them in moderation—and only after introducing berries—to ensure that they don't stimulate cravings for more sweet things. All fruits should be regarded as garnishes, not major components of a meal or snack.

Have fresh berries with a little cheese, cream, sour cream, or whole milk yogurt to mute the impact on your blood sugar. Add some berries to a breakfast smoothie. Toss them into a green salad or blend them into a vinaigrette dressing. You may also have small (1-tablespoon) portions of preserves made without added sugar. Each tablespoon should provide no more than 2 grams of Net Carbs.

| Fruit | Serving Size | Grams of Net Carbs |
|---|---|---|
| Blackberries, fresh | ¼ cup | 2.7 |
| Blackberries, frozen | ¼ cup | 4.1 |
| Blueberries, fresh | ¼ cup | 4.1 |
| Blueberries, frozen | ¼ cup | 3.7 |
| Boysenberries, fresh | ¼ cup | 2.7 |
| Boysenberries, frozen | ¼ cup | 2.8 |
| Cherries, sour, fresh | ¼ cup | 2.8 |
| Cherries, sweet, fresh | ¼ cup | 4.2 |
| Cranberries, raw | ¼ cup | 2.0 |
| Currants, fresh | ¼ cup | 2.5 |
| Gooseberries, raw | ½ cup | 4.4 |
| Loganberries, raw | ¼ cup | 2.7 |
| Melon, cantaloupe balls | ¼ cup | 3.7 |
| Melon, Crenshaw balls | ¼ cup | 2.3 |
| Melon, honeydew balls | ¼ cup | 3.6 |
| Raspberries, fresh | ¼ cup | 1.5 |
| Raspberries, frozen | ¼ cup | 1.8 |
| Strawberries, fresh, sliced | ¼ cup | 1.8 |

| Fruit | Serving Size | Grams of Net Carbs |
|---|---|---|
| Strawberries, frozen | ¼ cup | 2.6 |
| Strawberry, fresh | 1 large | 1.0 |

## CHEESE AND DAIRY PRODUCTS

You can now also reintroduce the remaining fresh cheeses, which are slightly higher in carbs than the ones you could eat in Induction. A half cup of either cottage cheese or ricotta with an ounce or two of nuts provides plenty of protein for one meal. Avoid low-fat and fat-free cottage cheese and ricotta products, which are higher in carbs. Top some salad greens with either one for a quick lunch or some berries for breakfast. Yogurt lovers can now savor plain, unsweetened, whole milk yogurt. Greek yogurt is even lower in carbs. Do make sure you buy the "original" whole milk, unflavored kind. Sprinkle on some sweetener or stir in a tablespoon of sugar-free fruit syrup or no-added-sugar preserves, if you prefer. Berries, either fresh or frozen, and yogurt are natural partners. But steer clear of processed yogurt made with fruit or other flavorings or with any added sugar. Likewise, avoid low-fat and no-fat yogurt products, which invariably deliver a bigger carb hit. Once more with feeling: "low calorie" doesn't necessarily mean low carb.

| Cheese or Dairy Product | Serving Size | Grams of Net Carbs |
|---|---|---|
| Cottage cheese, 2% fat | ½ cup | 4.1 |
| Cottage cheese, creamed | ½ cup | 2.8 |
| Milk, whole, evaporated | 2 tablespoons | 3.0 |
| Ricotta, whole milk | ½ cup | 3.8 |
| Yogurt, low carb | 4 ounces | 3.0 |
| Yogurt, plain, unsweetened, whole milk | 4 ounces | 5.5 |
| Yogurt, Greek, plain, unsweetened whole milk | 4 ounces | 3.5 |

## LEGUMES

Most members of the bean family, including lentils, chickpeas, soybeans, split peas, navy beans, black beans, and dozens of others (but not snap beans or snow peas, which are fine in Induction) are known as legumes. Many of them are dried; a few, such as lima beans and edamame, are also available fresh or frozen. Vegans and many vegetarians rely on legumes to help meet their protein needs. Their high fiber and protein content make legumes filling. Despite their fiber, they're significantly higher in carbs than the foundation vegetables you've been eating in Induction. There's also a wide range in their carb counts, as you'll see below. If and when you do begin to reintroduce legumes, use small portions and regard them as a garnish. Avoid baked beans, which are full of sugar, and other products such as beans in tomato sauce made with sugar or starches and bean dips. Always check carb counts and the ingredients list before purchasing any product.

*Tip:* Black soybeans are far lower in carbs than black (or turtle) beans (1 gram of Net Carbs per half cup of cooked beans, compared to 12.9 grams for black beans), with no trade-off in taste.

| Legume | Serving Size | Grams of Net Carbs |
|---|---|---|
| Black/turtle beans | ¼ cup | 6.5 |
| Black-eyed peas | ¼ cup | 6.2 |
| Cannellini beans | ¼ cup | 8.5 |
| Chickpeas/garbanzo beans | ¼ cup | 6.5 |
| Cranberry/Roman beans | ¼ cup | 6.3 |
| Fava beans | ¼ cup | 6.0 |
| Great Northern beans | ¼ cup | 6.3 |
| Hummus | 2 tablespoons | 4.6 |
| Kidney beans | ¼ cup | 5.8 |
| Lentils | ¼ cup | 6.0 |
| Lima beans, baby | ¼ cup | 7.1 |
| Lima beans, large | ¼ cup | 6.5 |
| Navy beans | ¼ cup | 9.1 |
| Peas, split | ¼ cup | 6.3 |
| Pigeon peas | ¼ cup | 7.0 |
| Pink beans | ¼ cup | 9.6 |
| Pinto beans | ¼ cup | 7.3 |
| Refried beans, canned | ¼ cup | 6.5 |
| Soybeans, black | ½ cup | 1.0 |
| Soybeans, green edamame | ¼ cup | 3.1 |

*Note:* Serving sizes for dried legumes are after cooking. Serving sizes for fresh legumes are for shelled beans.

### VEGETABLE AND FRUIT JUICES

Most fruit juices might as well be liquid sugar, making them completely off limits. The exceptions are lemon and lime juice, a couple of tablespoons of which are acceptable each day in Induction. In OWL, you can double that amount to serve over fish or make beverages or low-carb desserts. It's amazing how much flavor you can get from 4 tablespoons of these juices, but that amount does contain more than 5 grams of Net Carbs. You can now also introduce small portions of tomato juice or tomato juice cocktail.

| Juices | Serving Size | Grams of Net Carbs |
|---|---|---|
| Lemon juice | ¼ cup | 5.2 |
| Lime juice | ¼ cup | 5.6 |
| Tomato juice | 4 ounces | 4.2 |
| Tomato juice cocktail | 4 ounces | 4.5 |

## LOW-CARB PRODUCTS SUITABLE FOR OWL

Not all low-carb foods are created equal. Manufacturers use a host of different sweeteners and other ingredients, some of which may give you gastric distress, tempt you to overeat, or reawaken cravings you thought you'd put to rest. In addition to the bars and shakes you can enjoy in Induction, you may be able to handle some other low-carb products in OWL. In each case, we've provided the *maximum* acceptable carb count for a single serving. Always read the Nutrition Facts panel and list of ingredients before purchasing any product. Any sweet or salty food may stimulate you to overindulge. Deluding yourself that you can eat large quantities of a certain food just because a small portion of it is low in carbs is, well, delusional. Purchase and use these products with care. Low-carb products can be very convenient, but they're no substitute for vegetables and other unprocessed foods. Try products one at a time, and limit yourself to two servings a day of such foods. Again, if the carb count of a specific product exceeds the amount listed below, pass it up.

| Low-Carb Product | Serving | Maximum Grams of Net Carbs |
|---|---|---|
| Low-carb bagels | 1 | 5.0 |
| Low-carb bake mix | ¾ cup | 5.0 |
| Low-carb bread | 1 slice | 6.0 |
| Low-carb chocolate/candy | 1.2 ounces | 3.0 |

| Low-Carb Product | Serving | Maximum Grams of Net Carbs |
|---|---|---|
| Low-carb dairy drink | 8 ounces | 4.0 |
| Low-carb pancake mix | 2 pancakes | 6.0 |
| Low-carb pita | One 6-inch | 4.0 |
| Low-carb rolls | 1 | 4.0 |
| Low-carb soy chips | 1 ounce | 5.0 |
| Low-carb tortillas | One 7-inch | 4.0 |
| No-added-sugar ice cream | ½ cup | 4.0 |

## TO YOUR HEALTH—IN MODERATION

*Say cheers!* Now that you're in OWL, you can have alcohol if you wish—and if experience shows that you can handle it. There are several things to consider about consuming alcohol while losing weight. Most mixers, including tonic water, are wildly high in carbs, especially any made with fruit juice. (Sugar-free tonic water is acceptable.) So are flavored brandy and other cordials (although aged brandy and Cognac are low in sugar). Although most spirits contain no carbs, your body will metabolize alcohol before fat (in this respect, alcohol is a macronutrient), so drinking slows down fat burning and may slow your weight loss. And, of course, be sure to count the carbs.

Drink spirits neat or on the rocks with a lemon twist. A 12-ounce serving of regular beer contains up to 13 grams of carbs, which is clearly too high for OWL. A single light beer or, better yet, low-carb beer should be your brew of choice in this phase, and keep it to one. A glass of wine with dinner can make a basic meal a special occasion, but steer clear of sugary wine coolers and sweet dessert wines. You may find that you're more susceptible to the effects of alcohol while doing Atkins. And because alcohol can make you drop your inhibitions, you may find it more difficult to stay away from chips and other high-carb snack foods that often accompany alcohol. For all these reasons, the best advice we can give you is to go easy. If you have trouble reining yourself in, you might be better off avoiding alcohol until you're more in control.

| Beverage | Serving size | Grams of Net Carbs |
|---|---|---|
| Beer, "light" | 12 ounces | 7.0 |
| Beer, low-carb | 12 ounces | 3.0 |
| Bourbon | 1 ounce | 0.0 |
| Champagne | 4 ounces | 4.0 |
| Gin | 1 ounce | 0.0 |
| Mixers, sugar free | 1 serving | 4.0 |
| Rum | 1 ounce | 0.0 |
| Scotch | 1 ounce | 0.0 |

| Beverage | Serving size | Grams of Net Carbs |
|----------|--------------|--------------------|
| Sherry, dry | 2 ounces | 2.0 |
| Vodka | 1 ounce | 0.0 |
| Wine, dry dessert | 3.5 ounces | 4.0 |
| Wine, red | 3.5 ounces | 2.0 |
| Wine, white | 3.5 ounces | 1.0 |

## TROUBLESHOOTING

Sooner or later almost everyone finds that his/her weight loss temporarily halts. As you become increasingly accustomed to eating the low-carb way, it's all too easy to get sloppy about tracking your carbs. Instead of the 35 grams of Net Carbs you *think* you're consuming, for example, you might actually be closer to 55 (or even 75). Whether as a result of sloppiness, cockiness, overconfidence, or testing the limits, "carb creep" can stop weight loss in its tracks. Worse, you may lose your body's adaptation to burning primarily fat—the Atkins Edge. It's tempting to call this a plateau. But the first thing you should do is look carefully at your recent behavior and make course corrections if necessary. Ask yourself these questions:

- Have you truly been eating the right foods, or have you been tempting fate with inappropriate ones? Eliminate any questionable foods.
- Are you actually counting carbs? If you've been careless or stopped counting, go back to the carb level at which you were losing weight and remain there until weight loss resumes.
- Have you been too enthusiastic about adding back fruit? If so, eliminate fruit other than berries and, if necessary, cut back on the size of your berry portions.
- Are you eating excessive amounts of protein? Cut back to the midrange for your height but maintain your intake of fat.

## HITTING A PLATEAU

The pace of weight loss is always erratic, but the definition of a plateau is when you lose nothing—*nada*—despite doing everything right, over a period of at least *four* weeks. If your clothes are fitting better and you've lost inches, if not weight, you're not truly on a plateau. Keep on doing what you're doing. A plateau can try the patience of a saint. But patience is exactly what you need plenty of. To get things moving, in addition to the suggestions above, try some or all of these modifications:

- Tighten up your journal discipline. Write everything down.
- Decrease your daily intake of Net Carbs by 10 grams. You may have exceeded your tolerance for carbs while losing and inadvertently stumbled upon your tolerance for maintaining your new weight. Once weight loss resumes, move up in 5-gram increments again.
- Count all your carbs, including lemon juice, sweeteners, and so on.
- Find and eliminate "hidden" carbs in sauces, beverages, and processed foods that may contain sugar or starches.
- Increase your activity level; this works for some but not all people.
- Increase your fluid intake to a minimum of eight 8-ounce glasses of water (or other noncaloric fluids) daily.
- Cut back on artificial sweeteners, low-carb products, and fruit other than berries.
- Do a reality check on your calorie intake. (See page 107 in chapter 7.)
- If you've been consuming alcohol, back off or abstain for now.

If none of these modifications makes the scale budge for a month, you're truly on a plateau. Frustrating as it is, the only way to outsmart it is to wait it out. Continue to eat right and follow the other advice above, and your body (and the scale) will eventually comply.

## PUSHING THE LIMITS

Let's look at another all-too-common reason for a slowdown or stall. Call it a form of self-delusion. This is a conscious form of behavior, unlike carb creep. You may have found that you could have an occasional slice of regular bread or even sneak in a bowl of your favorite ice cream and still continue to pare off the pounds. "I have a really high metabolism," you might tell yourself, "so I can push the limits and still have Atkins work for me." Sooner or later—probably sooner, however—your weight loss will grind to a halt and you may experience renewed hunger and carb cravings, which then leads to eating more of the very foods you should stay away from.

Both carb creep and knowingly eating inappropriate foods can sabotage weeks or even months of hard work. Whether conscious or unconscious, such actions may conspire to make you think you cannot stick to the program and throw in the towel. Don't do it! You now know you can trim down on Atkins. You just need to use the knowledge that you've gained. If certain foods—low-carb bread or fruit, for example—appear to be setting you up for cravings or you simply can't stop eating them, eliminate them for a few weeks and then try to reintroduce them. Or not. There's no rule saying that you have to push your Net Carb intake beyond 30 or 40 grams a day.

But first, don't hate yourself for having fallen off the wagon. Such things happen. Have a talk with yourself about what made you vulnerable. Were you at a social gathering? Did you come back from a bike ride or the gym and feel entitled? Were you ravenous and the right foods weren't in the fridge? Were you feeling sorry for yourself for some reason and needed a "treat"? Whatever the reason, note it in your journal along with your plan of how to avoid getting into this fix again. Remember, the ability to burn off your own body fat is a valuable gift you've given yourself. Don't abuse it.

If you've had a bad day carbwise, simply eat properly the next day—and the following days. Your weight loss will likely slow down, and you may feel some cravings. If you've been completely out of control for more than a few days, you may need to return to Induction for a week or two until you get your appetite and cravings under control. If you eat a high-carb meal and are particularly sensitive to carbohydrates, it could take up to a week to return to burning primarily fat for energy. That's a high price to pay for the pleasure of eating a plate of French fries.

## TRIGGER FOODS

Okay, admit it. Like most of us, you've probably at one time eaten a whole box of cookies, a supersize bag of chips, or an entire cheesecake. The specifics may differ, but the guilt, self-disgust, physical discomfort, and overall sense of having lost control are similar. This behavior is not to be confused with having a craving for more carbs several hours after a high-carb meal. With a trigger food, it's a more immediate thing. You can't stop with one. The next thing you know, you're back for just another taste, and then more, again and again, until it's gone. When the box or bag is almost empty, you think, "What the heck, I might as well finish it off," even though the physical desire for it may have passed.

If you live alone or with an understanding partner, you may be able to simply banish your trigger foods from the house. But until you deal with the underlying reason why they provoke an uncontrollable reaction, you're at their mercy when you do come across them. In many cases trigger foods are associated with pleasurable past experiences. Chocolate chip cookies may remind you of coming home after school and finding the house filled with their sweet aroma. You may associate those cookies with the love and the security that you may feel is now missing in your life. Perhaps pistachio ice cream reminds you of stopping at a certain restaurant chain in happier days before your parents got divorced. Understanding why certain foods hold a power over you may help you take control.

## THE URGE TO BINGE

The Atkins Edge can also be your ally in controlling such urges. So here's the test: if you're at or just below your carb threshold, it's normal to feel comfortably empty at times without having to feel hungry. But if you're above your carb threshold, feeling empty *always* triggers hunger. If you feel overly hungry before meals, or if you experience binge eating, try reducing your average daily carb intake until the hunger or urge to binge goes away. In the simplest terms, bingeing can be a symptom of consuming excess carbs, so that you're no longer able to burn your own fat reserves and experience the appetite control that comes with shifting your metabolism.

Here are more practical ways to head off binges.

- Never shop for food when you're hungry.
- Don't wait until you're ravenous to eat.
- Don't buy food you know you'll eat in the car on the way home. (Better yet, don't eat while driving!)
- Understand when you're eating for emotional reasons rather than hunger.
- Call your diet buddy immediately when in the grip of a trigger food.
- Ask your spouse or housemate for help when you feel out of control.
- Eat mindfully. Don't eat in front of the television or at the movies, when you may lose track of how much and what you're eating.
- Always have suitable snacks in the house. If chocolate is a problem for you, have a substitute such as a low-carb bar always on hand.

## WHAT WILL OWL BE LIKE FOR YOU?

Though everyone's experience is unique, following are two possible scenarios for the first couple of months in OWL. Individuals with less weight to lose typically spend a shorter time in this phase, compared to others with many pounds to lose.

## SCENARIO 1

- Week 1: You move to 25 daily grams of Net Carbs, continuing to consume 12 to 15 grams of carbs in the form of foundation vegetables and reintroducing one type of nuts or seeds, then another, each day or every few days. You lose another 3 pounds.
- Week 2: You move up to 30 grams of Net Carbs, branching out into berries, one type at a time, and perhaps some melon. By the end of the week, you've lost 2 pounds but find that you're craving more fruit.
- Week 3: You move to 35 grams of Net Carbs and back off the berries and melon. Instead, you try some Greek yogurt one day, ricotta another day, and then cottage cheese. Another 2 pounds say good-bye to your bod.
- Week 4: You advance to 40 grams of Net Carbs, reintroducing small portions of berries, without stimulating cravings this time. You lose another 2 pounds.
- Week 5: You move to 45 grams of Net Carbs, treating yourself to a small alcoholic beverage over the weekend to celebrate the loss of another 2 pounds.
- Week 6: You advance to 50 grams of Net Carbs but don't add another new food group. You're surprised and pleased to lose another 3 pounds.
- Week 7: You move up to 55 grams of Net Carbs and have a small portion of lentil salad one day, some edamame another day, and a cup of split pea soup another day. You lose another couple of pounds.
- Week 8: You increase your intake to 60 grams of Nets Carbs and introduce low-carb bread as a "shelf" for your egg or tuna salad lunches. Nonetheless, you trim off another 2 pounds.

## SCENARIO 2

- Week 1: You move to 25 grams of Net Carbs a day, reintroducing nuts and seeds, one kind at a time. Your weight loss stalls for the week.
- Week 2: You stay at 25 grams of Net Carbs but lay off the nuts and seeds and replace them with more foundation vegetables. By the end of the week, you've lost 2 pounds.
- Week 3: You remain at 25 grams and try the nuts and seeds again. This time, you seem to be able to tolerate them, but you lose only a pound.

- Week 4: Frustrated with your slow progress, you remain at 25 grams of Net Carbs. You lose 2 pounds by week's end.
- Week 5: You increase your carb count to 30 grams but add no new foods. Another pound vanishes.
- Week 6: Encouraged by your ability to handle the nuts and seeds, you try introducing berries without changing your Net Carb count. You find that the berries provoke cravings, making it hard to be compliant. Although you lose another pound, it is a struggle.
- Week 7: You decide to forgo berries for the time being but go up another 5 grams to 35 grams of Net Carbs. You find yourself struggling with hunger again and lose nothing for a week.
- Week 8: You drop back to 30 grams of Net Carbs, having a small serving of berries every other day. You drop another pound and your cravings retreat.

If your experience resembles Scenario 1, you'll find it relatively easy to introduce new foods and increase your overall intake of carbs. Scenario 2 is clearly a different situation. Your own experience could be anywhere along this spectrum or you might lose at a faster rate, even into the second or third month on Atkins. You might be able to increase your Net Carb intake week by week without a slowdown, or you may find you need to move at a snail's pace so as to not interfere with weight loss or reactivate hunger and cravings. Progressing slowly also allows you to identify trigger foods you may find hard to eat in moderation. (Review the discussion of trigger foods on page 130.)

Not everyone will be able to reintroduce all Acceptable Foods for OWL, and some folks will be able to tolerate some only occasionally and/or in small amounts. This is particularly true of legumes and low-carb grain products, which many people find that they cannot reintroduce until they're in a later phase or possibly never. Sometimes a food that initially gives you trouble can be reintroduced later without adverse consequences.

## YOUR PERSONAL TOLERANCE FOR CARBS

As the two scenarios demonstrate, your objective in OWL is to determine how many carbs you can consume and continue to lose weight, keep your appetite under control, and feel energized. If relevant, you'll also want to see an improvement in various health markers. Phase 2 also enables you to explore and decide which foods you can and cannot handle. All this is part of the process of finding your personal tolerance for carbs, known as your Carbohydrate Level for Losing (CLL).

Think of it as exploring your dietary neighborhood while avoiding the metabolic bully's turf. People doing Atkins report a broad range of CLLs. Those with a higher tolerance may have a CLL of 60 to 80 grams or even higher. Still others find that they can't move much beyond the 25 grams of Net Carbs that initiate OWL. If you're losing less than a pound a week on average, you're probably close to your CLL and should not increase your carb intake. If your weight loss rate picks up, you may be able to raise your carb intake slightly. Your goal should be to enjoy as broad a range of foods as possible, but not at the risk of losing the benefits of carb restriction, namely continued weight loss, appetite control, the absence of obsessive thoughts about food, high energy, and a general sense of well-being.

It's always better to stay slightly below your carb tolerance level than to overshoot it and then have to back up. The delicate balancing act of finding your personal CLL is crucial to truly understanding your metabolism so you can ultimately maintain a healthy weight. That said, it may take a bit more "backing and forthing" until you identify your CLL. As long as you stay in OWL, you'll remain at or around that number, and both pounds and inches should continue to disappear.

Your CLL is influenced by your age, gender, level of physical activity, hormonal issues, medications you may be taking, and other factors. Again, younger people and men tend to have an advantage. Increasing your activity level or exercise program may or may not raise it. No matter what your tolerance for carbs, however, it's perfectly normal to lose in fits and starts. And, as you know, the scale isn't a perfect tool to measure the positive changes you're experiencing.

After a month or two in OWL, you should have a pretty good idea of where your CLL will land. This in turn will likely predict the path that you'll follow after this phase. If your experience is like Scenario 1, you'll most likely find you can add back a variety of carbohydrate-containing foods and exceed 50 grams of Net Carbs a day without losing the Atkins Edge. However, if your experience is more like Scenario 2, you may find that you have difficulty introducing carbohydrate foods higher on the carb ladder and have a CLL of somewhere between 25 and 50. In chapter 10, we'll detail two different approaches that allow you to customize your permanent diet to your individual needs.

## PERSONALIZE OWL

Once you have the basics of Ongoing Weight Loss under your belt—that same belt that you've probably had to tighten a notch or two—it's time to learn how to customize OWL to suit your needs, culinary heritage or preferences, and metabolism. Assuming that you're continuing to slim down steadily, you may be able to change the order established in the carb ladder, as long as you stick to your daily quota of carbs. So if you prefer to add berries before nuts or yogurt before berries, give it a try. But don't try this with legumes (unless you're a vegetarian or vegan), which are higher in carbs. What is not negotiable is continuing to get at least 12 to 15 grams of Net Carbs from foundation vegetables. Also, be sure to:

- Discontinue any new food if cravings result.
- Keep portions small.
- Count—don't estimate—your carbs.
- Record any reactions such as weight gain, change in energy level, or cravings in your diet journal and modify your choices accordingly.

## OWL FOR VEGETARIANS

See part III for Ongoing Weight Loss vegetarian meal plans, which start at 30 grams of Net Carbs, allowing you to eat all unsweetened dairy products except milk (whether whole, skim, low fat, or no fat) and buttermilk. If you're one of the many people who opt for the occasional meatless meal or even a meatless day or two each week, these guidelines and meal plans will help you as well.

Meat substitutes may be made from textured vegetable protein (TVP), soy protein (tofu and tempeh), wheat gluten (seitan), and even fungi (Quorn) among other ingredients. (See Acceptable Induction Foods: Soy and Other Vegetarian Products on page 84 for a more comprehensive list.) Some of these products contain added sugars and starches and some are breaded, so read the list of ingredients carefully. In OWL, avoid tempeh products that include rice or another grain. Others contain eggs, which place them off limits for vegetarians who eschew eggs. Many products have suitable carb counts—aim for no more than 6 grams of Net Carbs per serving so you can continue to get most of your carbs from foundation vegetables. Other tips for vegetarians:

- Most nonanimal protein sources (except for tofu and nut butters) are low in fat. Continue to get enough healthy fats in other dishes by dressing vegetables and salads with olive oil and other monounsaturated oils and eating high-fat snacks such as half a Haas avocado or some olives.
- Add back nuts and seeds before berries. Nuts and seeds contain fat and protein that will make Atkins easier to do and more effective.
- Tempeh, made with fermented soybeans, is higher in protein than tofu and more flavorful. Sauté tempeh with veggies in a stir-fry, crumble it into chili, soup, or sauces, or marinate and grill it.
- If you don't eat eggs, simply ignore the egg recipes on the meal plans and substitute crumbled tofu for scrambled eggs—a pinch of turmeric provides an appealing yellow hue. For baking, use an egg substitute product. A number of eggless breakfast suggestions appear on page 99.
- Vegetarians may add back legumes before other OWL Acceptable Foods, but do so in extreme moderation (2-tablespoon servings), using them as garnishes on soups or salads.

The following suggestions apply to vegans as well as vegetarians. Shakes made with plain unsweetened soy milk (or almond milk), soy (or hemp) protein, berries, and a little sweetener can make a tasty breakfast. Use tofu in shakes (try it puréed with peanut or almond butter for added protein) or sautéed with vegetables to stand in for scrambled eggs. Mayonnaise made with soy instead of eggs, mixed with crumbled tofu, chopped celery and onions, and a little curry powder makes a tasty eggless salad. Silken tofu and soy creamer can be used in desserts, as can agar-agar in jellied desserts.

There are numerous soy and rice cheeses, soy burgers, and other analogues described above, as well as nondairy "sour cream" and "yogurt." Dairy substitutes tend to be lower in carbs than their counterparts, although some cheeses are actually higher. Read the labels, as always. As long as these products don't contain added sugar or fillers, they're acceptable in Atkins. Products such as "bacon," "sausage," "burgers," and "meatballs" usually contain just a few carbs per serving.

Seitan is made with wheat gluten (the protein component of wheat) and is used for many meat analogues. It can be stir-fried, but its texture improves when it is simmered, braised, or oven-baked. Vegans should avoid Quorn products, made from fungi, which include milk solids and egg protein.

## OWL FOR VEGANS

It's clearly more challenging for vegans to do Atkins, but not impossible. If you're a vegan, you probably rely heavily on beans and other legumes, whole grains, and nuts and seeds as protein sources. Because you don't eat any dairy products, eggs, meat, or fish, it's not possible to satisfy your protein needs in Induction. By beginning in OWL, at a higher carb intake than vegetarians or omnivores, however, it's possible to do a version of Atkins that's free of all animal products.

- Start in OWL at 50 grams of Net Carbs, advancing by 5 grams of Net Carbs each week or every few weeks, as long as you continue to shed pounds, until you're 10 pounds from your goal weight.
- You can eat Induction-acceptable vegetables and OWL-acceptable nuts and seeds and their butters, berries, and other OWL-acceptable fruits, and legumes from the start.
- Consume enough soy products and other analogues to meet your protein guidelines, being sure to have at least two different types of protein a day so as to get a mix of essential amino acids.
- Be sure to add extra flaxseed, olive, walnut, and other natural oils to salads and vegetables to make up for the minimal amount of fat in most of your protein sources.

Follow the initial Ongoing Weight Loss Meal Plan for Vegans in part III. It may take you longer to get into a primarily fat-burning mode, as your initial carb intake is more than twice that of Induction's 20 grams of Net Carbs. You also need to be especially alert to cravings and unreasonable hunger at the higher level of carb intake. After a week at 50 grams of Net Carbs, assuming that you're losing weight and not experiencing cravings, you can move up to 55 grams, adapting the vegetarian meal plans to your needs.

## OWL WITH A LATIN BEAT

Now that you're in OWL, follow the general guidelines for the phase, and continue to focus on eating simply prepared protein dishes. Keep the following in mind.

- Reintroduce legumes only after you've reintroduced nuts and seeds, berries, and additional dairy products.
- If you feel you must have legumes earlier, try adding one type of bean at a time—and always in moderation—as a garnish (2 tablespoons cooked). Stop eating them if they arouse cravings or slow your weight loss.
- You may try to introduce low-carb tortillas (or make your own, using Atkins All Purpose Baking Mix), but back off if they cause cravings or you can't stop at two.
- If beans or low-carb tortillas turn out to be trigger foods and you can't stop with a small portion, cease and desist.
- Hold off on trying to reintroduce grains (including corn and rice) and starchy vegetables until you reach Phase 3, Pre-Maintenance.
- Remember that legumes, grains, and starchy vegetables are among the foods that have gotten you in trouble in the past, and it's likely that they'll never again become the mainstay of your diet even when you reach Phase 4, Lifetime Maintenance.

## WHAT'S FOR BREAKFAST IN OWL?

Once you're again eating nuts, seeds, and berries, a whole new array of breakfast options is at your fingertips. In addition to our Induction ideas (see page 98) and numerous egg options, here are a week's worth of ideas to tickle your taste buds. With one exception, each contains no more than 6 grams of Net Carbs per serving. Unless indicated, each recipe serves one.

*Granola-Topped Cheese:* Top ½ cup ricotta or cottage cheese (not low fat) with a mixture of 1 tablespoon chopped walnuts and 2 tablespoons flaxseed meal. Add a packet of sweetener, if desired.

*Almost Muesli:* This classic Swiss breakfast gets a low-carb update. Mix 2 tablespoons flaxseed meal and 1 tablespoon chopped almonds with ½ cup plain whole milk Greek or low-carb yogurt. Add 1 packet sweetener and cinnamon to taste. Top with berries, if desired.

*Strawberry Smoothie:* In a blender, add 2 tablespoons of unsweetened whey protein powder, 6 ounces plain unsweetened chilled almond milk, 1 packet sweetener, 2 tablespoons heavy cream, ¼ cup frozen strawberries, and ¼ teaspoon pure vanilla extract. Blend until smooth, adding a little water if too thick.

*Tropical Green Smoothie:* It sounds weird, but it's delicious. In a blender, add 2 tablespoons unsweetened whey protein powder, ¼ Haas avocado, 2 ounces unsweetened coconut milk, 2 ice cubes, and 4 ounces unsweetened chilled almond milk. Blend until smooth, adding a little water if too thick.

*Pumpkin Smoothie:* This recipe is slightly higher in carbs than the others. In a blender, add ¼ cup pumpkin purée (not pumpkin pie mix), 2 tablespoons unsweetened whey protein powder, 6 ounces plain unsweetened soy milk, 2 tablespoons heavy cream, 1 packet sweetener, ¼ teaspoon nutmeg or pumpkin pie spice, and 2 ice cubes. Blend until smooth, adding water if too thick.

*Nutty Blueberry Pancakes:* Beat 2 medium eggs with 1 tablespoon heavy cream and 1 tablespoon canola or high-oleic safflower oil. In another bowl, mix ½ cup almond flour and ½ cup flaxseed meal with ¼ teaspoon salt and 2 teaspoons cinnamon. Add ¼ to ⅓ cup seltzer water or club soda. Combine with the egg mixture. Ladle onto a hot skillet, dot with a few blueberries each, and flip when the underside is pale brown. Serve with sugar-free syrup. Makes six 4-inch pancakes. Serves 2.

*Avocado Boat:* Top half a Haas avocado with ¾ cup of cottage cheese and garnish with no-added-sugar salsa.

## SNACK TIME

You'll continue your midmorning and midafternoon snack habit in OWL, but in addition to the snacks suitable for Induction, most people can now branch out a bit more. None of these ten sweet and savory snacks contains more than 5 grams of Net Carbs:

- A half cup of unsweetened whole milk yogurt mixed with 2 tablespoons no-added-sugar grated coconut and 1 packet sweetener.
- Celery sticks stuffed with peanut or another nut or seed butter.
- Cucumber "boats" filled with ricotta and sprinkled with seasoned salt.
- 2 chunks of melon wrapped in slices of ham or smoked salmon.
- "Kebab" of 2 strawberries, 2 squares Swiss cheese, and 2 cubes jicama.
- *Nutty Cheese Dip:* Blend 2 tablespoons cream cheese, 1 tablespoon grated sharp Cheddar, a few drops of hot pepper sauce, a pinch of paprika, and 1 tablespoon chopped pecans. Serve with red pepper strips.
- *Blue Cheese Dip:* Blend 2 tablespoons blue cheese into 3 tablespoons unsweetened plain whole milk yogurt. Serve with zucchini spears or another vegetable.

- A scoop of cottage cheese topped with 2 tablespoons no-sugar-added salsa.
- Mix 4 ounces tomato juice and 1 tablespoon sour cream in a bowl, and you've got yourself a refreshing cold creamed soup. Top with chunks of avocado if desired.
- Mash ¼ cup blueberries with 2 tablespoons mascarpone cheese and top with flaxseed meal.

## WHAT'S FOR DESSERT IN OWL?

Once you're eating nuts and berries, your dessert options increase exponentially, but dessert needn't be an every-night occasion. If you've planned for it during the day by setting aside the roughly 6 grams of Net Carbs or less that these treats include, that's fine. Most of the Induction minirecipes on page 102 can be garnished with nuts or berries. (Also see the recipes at www .atkins.com/recipes.) Each recipe serves one unless otherwise indicated.

- *Chocolate-Peanut Whip:* Using a spatula, blend together 1 tablespoon unsweetened cocoa powder, 1 tablespoon smooth peanut butter, and 1 packet sweetener. Whip 2 tablespoons of heavy cream into soft peaks and gently fold into the peanut butter mix. Also delicious with almond butter.
- *"Blue" Cheese:* Mash ¼ cup blueberries with 1 packet sweetener. Mix with 2 tablespoons cream cheese and 1 tablespoon heavy cream.
- *Raspberry Parfait:* Beat ½ cup heavy cream until soft peaks form. Add 4 ounces mascarpone and 2 packets sweetener. Beat just until smooth. Using ½ cup raspberries, layer with the dairy mixture in 2 parfait glasses. Serves 2.
- *Nutty Rhubarb Parfait:* Make the Rhubarb Compote on page 102. Cool before layering with the whipped cream–mascarpone mixture above. Top with chopped nuts. Serves 2.
- *Strawberry-Rhubarb Compote:* Follow the recipe for Rhubarb Compote on page 102, but add ½ cup sliced strawberries and cook briefly with the rhubarb. Serves 2.
- *Cantaloupe-Orange Smoothie:* In a blender, mix 1 scoop unsweetened whey protein powder, ½ cup unsweetened soy milk, 1 packet sweetener, 1 cup cracked ice, ¼ cup cantaloupe balls, and ¼ teaspoon orange extract. Pulse until the mixture is the consistency of soft ice cream.

- *Lime-Coconut Mousse:* Using an electric mixer, beat together 2 ounces soft cream cheese and 4 packets sweetener until smooth. Slowly add ¼ cup lime juice, beating until creamy. Beat in 1 teaspoon coconut extract and 1 cup heavy cream until fluffy. Place in four bowls, sprinkle with unsweetened coconut flakes, and refrigerate until serving. Serves 4.

## PHYSICAL ACTIVITY: YOUR PARTNER IN ACHIEVING HEALTH AND GOOD LOOKS

Now that you're out of Induction, are feeling energized, and have shed some pounds, consider adding physical activity to your shape-up and health improvement program if you haven't already done so. If you're not accustomed to being physically active, build slowly. There's no need for expensive gym or club memberships, lessons, machines, weights, or workout gear. All you really need are a good pair of walking shoes or a yoga mat, some loose clothes, and perhaps some empty gallon milk bottles you can fill with water to use as weights and a resistance band, which might set you back a few dollars. If you have a stationary bike or other machine sitting unused in the basement or garage, dust it off and climb aboard. If you're embarking on a walking program, it's worth investing in a pedometer. No, it's not essential, but it sure is empowering to tally your weekly miles in your journal.

Not sure how to fit activity into your already busy schedule? Try devoting half an hour of the time you usually spend watching television or surfing the Web to physical activity. Or multitask by watching the news while doing leg lifts. Get up half an hour earlier to do yoga or stretches. Walk up and down the stairs for 10 minutes before breakfast. Take a walk on your lunch break. If you live near your job, walk or bike to work rather than take the car or bus. Or walk your kids to school rather than driving them if you live close by. (With childhood obesity on the rise, you could be doing them a favor.) There has to be a half hour in the day that you can devote to exercise if you put your mind to it. If weekdays are truly impossible, schedule time on the weekends, when you can make it a family activity. Once you begin to feel its myriad good effects, as with your new way of eating, physical activity will likely become a habit.

## TIME TO MOVE TO PRE-MAINTENANCE?

Our usual recommendation is that you proceed to Phase 3 when you're about 10 pounds from your goal weight. To decide when and if it's time for you to move to Phase 3, ask yourself the following questions:

**Have you been losing steadily and are now 10 pounds from your goal weight?**
If so, it's time to segue into your new permanent way of eating, which is the purpose of Pre-Maintenance.

**Do you have more than 10 pounds to go but are continuing to lose weight at a CLL of 50-plus without cravings and nagging hunger, but are champing at the bit for more food choices?**
You can try going directly to Pre-Maintenance, but return to OWL quickly if weight loss ceases and any previous symptoms return.

**Do you still have more than 10 pounds to lose and . . .**

- Your weight loss is stalled?
- Certain foods still trigger cravings?
- You're eating inappropriate foods on occasion?
- Your blood sugar and insulin levels are not yet normalized?

In such a case, you're better off staying in OWL for the time being.

**Alternatively, does this describe your situation?**

- You were able to lose weight in Induction but can't seem to budge in OWL.
- The greater choice of foods is creating problems with cravings and unreasonable hunger.
- You may have even regained some lost pounds in OWL.

If so, you may be someone who is particularly sensitive to carbohydrates and has to keep his/her carb intake low indefinitely. If your weight loss has stalled for more than four weeks and you're experiencing symptoms that are making it difficult to stay with OWL, this is not the time to consider moving to another phase. You've probably reached your Atkins Carbohydrate Equilibrium (ACE)—or exceeded it—sooner than you expected. Just to be clear, your CLL is the daily carb intake level that lets you keep losing weight, and your ACE is the level that lets you hold your weight stable. For some people, these two numbers can be pretty low and close together, 30 and 45 grams, for example. Say you've reached a daily intake of 40 grams of Net Carbs. If you're still losing weight but are experiencing hunger, this level may be destabilizing indicators that you'd recently brought under control.

When you bump up against your ACE before reaching your goal, it means that the metabolic bully is back and needs to be dispatched. Here's how. Drop back 5 grams for one or two weeks. If you feel no better and are still not losing, drop back another 5 grams. A better CLL for you may be 35 or even 30 grams or less. Look at your foods as well. If, for example, you've recently added berries and suspect that they may be the culprit, eat them a couple of times a week instead of every day. Add no new food groups until you feel better. Once you stabilize, you can continue to try to add new OWL foods as long as both your weight loss and your overall feelings of well-being remain. When you're 10 pounds from your goal weight, move to Pre-Maintenance.

However, if you're consuming somewhere between 25 and 50 grams of Net Carbs, cannot increase your CLL, and are 10 pounds from your goal weight, there's no point in trying to introduce foods higher on the carb ladder. Instead, stay in OWL until you reach your goal weight, maintain it for a month, and then follow the lower-carb approach to Lifetime Maintenance designed for people who are more sensitive to carbs. You may need to back down on carbs and increase your fat intake. Don't feel bad if you find that your CLL is quite low. Instead, be grateful that Atkins allows you to find the individualized level that will allow your body to correct or stabilize the underlying condition and keep the bully at bay.

We'll conclude this chapter with a brief recap of OWL.

- Begin OWL at 25 grams of Net Carbs per day.
- Increase your intake in increments of 5 grams at the pace that is comfortable for you, listening carefully to your body's signals as well as charting your weight loss progress.

- Reintroduce carbohydrate foods in the following order: nuts and seeds, berries and a few other low-carb fruits, additional dairy products, vegetable juices, and legumes, understanding that not everyone can reintroduce all these foods.
- Continue to consume the recommended amounts of protein and plenty of natural fats and to count your carbs.
- Continue to drink about eight glasses of water and other acceptable fluids and to maintain your sodium intake with sufficient broth, salt, or soy sauce as long as you are consuming 50 grams or less of Net Carbs per day.
- Use certain low-carb products in moderation if you can handle them.
- Continue to take your daily multivitamin/multimineral and omega-3 supplements.
- Continue or begin to be active or exercise if you can do so comfortably.
- Understand that weight loss moves erratically and you may experience plateaus.

Even if you're not moving on to Pre-Maintenance yet or at all, do make a point of reading the next chapter. Meanwhile, read about Jessie Hummel's return to health and vigor thanks to losing weight on Atkins.

# BACK IN SHAPE

When he couldn't squeeze into an old suit, Jessie Hummel realized it was time to do something about his weight. Three years later, both his excess weight and his bad habits are history.

## VITAL STATISTICS

Current phase: Lifetime
  Maintenance
Daily Net Carb intake:
  60–70 grams
Age: 65

Height: 6 feet
Before weight: 228 pounds
Current weight: 194 pounds
Weight lost: 34 pounds

**Had you always had problems with your weight?**
No. Until I reached my 60s, I had never dieted a day in my life. But when I turned 60, my metabolism changed and I retained weight. The hardest part of being heavy was looking in the mirror, but the defining moment came when I wanted to wear my black suit to funeral services for one of my brothers-in-law and found that I couldn't squeeze into it. At the service some people who hadn't seen me in years commented to my wife, "Jessie looks the same except he's fatter."

**What made you decide on Atkins?**
When I was younger, I knew about Atkins, but it was my wife who suggested I try it because she knows how much I enjoy my evening cocktail. Even though you can add alcohol in Ongoing Weight Loss, I didn't have a drink until I reached my goal weight. And I haven't had any sugar or bread since I've been on the Atkins Diet.

**Did you have any health issues that were factors?**
Several years back, carrying around the extra pounds, my left knee went chronic on me with pain and discomfort. My "saw bones" said, "Welcome to arthritis," which I could trace back to my youth. Well, once I had lost the weight, which took about four months, my knees no longer hurt. My doctor was fine with my doing Atkins, but he did

want to check my cholesterol every six months, and my readings have been fine. Now he tests it just once a year.

**What was the most difficult thing for you?**
This will sound strange, but it was hard for me to eat three times a day. I never used to eat breakfast or even lunch unless I had a business meeting. I just wasn't hungry, but I knew it was important to eat regularly. Even now, I usually just have an Atkins bar for lunch.

**How about exercise?**
After losing weight, I started a daily aerobic fitness program that works about 80 percent of my body. Now that I'm retired, my passion is swimming, which is excellent exercise. I have to swim every day. Fortunately, we live in Florida and have a heated pool, but getting in and out of it in the winter is still a challenge. I'm in as good shape as when I was in the military years ago.

**What inspired you to stick with the program?**
I'm a self-motivator, but while I was losing pounds, weighing myself once every week helped. I also changed my habits so that things I did for years like late-night snacking are no longer a part of my life. Now that I'm at my goal weight, wearing trousers with a 36-inch waist, down from 42, is a daily reminder of what I've achieved. Even though my wife is a terrific cook and from time to time she tempts me with certain dishes, I just say no.

**Have you had any trouble maintaining your weight?**
No. Based upon my weekly weigh-in, I adjust my carb intake within a 10-gram range so that I never put on more than a couple of pounds, which I then take off immediately.

**What advice can you offer other people?**
Give away your old clothes that no longer fit. Establish new habits. Find a form of exercise you love to do and do it.

# Chapter 9

# INTO THE HOME STRETCH: PRE-MAINTENANCE

The last few pounds and inches are often the most stubborn to let go, particularly if you try to advance your carb intake too quickly. This phase could take as long as three months or even more, but that's fine. Now is the time to think like a tortoise, not like a hare.

For those of you who began Atkins in Induction or Ongoing Weight Loss (OWL), the end is in sight. (Of course, you know that "the end" is really only the beginning of your new lifestyle.) If your goal was to slim down, it's within your grasp. If you were determined to lower your blood pressure and your blood sugar and insulin levels or improve your cholesterol and triglyceride levels, your indicators should show marked improvement. Just for fun, flip back through some of the entries in your diet journal to remind yourself of how far you've come in the last several months (or weeks, if your objectives were small). Your achievements are the result of keeping your eye on the big picture, feeding your body in a way that minimizes temptation, and not letting minor setbacks derail you.

Let's put one issue to rest. Many people don't understand why Atkins is made up of four phases instead of three. Once you reach your goal, you're done, right? Wrong! Difficult as losing weight is, it pales in comparison to the challenge of maintaining your healthy new weight. Almost anyone can stick with any diet for weeks—or even months. But permanently changing your way of eating is much more difficult. That's why Phase 3, Pre-Maintenance, and Phase 4, Lifetime Maintenance, are distinct. In Phase 3, you'll attain your goal weight and then make sure that you can stay right there for a month. (Some people remain in Ongoing Weight Loss, or OWL, until they reach their goal weight, as discussed in the last chapter.) This dress rehearsal prepares you for the real show, the rest of your life in

Lifetime Maintenance. Regard Pre-Maintenance as the beginning of your transition to a permanent and sustainable way of eating.

Whether the Carbohydrate Level for Losing (CLL) that you found in OWL is 30 or 80 grams of Net Carbs, you've obviously hit upon a mix of nutrients that works for you, at least for weight loss. Give yourself a round of applause as you begin to whittle away those last few pounds and inches and normalize your health indicators. Check out the Phase 3 meal plans in part III to get an idea of how you're likely to be eating in Phase 3, in which many of you will have the opportunity to test the waters with the remaining carbohydrate food groups. These include fruits other than berries, starchy vegetables, and whole grains. Which is not to say that you *have* to eat these foods or even that you *can* eat them.

You'll explore your tolerances for foods higher on the carb ladder as you increase your overall carb intake (generally in 10-gram increments) until you reach and maintain your goal weight for a month. Although this seems like a relatively small goal, particularly if you've already trimmed a substantial amount of extra weight, the last few pounds and inches are often the most stubborn to let go, particularly if you try to advance your carb intake too quickly. This phase could take as long as three months or even more, but that's fine. Now is the time to think like a tortoise, not like a hare. But first, time for a reality check.

### Are you impatient to reach your goal?

Of course you are. It's natural to want to cross the final hurdles when the finish line is in sight. But it's important to understand that achieving your goal weight is only one battle in the war that you'll be waging for permanent weight management. In addition to saying good-bye to those final 10 pounds of excess fat, you want to identify your overall tolerance for carbohydrates, as well as which foods you can and cannot handle. In this phase you'll fine-tune those two concepts. Hard as it may be at this crucial time, keep your focus on the process, which will naturally lead to your desired results. If you rush to shed those last pesky pounds, you may never learn what you need to know to keep them off for good.

### Are you champing at the bit to get back to your old way of eating?

If you're feeling deprived and looking forward to revisiting all your old food friends as soon as possible, you're cruising for a bruising. Unless you're blessed with superhuman powers of self-control or the metabolism of a superhero—in which case we doubt you'd be reading this book—it's simply unrealistic to think you can drop weight and/or get your blood sugar, blood pressure, and lipids under control and then return to your old way of eating without repercussions. In fact, no matter how you lose weight, abandoning your new way of eating once you reach your goal almost inevitably leads to weight regain. If you return to a high-carb diet—usually laden with heavily processed foods—you'll also likely experience the attendant health problems we've already mentioned and will discuss in detail in part IV. In this chapter, we'll help you define a *reasonable* way to eat on a regular basis. If you plan to celebrate reaching your goal with pasta, French fries, and jelly doughnuts, why are you wasting your time slimming down on Atkins? You'll simply be hopping back onto the diet seesaw. Those of you who previously achieved your goal weight on Atkins only to gain back the weight have learned this lesson the hard way. Again, Pre-Maintenance trains you for a lifetime way of eating.

**Have you achieved good results to date, but only with considerable effort?**
You may have lost pounds, only to gain some of them back. If you've followed the program to the letter and found that certain foods reawakened cravings, you may have moved beyond your Carbohydrate Level for Losing (CLL). Or you may have progressed too quickly. As you now know, both can reawaken the sleeping metabolic bully. Frustrating as these experiences have surely been, the silver lining is that they've given you valuable information on what you can and cannot eat. Knowledge is power. Even if you don't like everything you've learned, your hard-earned education about your body's response to carbohydrates will allow you to work within its comfort range—and put you, not that box of cookies or slice of pizza, in control.

**Was your experience in OWL an exercise in frustration?**
You may have found that reintroducing certain foods stalled your weight loss or actually made you regain a few pounds. Perhaps you became reacquainted with some of the old familiar demons: cravings, out-of-control appetite, and midafternoon fatigue. Maybe you felt that you'd jumped back on that blood sugar roller coaster. Like it or not, it may be that your body is particularly sensitive to carbohydrates and you'll have to continue to keep

your intake low to avoid regaining weight and experiencing other harmful metabolic effects. You may need to heal your metabolism by continuing at a relatively low-carb level for the foreseeable future. As you'll learn in the next chapter, we've tailored Lifetime Maintenance to provide a version that allows you to safely keep your carb intake at no more than 50 grams of Net Carbs.

## BEGINNING IN PRE-MAINTENANCE

If you're starting out with 10 to 20 pounds to lose or are presently happy with your weight and are changing your diet for health reasons, you may start in this phase at 40 grams of Net Carbs a day, increasing by 10-gram weekly increments until you approach your Atkins Carbohydrate Equilibrium (ACE), discussed below. If weight is not your issue, you'll know that you've exceeded your ACE when you develop cravings or unreasonable hunger, your energy level drops, or your health indicators stop improving or revert to previous levels. Read the preceding chapters on Induction and Ongoing Weight Loss (OWL), and follow the guidelines described above. If you have more weight to lose but are unwilling to limit your food choices and willing to trade off with a slower pace of weight loss, you can also start in this phase. Understand, however, that moving through the four phases maximizes fat burning, even if you spend relatively little time in the earlier ones. If you see no (or unsatisfactory) results on Pre-Maintenance after two weeks, you should probably start over in OWL at 30 grams of Net Carbs.

Vegans or vegetarians with modest weight loss goals or those who simply want to feel better and more energetic may also start Atkins in Pre-Maintenance, as discussed below.

## WHAT TO EXPECT IN PRE-MAINTENANCE

As you increase your carb intake and home in on your goal weight, you may lose an average of as little as a half pound a week, which is perfectly natural. All the while, you'll be learning the eating habits that will guide you for the rest of your life. As in OWL, you'll experiment as you figure out what you can and can't eat. This process of testing your limits or even temporarily backing off—using your weight change as the imperfect indicator you now know it is—is all part of the learning curve.

There's a good likelihood that at some point you'll find yourself on a plateau. If you experienced one or more of the inexplicable cessations of weight loss in OWL, you'll know what to do. If you haven't plateaued before, go back to "Hitting a Plateau" on page 128 and carefully reread that section. Dealing patiently with and learning from a plateau is essential to your continued success. (If you seem to be getting nowhere despite following these suggestions, it's likely that you've happened upon your ACE prematurely and need to drop back 10 to 20 grams of Net Carbs to continue losing.) After all, your ultimate success in Lifetime Maintenance is achieving a permanent plateau—aka your goal weight. You may get discouraged and be tempted to revert to OWL (or even Induction) to banish those last pesky pounds ASAP. Don't do it! Pre-Maintenance is where you learn how to eat in the real world of family dinners, business lunches, holiday gatherings, vacations, and myriad other occasions in which food plays a major role.

## THE BASICS OF PRE-MAINTENANCE

Now that you're in Phase 3, you'll still follow pretty much the same drill you have until now to stay in a fat-burning mode. You must know it by heart by now: count your carbs, and be sure that 12 to 15 grams of your total daily Net Carb intake is made up of foundation vegetables. They'll continue to be the platform upon which you build as you add back new carbohydrate foods. Also, keep eating the recommended amounts of protein and sufficient natural fats to feel satisfied at the end of each meal. Continue to drink plenty of water and other acceptable beverages, consume enough salt, broth, or soy sauce (unless you take diuretics) if your Net Carb intake is 50 grams or less, and take your supplements.

So what's different? You'll slowly increase your daily Net Carb intake in 10-gram increments as long as weight loss continues and follow the Pre-Maintenance meal plans in part III. In effect, you're swapping the pace of your weight loss for a slightly higher CLL. But if this brings your weight loss to a grinding halt or you gain back a pound or so that remains longer than a week, simply drop back 10 grams. Stay there for a couple of weeks, and if slight weight loss resumes, try increasing your carb intake by 5 grams to see if you get the same reaction you did with a 10-gram increase. You may wind up remaining at the same CLL that you were at in OWL, even as you reintroduce some of the acceptable foods for this phase. Once you exceed 50 grams of Net Carbs, you need not continue to consume salty broth, soy sauce, or a half teaspoon of salt each day.

## ACCEPTABLE FOODS FOR PRE-MAINTENANCE

In addition to the foods you can eat in Induction and OWL, the following foods are acceptable in Pre-Maintenance—if your metabolism can tolerate them. You can also add small portions of whole milk (4 ounces contain almost 6 grams of Net Carbs) or buttermilk, but not skim, nonfat, or low-fat types. If you're lactose-intolerant, you can have lactose-free dairy products or buttermilk (also in 4-ounce portions). Eat nothing that isn't on these three lists unless you know the carb count and the ingredients (including added sugars). Follow the carb ladder (page 120), starting with legumes, unless you've already reintroduced them in OWL—as vegetarians and vegans almost certainly have.

### LEGUMES

Though legumes are relatively high in carbs, they also contain lots of fiber and contribute protein to meals. Introduce them one by one and in small portions. If you love a bowl of lentil soup on a chilly day, a side dish of steamed edamame, or a snack of hummus, this step will make you a happy camper. If beans are not your thing, simply skip this group of carbohydrate foods. (For a list of legumes with carb counts, see page 125.)

### OTHER FRUITS

Assuming you didn't have trouble reintroducing moderate portions of berries, cherries, and melon in OWL, you can now experiment with other fruits. As you'll see below, carb counts vary significantly. Remember that all fruit is high in sugar and should be treated as a garnish. Start by introducing portions of no more than a half cup of such relatively low-carb fresh fruits as plums, peaches, apples, tangerines, and kiwis. One small ripe banana, on the other hand, packs about 21 grams of Net Carbs and its close relative, the plantain, even more. Avoid canned fruit. Even fruit packed in juice concentrate or "lite" syrup is swimming in added sugar.

Continue to stay away from fruit juice, other than lemon and lime juice. A cup of *unsweetened* apple juice, for example, racks up 29 grams of Net Carbs, and orange juice (even freshly squeezed) is a close runner-up. Without the fiber to slow its absorption, fruit juice hits your metabolism like a sledgehammer. Likewise, drying fruit, including apricots, raisins, prunes, and apple slices, concentrates the sugars, elevating their carb count. But as you can see in this table, there are lots of fruit choices that come in at less than 10 grams of Net Carbs per portion. The following carb counts are for fresh fruit.

| Fruit | Serving Size | Grams of Net Carbs |
| --- | --- | --- |
| Apple | ½ medium | 8.7 |
| Apricot | 3 medium | 9.2 |
| Banana | 1 small | 21.2 |
| Carambola (Star fruit) | ½ cup sliced | 2.8 |
| Cherimoya | ½ cup | 24.3 |
| Figs, fresh | 1 small fruit | 6.4 |
| Grapes, green | ½ cup | 13.7 |
| Grapes, purple Concord | ½ cup | 7.4 |
| Grapes, red | ½ cup | 13.4 |
| Grapefruit, red | ½ fruit | 7.9 |
| Grapefruit, white | ½ fruit | 8.6 |
| Guava | ½ cup | 5.3 |
| Kiwi | 1 fruit | 8.7 |
| Kumquat | 4 fruits | 7.5 |
| Loquat | 10 fruits | 14.2 |
| Lychee | ½ cup | 14.5 |
| Mango | ½ cup | 12.5 |
| Orange | 1 medium fruit | 12.9 |
| Orange sections | ½ cup | 8.4 |
| Nectarine | 1 medium fruit | 13.8 |
| Papaya | ½ small fruit | 6.1 |
| Passion fruit | ¼ cup | 7.7 |
| Peach | 1 small fruit | 7.2 |
| Pear, Bartlett | 1 medium fruit | 21.1 |
| Pear, Bosc | 1 small fruit | 17.7 |
| Persimmon | ½ fruit | 12.6 |
| Pineapple | ½ cup | 8.7 |
| Plantain | ½ cup | 21.0 |
| Plum | 1 small fruit | 3.3 |
| Pomegranate | ¼ fruit | 6.4 |
| Quince | 1 fruit | 12.3 |
| Tangerine | 1 fruit | 6.2 |
| Watermelon | ½ cup balls | 5.1 |

## STARCHY VEGETABLES

Vegetables such as winter squash, sweet potatoes, and root vegetables such as carrots, beets, and parsnips have their virtues. All root vegetables are rich in minerals, and brightly colored ones are full of antioxidants. But the flip side is that these same vegetables are significantly higher in carbs than foundation vegetables are. You'll want to keep your portions of these starchy vegetables small unless you have a very high tolerance for carbs. Even within this grouping, carb counts vary greatly. Carrots and beets, for example, come in well below corn on the cob and potatoes. And a single serving of cassava exceeds the total carb intake for a day in Induction, with taro a close runner-up.

| Vegetable | Serving Size | Grams of Net Carbs |
|---|---|---|
| Beets | ½ cup | 6.8 |
| Burdock | ½ cup | 12.1 |
| Calabaza (Spanish pumpkin), mashed | ½ cup | 5.9 |
| Carrot | 1 medium | 5.6 |
| Cassava (yuca), mashed | ½ cup | 25.1 |
| Corn | ½ cup | 12.6 |
| Corn on the cob | 1 ear | 17.2 |
| Jerusalem artichoke* | ½ cup | 11.9 |
| Parsnips, cooked | ½ cup | 10.5 |
| Potato, baked | ½ potato | 10.5 |
| Rutabaga | ½ cup | 5.9 |
| Squash, acorn, baked | ½ cup | 7.8 |
| Squash, acorn, steamed | ½ cup | 7.6 |
| Squash, butternut, baked | ½ cup | 7.9 |
| Sweet potato, baked | ½ potato | 12.1 |
| Taro | ½ cup | 19.5 |
| Yautia (arracache), sliced | ½ cup | 29.9 |
| Yam, sliced | ½ cup | 16.1 |

*All vegetables are measured after cooking except for Jerusalem artichoke.

## WHOLE GRAINS

This is usually the last food group to reintroduce (if at all), and with good reason. Ounce for ounce, grains are generally the highest in carb content of any whole food. You'll note that we refer to this category as *whole* grains, not simply grains. Oats, buckwheat, brown rice, and other whole grains are good sources of fiber, B vitamins, vitamin E, and minerals such as zinc and magnesium. But they and products made with them—whole grain bread, for one—come with a high-carb price tag. Even for people with a relatively high ACE, these foods could bait the metabolic bully. Introduce them with care and, if tolerated, consume them in moderation.

| Whole Grain | Serving size | Grams of Net Carbs |
| --- | --- | --- |
| Barley, hulled | ½ cup | 13.0 |
| Barley, pearled | ½ cup | 19.0 |
| Bulgur wheat | ½ cup | 12.8 |
| Cornmeal* | 2 tablespoons | 10.6 |
| Couscous, whole wheat | ½ cup | 17.1 |
| Cracked wheat | ½ cup | 15.0 |
| Hominy | ½ cup | 9.7 |
| Kasha (buckwheat groats) | ½ cup | 14.0 |
| Millet | ½ cup | 19.5 |
| Oat bran* | 2 tablespoons | 6.0 |
| Oatmeal, rolled* | ⅓ cup | 19.0 |
| Oatmeal, steel cut* | ¼ cup | 19.0 |
| Quinoa | ¼ cup | 27.0 |
| Rice, brown | ½ cup | 20.5 |
| Rice, wild | ½ cup | 16.0 |
| Wheat berries | ½ cup | 14.0 |

*With these exceptions, all measurements are for cooked grains.

## PROCEED WITH CAUTION

Refined grains and processed foods made with them are a very different story. Their high carb count is accompanied by scant nutritional value. As much as possible, continue to stay away from refined grains such as white flour and bread and crackers made from them. Refined grains, including white rice, have been stripped of their valuable bran and germ (the seed embryo, which is rich in antioxidants, fatty acids, and other micronutrients).

You'll note that the list of Acceptable Foods for Pre-Maintenance doesn't list processed foods such as bread, pasta, pita breads, tortillas, crackers, breakfast cereals, and the like, as carb counts vary significantly from one manufacturer to another. While you should continue to check the Nutritional Facts panel on all processed products, foods that incorporate grains particularly qualify as minefields. In addition to avoiding foods with trans fats and added sugar, watch out for white or "enriched" flour. Baked goods made with whole wheat or other whole grains—look for 100 percent whole grain—tend to be higher in fiber and thus lower in carbs, as well as higher in micronutrients. If white flour is the first item on the ingredients list, followed by whole grain flour, forget about it.

## SMALL CHANGES, BIG IMPACT

Even if you're able to incorporate most or all carb foods into your diet, here are some tips to avoid sparking weight regain and the return of symptoms indicating sensitivity to carbs.

- Instead of rice or pasta as a base for sauces, curries, and other dishes, use shredded lettuce or cabbage, mung bean sprouts, grated raw zucchini or daikon radish, spaghetti squash, or shirataki noodles (made from soybeans and a nonstarchy yam).
- Eat carrots raw instead of cooked, which pushes up the carb count.
- Certain fruits are lower in carbs before they're fully ripe. A few slices of a green pear make a tart addition to a tossed salad without adding too many carbs. Grated green papaya makes a great slaw dressed with unsweetened rice vinegar and sesame oil.
- Wrap sandwich fixings in nori, the sheet seaweed used for sushi, instead of wraps or tortillas. Avocado and either salmon or sliced chicken are a natural combo, as are tuna salad and shredded lettuce.
- Regard half a baked potato as a portion. Slice the potato lengthwise before baking, and when it's done, mash the pulp with blue cheese, pesto, or herb butter.
- Some whole grain flat breads are high in fiber and relatively low in Net Carbs, making them a good choice for open-faced sandwiches. Scandinavian bran crisps are even lower in carbs.
- Make your own muesli or granola with rolled oats, chopped nuts and seeds, and ground flaxseed. Serve a half cup portion with plain whole milk yogurt, some berries or half a chopped-up apple, and some sweetener, if you wish.
- Sprinkle small portions of barley, bulgur, buckwheat, wheat berries, or wild rice onto salads or soups for a texture treat without much carb impact.

# WHAT DOES PRE-MAINTENANCE LOOK LIKE?

As before, you'll add the acceptable new foods gradually, one group at a time as long as you can handle them, and one food at a time within each group. It's important to continue to record in your journal how you respond to each new food because you're now entering territory full of foods that may have triggered cravings and possibly binges in the past. So let's look at three scenarios of how your first several weeks of Pre-Maintenance might go.

### SCENARIO 1

Say that you've left OWL with a CLL of 50.

- Week 1: You move up to 60 grams of Net Carbs a day, sampling a few different kinds of legumes over the week, during which you lose another pound.
- Week 2: You move to 70 grams of Net Carbs and reintroduce small portions of new fruits. You lose no weight and struggle with cravings for more fruit.
- Week 3: You drop back down to 60 grams of Net Carbs and continue with small portions of fruit, being sure to have them with cream, yogurt, or cheese. The cravings diminish, and you lose half a pound over the week.
- Week 4: You remain at 60 grams of Net Carbs and reintroduce small portions of carrots, sweet potatoes, and green peas on alternate days. You lose another pound by week's end.
- Week 5: You move to 70 grams of Net Carbs and cautiously introduce tiny portions of whole grains every other day, shedding a half pound by week's end.
- Week 6: You move to 80 grams of Net Carbs and continue to carefully try different fruits, legumes, starchy vegetables, and occasionally whole grains. By the end of the week, you've lost another half pound.

### SCENARIO 2

Again assume you had a CLL of 50 upon leaving OWL.

- Week 1: You move up to 60 grams of Net Carbs a day. You couldn't care less if you ever eat another legume again, but you sample a few different kinds of fruit over the week. Your weight is unchanged at week's end.

- Week 2: You remain at 60 grams of Net Carbs and find yourself craving more fruit, so you make sure to always combine it with cheese, cream, or yogurt, and you manage to lose a half pound.
- Week 3: You move to 65 grams of Net Carbs and reintroduce small portions of carrots, sweet potatoes, and sweet peas on alternate days. By week's end, you've regained a pound.
- Week 4: You drop back to 55 grams of Net Carbs and continue to cautiously consume both fruit and some starchy vegetables. Although you don't regain weight, you don't lose any either.
- Week 5: You move up to 60 grams of Net Carbs but back off the starchy vegetables. By the end of the week, you've lost half a pound and wonder whether you're getting pretty close to your ACE.
- Week 6: You continue at this carb level and hold off on the starchy vegetables, losing half a pound that week.

## SCENARIO 3
Now let's assume that you left OWL with a CLL of 35.

- Week 1: You move to 45 grams of Net Carbs, adding small portions of legumes. Although your weight remains stable, by the end of the week, you've had some ravenous episodes and feel bloated.
- Week 2: You drop back to 35 grams of Net Carbs and back off the legumes. Your weight loss resumes, and the bloating and cravings disappear.
- Week 3: You're feeling good and slowly losing weight, so you decide not to push your luck and remain at 35 grams of Net Carbs for another week.
- Week 4: You move up to 40 grams of Net Carbs and try reintroducing small legume portions. You continue to feel good and lose another half pound.
- Week 5: You move up to 45 grams of Net Carbs and add small amounts of fruit, which produce cravings and stall weight loss.
- Week 6: Understanding that feeling good and in control is more important than trying to push things, you back down to 40 grams of Net Carbs, experimenting with new foods in small portions, until you've achieved your goal weight.

As you can see, there is a tremendous variation in how individuals respond to increases in carb intake and to different foods. Your own scenario will undoubtedly differ. Also remember that your weight can vary by a few pounds from day to day, independent of increments in carb intake and different foods. That's why it's important to continue to use the weight-averaging method described on page 77.

## YOUR CARB TOLERANCE

Like it or not, you may find that there are some foods you simply cannot handle or must eat very carefully in order to not regain weight and stimulate cravings. Likewise, if elevated blood sugar or metabolic syndrome has been an issue for you, it's likely that you'll need to be very careful about introducing higher-carb foods. (For more on metabolic syndrome, see chapter 13.) Knowing your limits will enable you to have a realistic approach to meal planning once you're in Lifetime Maintenance. Anxious as you may be to reach your goal weight, achieving it in a way that's close to the way that you'll be eating to sustain that new weight makes it more likely you'll succeed long term.

Once you've achieved your goal weight but before you move to Lifetime Maintenance, you'll have to find your Atkins Carbohydrate Equilibrium (ACE). In contrast to your CLL, which relates to weight loss, your ACE is the number of grams of Net Carbs you can eat each day, while *neither losing nor gaining* weight. Many people wind up with an ACE of 65 to 100 grams of Net Carbs, but some people have a considerably lower ACE and a very few people an even higher one.

It's important to understand that looking merely at weight loss can oversimplify the issue of carb tolerance. Your energy level, ability to concentrate, tendency to retain fluid, and, of course, the old signals of unreasonable hunger and carb cravings must also be considered. For example, even if you're losing weight at a CLL of say, 50 grams of Net Carbs a day, you might still be reawakening food cravings or blood sugar swings or experiencing low energy, which could make maintaining that level of carb intake problematic long term. Why are we bringing this up? Because some people, for a variety of reasons, find that they do best at 25 to 50 grams of Net Carbs in either the weight loss or weight maintenance phases. Your objective is not to push your carb intake to the absolute limit but to advance to the point where you're comfortable and don't stimulate the return of any of the old symptoms that originally got you into trouble. Bottom line: finding your ACE is not just a matter of getting to the right weight; if you're pushing your ACE too high, it is probably not sustainable.

What's unique about the low-carb way of eating compared to other diets is that adhering first to your CLL and later your ACE results in profound changes in your metabolism, enabling you to better control your intake of calories. The flip side is that if you exceed your ACE, you're forcing your body to burn more glucose while inhibiting fat breakdown and utilization. This makes it harder to control appetite and feel satiated, with the result that you'll almost certainly regain lost pounds. You'll lose the Atkins Edge and the metabolic bully will rear its ugly head again, blocking fat burning.

## CUSTOMIZING PRE-MAINTENANCE

We generally recommend that you introduce carbohydrate foods in the sequence shown by the carb ladder in both OWL and Pre-Maintenance. But if you're continuing to lose weight at a reasonably regular pace and the foods you've reintroduced recently haven't sparked uncontrollable hunger or other symptoms, you may be able to change the order. If you'd rather have a small serving of brown rice with your chicken curry than sink your teeth into a crisp apple, that's your choice. But be alert to the dangers. The desire for a certain food, particularly one higher in carbs, may be a sign that you'll have trouble handling it in moderation. As always, count carbs to make sure you're not exceeding your revised CLL and watch for those familiar warning signals.

## GETTING (THE FAT) UP THERE

From everything we've told you so far, you'd think that it's the carbs in your diet that stop weight loss at your goal. That's partially true, because carbs do exert a strong control over your metabolism—the bully thing. But when you move from losing weight to maintaining weight, you need to increase your consumption of healthy, natural fats slightly to meet your maintenance energy needs. No, you don't need to measure or count your intake of fatty foods. With your appetite as your guide, you just need to let it happen. We'll tell you how in the next chapter. All you need to know for now is that as you approach your goal weight, you may become aware of something that hunting peoples have known about for centuries: "fat hunger." It's a different and subtler feeling than having the bottom drop out on you after a sugar rush. But if you find yourself staring into the fridge and eyeing the butter, cheese, or salad dressing, you've probably been skimping on fat. Learning to recognize and respond appropriately to fat hunger is an important skill for success in Lifetime Maintenance.

## THE RIGHT WEIGHT FOR YOU

When you began your journey on Atkins, we advised you to establish your goals, including a target weight. Undoubtedly, you've kept this number and the image of yourself at that size in your mind's eye. You may be zeroing in on that figure (pun definitely intended) at this very moment. But setting a goal weight is more of an art than science. Following the Atkins Diet seems to allow people to find their natural healthy weight, which might be higher or lower than the one you'd originally envisioned.

It's not uncommon at this point for people to find themselves shy of their initial goal. So what do you do if you work your way through Pre-Maintenance and reach a point where you're able to stabilize your weight but it's slightly higher than the number you were targeting? If it's merely a matter of a few pounds and you're pleased with how you look and feel, this is the right weight for you. After all, wouldn't you rather be at a weight that you can maintain relatively easily instead of waging an ongoing struggle to be three or four pounds thinner?

But what if it's more than a few pounds? If you haven't already jumped onto the activity wagon, one option is to finally climb aboard. Do keep in mind that not everyone is genetically programmed to lose a lot of weight by exercising. Nonetheless, even if you don't shed a few more pounds, you may be able to shape your body with weight-bearing exercise. The other option is to be patient, hone your maintenance skills, and give your mind and body a break for six months or so. If you find that you're unduly stressing yourself by trying to lose 50 pounds in one fell swoop, sometimes it's better to lose say, 30 pounds, and then move to Lifetime Maintenance to stabilize your weight by practicing your new habits. After at least six months—your body is likely to resist further weight loss before that rest period—you can return to OWL to lose some or much of the remaining excess pounds, before returning to Pre-Maintenance to shed the last 10.

What about the opposite scenario? You've lost the 25 pounds you set as your goal but now realize that you could probably pare off another 5. Just stay at the same level of carb intake you're presently at, and the rest of the pounds should drop off slowly.

# PRE-MAINTENANCE FOR SPECIAL GROUPS

Whole grains usually loom large for vegetarians and vegans, and starchy vegetables are often important components of their meals. However, they're
among the very foods that may have gotten you in trouble in the past. Follow the general guidelines for reintroduction and think of these foods, as
well as legumes, as side dishes, rather than the mainstays of a meal. You may
find that over time you can tolerate larger portions as long as you steer clear
of refined grains and most processed foods. Both vegetarians and vegans
should add back starchy vegetables followed by whole grains before higher-
carb fruits (other than the berries and melon acceptable in OWL).

Likewise, legumes, starchy vegetables, grains, and tropical fruits are key
components of all Hispanic cuisines. Again, it is this very combination of
foods (often in the context of the American junk-food culture) that's likely
led to weight gain and other metabolic danger signals. If you're able to reintroduce all these foods, we recommend the following ways to minimize
weight regain and elevated blood sugar and insulin levels.

- Continue to season protein dishes with traditional seasonings, but avoid
  carb-laden sauces.
- Continue to focus on foundation vegetables such as garlic, sweet and chili
  peppers, chayote, jicama, nopales, tomatillos, pumpkin, cauliflower, and
  white turnips—along with that delicious source of fat: avocado.
- Reintroduce such starchy vegetables and tubers as calabaza, yuca (cassava
  root or manioc), potatoes, taro, arracache, yams (ñame), and yautia, in
  small amounts and one by one. Have them rarely, and be on the alert for
  signals that you cannot tolerate the carb load. Gram for gram, they're
  among the highest-carbohydrate foods.
- Use brown rice instead of white rice, and keep serving sizes small. Do the
  same with corn (maize).
- Use legumes that are relatively low in carbs, such as black soybeans, pinto
  beans, and red kidney beans.
- Treat all fruits, but particularly bananas, plantains, cherimoya, and
  mangos, as garnishes, rather than major components of a meal.
- Continue to eat low-carb or corn (maize) tortillas in moderation. (A
  conventional 6-inch corn tortilla contains about 11 grams of Net Carbs
  compared to 3 or 4 grams for a low-carb one; a low-carb 6-inch "flour"

tortilla is comparable in carb count, in contrast to the roughly 15 grams of Net Carbs in a conventional flour tortilla.)

Your long-term objective is to honor your culinary heritage without falling back into the same eating patterns that got you into trouble in the first place. This juggling act will inevitably involve some compromises.

## WOULDN'T YOU RATHER?

Paradoxically, the closer you get to your weight goal, sometimes the harder it is to stick to your resolve. This slowdown can leave you vulnerable to instant gratification. "I'm not losing much anyway, so why not have that chocolate cupcake?" you say to yourself. For a moment, that momentary pleasure seems more important than how you'll look in that new bathing suit or expensive suit. Assuming that you're continuing to eat enough fat, protein, and fiber to remain satiated, often the ability to stay the course is a matter of having a list of reasons to remind yourself why it's worth resisting temptation. These may reside in your head, on an index card, in your diet journal, or even on your PDA. Here are some ideas that should stimulate you to come up with your own list. Say to yourself, I love to:

- Be able to see my feet when I look down.
- Slide easily into my pants instead of waging a tug-of-war.
- Get admiring looks.
- Have a social life.
- Feel pleasantly full but not stuffed after a meal.
- Feel at ease in the buff.
- Feel sexually desirable.
- Wear clothes that show off, rather than hide, my body.
- No longer have to avoid mirrors.
- Feel full of energy.
- Participate in activities with my family.
- Know my size no longer embarrasses my spouse or children.
- Feel healthy and comfortable with myself.
- Know that I'm in control of my destiny.

## READY TO MOVE ON TO LIFETIME MAINTENANCE?

Of all the phases, the whether-to-move-on question is easiest in Pre-Maintenance. It's a simple black-and-white issue.

**Have you reached your goal weight and maintained it for a month?**
If so, it's time to move on to the rest of your life in Lifetime Maintenance.

**Have you not yet reached your goal weight? Have you not maintained it for a month? Have some newly reintroduced foods triggered cravings that are making it hard for you to stay in control and provoked other symptoms?**
If the answer to any of the above questions is yes, you're clearly not ready to move on. (The exception is the decision to take a vacation from weight loss and go to Lifetime Maintenance, resuming weight loss after at least six months, described above.) Review this chapter, and proceed slowly. Yo-yo dieting can make you resistant to weight loss. You may need to reduce your ACE to lose and then maintain your goal weight.

**Have you reached your goal weight and your ACE is somewhere between 25 and 50? Did you have type 2 diabetes or did you have any signs of metabolic syndrome before you began Atkins?**
If many of the foods considered acceptable for Pre-Maintenance give you trouble and/or your ACE is close to the number of grams of Net Carbs (50 or less) that you were consuming in OWL, you should consider the lower-carb version of the Lifetime Maintenance program described in the next chapter. This is particularly the case if you still have metabolic syndrome (see chapter 13) or type 2 diabetes (see chapter 14).

In the next chapter, we'll look at how Lifetime Maintenance—which you can customize to your individual circumstances—will enable you to make your new weight permanent as you continue to retain your health and vitality. But first, read how Jennifer Kingsley finally adopted Atkins as her lifestyle after using it twice as a quickie diet.

# THE THIRD TIME'S A CHARM

After two experiences with Atkins and the loss of more than 100 pounds, Jennifer Kingsley gained much of it back during pregnancy. Once she "got it" that Atkins is more than a weight loss diet, she was able to finally say good-bye to foods that made her heavy, depressed, and subject to ailments.

## VITAL STATISTICS

Current phase: Lifetime
  Maintenance
Daily Net Carb intake: 120 grams
Age: 39

Height: 5 feet, 4 inches
Before weight: 230 pounds
Current weight: 117 pounds
Weight lost: 113 pounds

**Has your weight always been an issue?**
Growing up, I was definitely heavier than most of the other girls. In high school I was dealing with backaches, knee pain from an injury, nearly debilitating PMS symptoms, depression, etc. At 19, I was told I had high cholesterol. I began to slowly gain weight after my first son was born. Eventually, I just stopped weighing myself. I estimate that I was at least 230 pounds.

**What motivated you to try Atkins?**
Shopping for clothes was the most painful experience. I finally broke down crying in the middle of a department store after weeks of looking for a dress to wear to a special event. After that, I constantly made excuses not to accept invitations. Then in December of 2002, I learned that my boyfriend was to be best man in a wedding in February. I knew just the dress in my closet that I wanted to wear. Problem was, it was several sizes too small. So I started Atkins—and six weeks later I wore that dress to the wedding.

### Why didn't you stay with Atkins?

At the reception, I ate whatever I wanted. That night I felt really sick, and I realized that over the last few months on Atkins, I hadn't felt the old aches, pains, and bloated stomach. And I wasn't depressed. But it was really hard to start Atkins again. I didn't have the wedding to keep me motivated, and I could still fit into my old clothes. At first, that is. When they kept getting tighter and tighter, I realized I didn't want to be back where I was before—crying in the middle of a department store.

### What got you back on track?

A coworker was preparing for her wedding and I wanted to get back to a size 12 again, so we started Atkins together in July of 2003. By June of the following year, I reached what I *thought* was my goal. Then I wondered, "Maybe I could get into a size 10 again." When I reached a size 8, I went out and bought a new wardrobe. But it turned out that I was on a plateau. Suddenly I was wearing a size 6 and then a 4, and finally a 2. I weighed 120 pounds and happily stayed there until July of 2006.

### What happened then?

I realized I was pregnant. My weight gain was mostly normal at first. But I wasn't sure how to maintain my low-carb way of eating while pregnant—or even if I could. My doctor told me to get plenty of whole grains. So I did. Almost immediately, I wanted every simple carbohydrate I could get my hands on. My exhaustion returned, along with aches and pain. At one point, my doctor even tested me for gestational diabetes because of my excessive weight gain. After my son was born, I breast-fed him. People told me nursing helps shed pounds, but I was gaining a pound or two each week until I was back up to 170 pounds. I gained a bit more before I found the Atkins Web site and backed into Lifetime Maintenance, which got me down to 151 pounds. Once my son weaned himself in March of 2008, I decided to return to Induction.

**What was different this time?**

I spent several months reacquainting myself with the diet on the Atkins Web site and message board. I began to understand there was a lot more to Atkins than dieting. I realized that the only time I truly felt good in my life was while I was on Atkins. There was obviously a nutritional reason for many of those health problems. This time I focused on my nutritional needs—not just my weight loss. By September of that year, I had lost the "baby" weight and was back into my prepregnancy clothes.

**What did you learn about yourself in the process?**

On Atkins, my depression is gone. My chronic fatigue, yearly urinary tract infections, back and knee pain, and bloating are all gone too. And cholesterol? One doctor called my blood work "stellar." I also realized that I get ill when I eat gluten. I have two cousins with celiac disease, and once I researched it, I realized that whether or not I actually have celiac disease myself, gluten is a major problem for me. Now I avoid wheat altogether, but I can eat some other whole grains like oats and teff.

**What's your fitness routine?**

I do yoga regularly, but haven't been able to go to the gym as much as I would like. Having a three-year-old around is actually quite a bit of exercise!

**What advice can you offer other people?**

Visit the Atkins Community message board. The support I've received has been incredible, and I hope to return the favor by supporting others. I know that this is still a journey for me. I continue to learn and grow. There is no finish line.

# Chapter 10

# KEEPING IT OFF: LIFETIME MAINTENANCE

Long-term success with weight maintenance has both practical and psychological components. Fortunately, you've already learned and practiced many of the skills necessary for this momentous task.

You've done it! You've reached the goal for which you've striven long and hard and proved that you have the persistence to realize your dreams. You're now officially out of the weight loss phases of Atkins and into Phase 4, Lifetime Maintenance, aka the rest of your life. The very fact that you've found your ACE and reached your goal weight is proof that what you've been doing works for you. Keep it up—with certain modifications—and you should be able to extend that success. If you started Atkins to resolve such health issues as high blood sugar or insulin levels, hypertension, or unfavorable lipid levels, in addition to maintaining your new weight, you'll obviously want to maintain your improvements in these markers as well.

Regardless of your health when you began Atkins, now is the time to revisit your health care provider. (If your weight loss journey has lasted more than six months, you may have already done so.) You'll almost surely receive good news. Obviously you don't need your physician to tell you that you've lost 30 pounds (or whatever), but you'll likely discover that you've also scored some significant improvements in your health indicators. That news should relieve any lingering concerns you may have about the healthfulness of following a low-carb lifestyle.

As you well know, making these changes permanent is at least as challenging as achieving them. Success with weight maintenance has both practical and psychological components, and we'll help you deal with both. Fortunately, whether or not you realize it, you've already learned and practiced many of the skills necessary for this momentous task. Think about it:

- You've developed a whole set of new habits.
- You've experienced the empowerment that comes with controlling what you put into your mouth.
- You know how many carbs you can consume without regaining weight.
- You can distinguish between empty carbs and nutrient-dense carbs.
- You understand why eating sufficient fat is key to appetite control and the Atkins Edge.
- You've learned how to distinguish between hunger and habit and between feeling satisfied and feeling stuffed.
- You recognize the signs that a certain food or pattern of eating triggers cravings.
- You've experienced the exhilaration of feeling good and full of energy.

Before you started your weight loss journey, we asked you why you would consider *not* doing Atkins when its benefits are so obvious. Now we ask you a similar question. Knowing what you now know and succeeding as you have, why would you ever go back to your old way of eating—letting sugars and other processed carbs bully your metabolism—which is almost sure to result in weight regain and the reemergence of health problems and self-esteem issues?

## PROTECT YOUR WEIGHT LOSS, BUT MAINTAIN YOUR WEIGHT

Early in this book, we talked about the two definitions of the word "diet." Now that you've lost that extra padding, it's time to focus on the word's primary definition: a way of living. Because your weight loss diet has smoothly morphed into your permanent lifestyle, there shouldn't be any big surprises. The lessons that you've learned about which foods to eat in which amounts remain valid now that your goal is to hold steady.

You want to arrive at a place where you're mindful of your weight but not obsessed with it. Weigh and measure yourself once a week. As you know, the scale may "lie," thanks to natural day-to-day weight fluctuations within a four-pound range, but the measuring tape tends to be less variable. (For a review of weight averaging, see page 77.) If your measurements consistently increase and your clothes feel and look tight, it's time to act. As long as you've gained no more than 5 pounds, simply drop down 10 to 20 grams of Net Carbs below your ACE and the extra pounds should retreat. But it's not just a matter of weight. It's equally important to stay alert for cravings, unreasonable hunger, lack of energy, and other familiar indicators that you may be veering away from your fat-burning safety zone and losing the Atkins Edge. All these may signal that you're consuming too many carbs or that you're sensitive to the effects of one or more recently added foods. As you adjust your intake accordingly, with every passing week you'll get a better idea of your limits.

Now that you're no longer trying to trim pounds and inches, you clearly need more energy from food sources since you're no longer relying on your body fat for some of your fuel. Most people find that their appetite increases slightly as they approach their body's healthy natural weight, even as they stay within their ACE. It's important to understand that the extra fuel to keep your weight stable should come primarily from dietary fat so that you remain in a fat-burning mode. If you find that your weight is dropping below the desired level or experience fat hunger, you'll need to allow a little more fat into your diet.

## FAT REMAINS YOUR FRIEND

When you were losing, say, an average of 1 pound a week, each day you were burning about 500 Calories of your body fat for energy. As you transition into Lifetime Maintenance, your body doesn't really care where your favorite fuel comes from hour by hour: inside—your stores of body fat—or outside—dietary fat. Say that you're consuming 75 grams of Net Carbs per day (300 Calories) and 15 ounces of protein (roughly 400 Calories); together they add up to just 700 Calories. If you're a five-foot, four-inch-tall woman and your body is burning 1,800 Calories a day, the other 1,100 Calories have to come from fat. Why not simply increase your protein intake instead? Because, as you learned in chapter 5, the amount of protein you've been eating all along is close to optimal, and more isn't better. As for adding more carbs, once you've found your Atkins Carbohydrate Equilibrium (ACE), it's likely to remain your upper limit for the foreseeable future.

If you ignore this advice and continue to add carbs beyond your ACE, you'll soon be revisited by the same old demons of hunger and carb cravings. Overconsuming carbs only invites that metabolic bully back into your life. Your metabolism is already adapted to efficiently moving fat into your cells and using it for energy rather than storing it for later use, providing a sustained and predictable fuel supply. Perhaps you've noticed that once you've adapted to a low-carb diet and complying with your ACE, you can be an hour or two late for a meal and not feel desperate. How so? The answer is that even when you're at your goal weight, you still have a couple of months' worth of energy reserve tucked away as body fat. This means that your muscles, your liver, and your heart are getting a continuous, uninterrupted flow of energy directly from fat. Even your brain, which requires more than 500 Calories per day, gets much of its energy from fat. If you've banished 30 pounds of body fat since you started Induction, your body has burned off an awesome 100,000 Calories more than you ate. And there's no reason your metabolism can't continue that same burn rate for fat—keeping the Atkins Edge—as you maintain your new weight.

How can you add fat calories in a palatable way? Follow the meal plans for Pre-Maintenance, adding small portions of salad dressings, sauces, and spreads. Many cultures have used sauces, gravies, and meat drippings this way for millennia. For more ideas, see the sidebar "Delectable Choices" and check out the recipes for sauces in part III.) There's no need to count fat grams or calories. Just let your taste and appetite dictate, without letting fat phobia get in your way. It may take a while to learn to trust your instincts. Fat has an inherent ability to satisfy your appetite and to keep you feeling satisfied longer than the same amount of carbohydrate. You'll probably get a chuckle out of the fact that you, who once had a weight problem, now have to be careful not to go too far in the opposite direction.

## DELECTABLE CHOICES

Add some of the following healthy fats to those you've been eating throughout your weight loss journey to maintain your goal weight without fat hunger or carb cravings. Each portion provides 100 or so Calories of healthy fat. The difference in energy intake between OWL and Lifetime Maintenance for most people is somewhere between 300 and 500 Calories, so making this dietary transition is as simple as adding three to five of these portions to your existing daily intake. See the recipes in part III for more delicious choices.

- 1 tablespoon oil for dressing salads
- 1 tablespoon butter or herb butter/oil mix
- 1 ounce cream
- 2 ounces cheese
- 10 large ripe olives with a teaspoon of olive oil
- ½ Haas avocado

- 1 ounce almonds, walnuts, pecans, or macadamias
- 1 tablespoon mayonnaise (made with canola, high-oleic safflower, or olive oil)
- 2 tablespoons pesto
- 2 tablespoons nut butter

Here's one more issue *not* to worry about. You may be concerned that you can't digest all this fat. With the possible exception of someone who has had gallbladder surgery, this is not likely to be a problem. Why? Have you ever eaten a pint of ice cream at one time? Honestly now, the last thing on your mind back then was worrying that your digestive system couldn't handle 75 grams of fat in less than an hour, right? Given that experience, why would you worry about whether it can handle 50 to 60 grams of fat as part of a whole foods meal?

## CUSTOMIZING LIFETIME MAINTENANCE

Throughout this book, you've learned how the versatility of Atkins allows you to tailor the diet to your particular needs and preferences. You've already made many choices as you worked toward your goal weight. Likewise, there's no one-size-fits-all maintenance program. The single most important decision that you'll confront is this: What do I need to do to keep off the weight I've lost and maintain my health long term? From experience we've learned that you must do something different than you did in the past because maintenance doesn't just happen.

You already know about the tremendous variation among individual ACEs, which enables some people to consume considerably more carbs each day than others without regaining weight or seeing the return of cravings, low energy, and other symptoms. Others find that they just feel better with a lower intake of carbs. Just as we've advised you to increase your overall carb intake—and the variety of carb foods—slowly in the weight loss phases, we want you to think carefully about your carb intake in Lifetime Maintenance. Rather than push yourself to a level that makes maintenance hard to sustain, you may be happier and more successful at a lower level. In fact, you may even find you'll prefer to back down 5 or 10 grams from the ACE you achieved in Pre-Maintenance. Remember, the goal here is to banish the weight you've lost for good, not win some contest for having the highest ACE on the block!

## HEALTH AND YOUR ACE

If you have a condition such as hypertension, diabetes, a high triglyceride level, or low HDL cholesterol level, all of which indicate a risk of developing cardiovascular disease, you may find that they're better controlled if you remain at a lower level of carb intake than the ACE determined by your ability to maintain your weight. Rest assured, there's no risk in staying between 25 and 50 grams of Net Carbs. This is particularly worth considering if you previously needed medication to control any of these conditions. Ask yourself two interlocking questions:

- Do I feel safer and better on the medication(s)?
- Or do I feel safer and better on a diet that gives me equal or better control of this condition with less medication or none at all?

For some people, staying at or less than 50 grams per day of Net Carbs gives them a better long-term response to these conditions. If ongoing health issues require medication or you've experienced weight regain despite your best efforts, you may also want to reduce your ACE. In effect, your choice of foods can work like your medicine. (Depending upon how severe the condition, you may still be able to cut back on or eliminate your medication at a somewhat lower level of carb intake.) Your best approach to Lifetime Maintenance is to understand all of your options and keep them open as you move forward. If you have to work hard to maintain your weight at a higher ACE, you may later decide that it's too stressful to do so. Or you may find that some of your health indicators have worsened. At that point, you might choose to reduce your carb intake to improve your life. Alternatively, if you've been able to maintain your weight for some time and/or your blood pressure, blood sugar, blood lipids, or other metabolic indicators remain in the low-risk range, you may consider gradually increasing your carb intake. Your ACE is never carved in stone, and you can raise or lower it as experience dictates.

## TWO SUSTAINABLE PATHS

If you've done well with Atkins so far, you'll very likely continue to do so by following one of two Lifetime Maintenance options: one at 50 grams of Net Carbs or less and the other above 50 grams. In either case, with the exception of omega-3s (such as fish oil or flaxseed oil), it's best to continue to stay away from high-polyunsaturated-fat vegetable oils such as corn, soybean, sunflower, cottonseed, and peanut oils. Instead, focus on olive, canola, and high-oleic safflower oils. Also feel free to continue to eat saturated fats. Each option meets all of your energy and essential nutrient needs and can be tailored to your individual metabolism. It's likely that you already have a pretty good idea which path is the one for you, based upon your metabolism, your ACE, and your experiences in OWL and Pre-Maintenance.

### LIFETIME MAINTENANCE WITH AN ACE OF 50 OR LESS

The simplest description of this approach is Ongoing Weight Loss with a bit more variety and some additional fat. Here's how to do it.

- Remain at the ACE you identified in Pre-Maintenance.
- Continue to eat the same healthy whole foods you've come to rely on:
    - About 4 to 6 ounces of protein foods at each meal
    - Enough healthy fats to keep you satisfied
    - The right balance of fats
    - At least 12 to 15 grams of Net Carbs from foundation vegetables
- Continue to consume 2 servings of broth (not low sodium), 2 tablespoons of soy sauce, or half a teaspoon of salt each day unless you're taking a diuretic medication or your doctor has advised you to restrict salt.
- In addition to Acceptable Induction and OWL foods, continue to eat any Acceptable Pre-Maintenance foods you've been able to reintroduce.
- If you find it hard to eat moderate portions of any food, new or otherwise, or it causes cravings, stay away from it.
- If you still have indicators of metabolic syndrome or type 2 diabetes despite your weight loss, don't keep increasing your carb intake. Instead, if you're not satiated, try increasing your fat intake as described above. (For more on how Atkins addresses these health conditions, see part IV.)
- Follow the meal plans for OWL at the appropriate number of grams of Net Carbs, but add more healthy natural fats as your appetite dictates.
- Continue your multivitamin/multimineral and omega-3 supplements.

### LIFETIME MAINTENANCE WITH AN ACE ABOVE 50

This path can be best described as your last month of Pre-Maintenance, again with a bit more fat. The main difference from the lower-carb path described above is that you can select from a broader range of carbohydrate-containing foods. With greater variety, however, comes a greater risk of temptation, so you may need to exercise extra vigilance to conform to your ACE. Here's how to do it.

- Remain at the ACE you identified in Pre-Maintenance.
- Continue to eat the same healthy whole foods you've come to rely on:
  - About 4 to 6 ounces of protein foods at each meal
  - Enough healthy fats to keep you satisfied
  - The right balance of fats
  - At least 12 to 15 grams of Net Carbs from foundation vegetables
- Continue to add new foods as your ACE allows as long as they don't stimulate excessive hunger and cravings. If they do, back off and try to reintroduce them at a later date. Stay away from any foods that provoke old bad habits.
- If you drop below your desired goal weight, increase your fat intake as described above.
- Broth or other ways to introduce salt are no longer necessary, but you may continue to consume them, if you prefer.
- Follow the Pre-Maintenance meal plans at your ACE but add more healthy natural fats as your appetite dictates.
- Continue your multivitamin/multimineral and omega-3 supplements.

Perhaps the best way to think of the two paths in Lifetime Maintenance is like a pair of fraternal twins. They share many similarities but have some significant differences, as summarized below.

### DAILY INTAKE IN TWO LIFETIME MAINTENANCE PATHS

| ACE | Above 50 Grams of Net Carbs | Below 50 Grams of Net Carbs |
|---|---|---|
| Foundation vegetables | Minimum 12–15 grams | Minimum 12–15 grams |
| Total daily protein (meals plus snacks) | Women: 12–18 ounces Men: 16–22 ounces | Women: 12–18 ounces Men: 16–22 ounces |
| Healthy natural fats | As your appetite dictates | As your appetite dictates |
| Total grams of Net Carbs | 50–100 | 25–50 |
| Range of carbohydrate foods possible | Foundation vegetables Nuts and seeds | Foundation vegetables Nuts and seeds |

| ACE | Above 50 Grams of Net Carbs | Below 50 Grams of Net Carbs |
| --- | --- | --- |
| | Berries and other fruits | Berries |
| | Legumes | Other foods possible* |
| | Starchy vegetables* | |
| | Whole grains* | |
| Broth/bouillon/salt | Optional | 2 servings (unless you are hypertensive or on diuretic medication) |

*If your ACE allows.

## NEW TASTES, NEW HABITS

Now that you've slimmed down and shaped up, you may have found that other things are changing in your life as well. Perhaps your social life has improved. The downside, of course, is that social situations can test your resolve. As long as you don't exceed your ACE, you should have the Atkins Edge in your corner, but you also need to learn strategies for coping with situations that crop up at work, when dining out or traveling, and more. To a large extent, your carbohydrate threshold, aka your ACE, will influence how you'll address these "real-world" issues and situations, but don't underestimate the importance of your mind-set.

Whether your ACE is 30 or 100, as you develop new habits, they'll ultimately become second nature. You'll probably notice that you will increasingly gravitate to healthy foods and find it easier to stay away from problematic ones. Again, we advise you, as much as possible, to avoid table sugar, high-fructose corn syrup, other forms of sugar, and foods made with them, including fruit juice, energy drinks, and commercial smoothies. Once you get out of the sugar habit, you'll likely find that such foods lose their hold over you and may taste overly sweet. And now that you know that such foods wreak havoc on your body's ability to burn fat, sabotaging your efforts at weight control, you have good reason to steer clear of them.

The same goes for foods made with white flour or other refined grains. White bread, pasta, potatoes, grits, and other starchy foods may now not taste as wonderful as you remembered them. In fact, much of the flavor and satisfaction you associated with such foods comes from the herbs, spices, and fats served with them—not the food itself. You can savor olive oil, butter, cream, sour cream, Parmesan cheese, and a myriad of tasty condiments on salads, vegetables, meat, fish, and a variety of other foods without the downside of metabolic interference.

Does this mean you can never again enjoy another piece of Grandma's pumpkin pie or a bowl of pasta or a stack of pancakes with maple syrup? One should never say "never." We know as well as you do that it's darn hard to live on this planet and not be tempted to occasionally eat such foods. If your weight has stabilized and you aren't experiencing cravings, you might allow yourself an occasional exception to your low-carb diet. Just remember that such empty carbs take you out of fat-burning mode. On the other hand, there's a thin line between the "just one taste" mentality and carb creep. If you're regularly having a forkful of problem foods here and a spoonful there, you could be heading for trouble. It's not that you can't recover from the temporary metabolic shift away from fat burning given a few days of firm resolve, but you should understand what happens when you do. For many people, it's the equivalent of playing with fire. You've spent a lot of time and effort building your "metabolic house"—it would be a shame to burn it down.

## GOOD-BYE TO OLD HABITS

Even as you settle into your new lifestyle, it's all too common to find yourself caught up short as you find it hard to break habits you've had for years, perhaps even decades. Whether it's having a doughnut with coffee at break time or a jumbo container of popcorn at the multiplex, or eating comfort foods when you're lonely or depressed, these routines can exert a powerful influence on you. How can you change habits that may seem relatively innocuous in and of themselves but cumulatively can jeopardize all the new habits you've carefully developed over the last several months? Here's a four-step way to come to grips with the situation.

1.  Identify the habits that are threatening your commitment to weight maintenance and good health. List them in your diet journal.

2.  Check to see if you've eaten enough of the right foods in the twelve hours before you were tempted to revert to your old behavior. Habits and cravings can be a way your body says, "You're not feeding me enough."

3.  Look at both the short- and long-term risks these habits pose. For example, short term might be reawakening cravings that threaten your resolve and long term might be increasing your susceptibility to the type 2 diabetes in your family history.

4.  Come up with a replacement habit, and record it in your journal. For example, swap the doughnut for your favorite low-carb bar and make sure to always have a supply at work. Take a small bag of salted nuts and a bottle of water to the movies with you, and don't go near the snack bar. In fact, your new habit doesn't have to relate to food. Any eating that's motivated by anything other than hunger is a prime candidate for radical change. Maybe a short walk after dinner with your spouse can replace dessert. You can practice yoga rather than eat chocolate when you're feeling blue. Develop a plan of action for each new habit. If you spend too much time alone watching television in the evenings, join a book club or health club, or get involved in community activities. Look at both the long- and short-term benefits these new habits offer. Having a clear vision of how your new habit can help you maintain your healthy lifestyle, feel good about yourself, and increase the prospect of a long, healthy life is a strong motivator.

    Finally, don't beat yourself up if you occasionally fall back into an old habit. It takes a while to break old habits and make new ones.

## AVOIDANCE VERSUS EXPERIENCE

We talked about empty carbs above. But you can also all too easily exceed your ACE with carbohydrate foods on the three Acceptable Foods lists. Even with a relatively high ACE, you need to continue to be mindful of what you eat. Your approach may differ from how your best friend or spouse does it. For some people, the solution is to "just say no" to any carbs not on their personal list of suitable foods—basically a behavior pattern of avoidance. These individuals have decided that it just isn't worth trying out foods that aren't in their comfort zone. Others adopt this strategy after experimenting with how much and what kinds of carbs they can handle. Through hard-won experience, they've identified the line they cannot cross. For some people it's a distinct line, for others a buffer zone. The "distinct liners" behave the way a person who realizes that she/he can't handle alcohol does: experience leads to avoidance. People who find that they can be somewhat more flexible around foods with higher carb counts behave much like someone who can handle alcohol in moderation. To a large extent, the thickness of your line is likely to depend on your ACE. If you've found you do best at 40 grams of Net Carbs a day, you have a thin line and will probably find it wise to adopt a restrictive mind-set about stepping over it. But if your ACE is 90, you may have learned that your buffer zone can be a bit wider.

If experience tells you that you can handle it, knowing you can have a small portion of dessert at a dinner party or an occasional half bagel without endangering your hard-won goal weight is empowering. It's equally empowering to know that strict avoidance of anything on the other side of the "line" best protects your sense of control and physical well-being. In either case, you have to explore where you fit into this spectrum by carefully testing your response to different foods and backing away when you find that you've gone too far.

## STRATEGIZING YOUR SOCIAL LIFE

Advance planning is also key to not exceeding your limits. If you're going to be, say, at a wedding or holiday celebration that could prove to be a minefield of problematic foods, consider these survival tactics:

- Have a substantial snack or even a meal before the event to temper your appetite.
- Look at the various offerings, decide what you're going to have, and stick with them. If you do choose to eat a high-carb food, pick your poison. If you are going to splurge on pasta salad, pass on the dessert.
- Make only one trip to the buffet table.
- Eat only until you're satisfied but not stuffed.
- Drink alcohol in moderation, both because your body burns it before carbs and fat and so as not to let down your inhibitions and eat inappropriate foods. Pass on any drinks that contain fruit juice or sugar.
- If your host or hostess pressures you to have just one piece of pie or cake, politely say that you're too full. Or take a small taste, say it is delicious, and then claim that you're so full you can't eat any more.

What about when you're on vacation or a business trip to a dining mecca? After all, it would be a shame to go to New Orleans, San Francisco, or New York and not sample some of the local delicacies. Here are some ideas of how to enjoy the cuisine without overdoing it.

- Have eggs or a low-carb shake for breakfast and a salad with protein for lunch. That should leave a bit of a margin to enjoy the local specialty—in moderation, of course. (Also see the sidebar "Thumbs Down, Thumbs Up.")
- Explore the range of local foods. The seafood in San Francisco and New Orleans is justly famous. Choose a local specialty that's prepared without breading or starchy sauces.

- The moment you get home, return to your ACE if you've not gained weight.
- If you've put on a couple of pounds, drop back 10 to 20 grams of Net Carbs until you restore your goal weight.

## THUMBS DOWN, THUMBS UP

Your long-term success in maintaining your healthy new weight will depend in large part on the small choices you make every day. Here are just a few alternatives to foods that can get you into trouble.

| Thumbs Down | Thumbs Up |
| --- | --- |
| Tortilla chips | Salted nuts or seeds |
| Crackers | Bran crispbread |
| Potato chips | Soy chips |
| Glazed/honey-cured ham | Regular ham |
| Turkey loaf | Turkey breast |
| Tuna sandwich | Tuna salad plate |
| Meat loaf | Roast beef |
| Breaded shrimp | Sautéed or grilled shrimp |
| Stuffed clams | Steamed clams |
| Crab cakes | Steamed or sautéed crabs |
| Chicken nuggets | Grilled chicken |
| Smoothie | Atkins Advantage shake |
| Fruit juice | Berries or other fruit |
| Muffin | Atkins Day Break bar |
| Chocolate bar | Atkins Endulge bar |
| Brownie | Atkins Advantage bar |
| Flavored yogurt | Whole milk yogurt with fresh berries |
| Almost any dessert | Berries and cream |

## THE MIND GAME

In addition to developing new habits and eating filling foods in the form of protein, fat, and fiber, there's a third component that comes into play in order to stay in charge of your intake. We're talking about the relationship between your emotions and food. Find a time when you know you won't be disturbed and record in your journal your feelings about your accomplishments, your new looks, and your sense of what's possible. We know, we've said it before, but please pay special attention this time. If you're like many people who've recently transformed themselves, you may be on an emotional high, with all sorts of plans for the future. Now that you know you can take charge of your eating habits, your health, and your physical self, you realize that there are many other changes you can make as well. Consider how this empowering experience may help you open other doors in your life—if it hasn't already. List them as possible goals. Certainly, several of our Success Stories demonstrate that changing one's appearance or making health improvements often leads to major life shifts. What have you dreamed of doing but put aside because you didn't think you could achieve it? Now is the time to dust off those dreams and go for them.

Also record in your journal any disappointments that you may have experienced in the last few weeks. It's not uncommon to feel a complex mix of emotions upon reaching your goal weight. Among other things, you no longer have the ongoing reduction in your weight and measurements to reinforce your motivation. Also, it's all too easy to have blamed all your problems in the past on being overweight and then feel let down when certain issues remain after the pounds depart. For example, you may have assumed that once you subtracted all those pounds and inches, you'd see your career blossom. Or you may have thought that your social life would improve once you slimmed down. Guess what? You still have to work at making changes. If you were always shy because of your size, it's unrealistic to assume that you'll promptly become an extrovert as you shrink. After all, you've changed your body, not had a personality transplant! It may take you some time to achieve the confidence that goes with that terrific-looking person you see in the mirror.

Sometimes, however, it isn't just a matter of becoming comfortable with that changed person. All too often, formerly heavy people find that they have a hard time letting go of their old self-image. It's not that they don't want to, but they are so used to seeing themselves as unattractive, overweight, and unworthy that they continue to think of themselves that way. Some of this can be dealt with at the conscious level. For example, simply taping before and after photos of yourself to your mirror can provide a constant reminder of how much you've changed for the better.

## PERCEPTION AND REALITY

The part of your brain that enables you to touch your finger to your nose with your eyes closed also tells you, for example, how much space you occupy. Try this exercise if you've lost more than 30 pounds:

- Put two straight-back chairs back-to-back in the middle of the room.
- Stand by one chair and pull it out just far enough that your eye tells you there's enough space to pass between them with your hips barely brushing the chair backs.
- Now step between the chairs to see how good your eye was at judging your width.

We've found that most people who've recently lost a significant amount of weight pull the chair out too far, often by several inches. People who've been the same weight for more than two years, however, usually nail it to within an inch. This how-wide-am-I instinct apparently takes between six and twelve months to adjust after major weight loss. And this is only one sense-of-self instinct out of many, all of which take time to realign after you lose weight. In the meantime, you need to consciously tell yourself, "I'm doing great, and I'm proud of myself."

## LIFE GOES ON

The real risk here is that if you continue to hang on to your old image of yourself, sooner or later you may revert to that reality because it's familiar territory. The other image, the one expressed by your new physique, is still filled with uncertainty. And life goes on, with all its messiness. You may be looking and feeling great, but your kids will still get sick, talk back, break things, and bicker with their siblings. Your significant other will not always be a model of understanding and support. You may lose your job. Your car won't promise to never break down. You get the picture: you've made a major change in a big part of your life, but in case you haven't noticed, the world doesn't revolve around you.

It's important to find a way to air such concerns, whether in the Atkins online community or with your friends or family members. Don't let setbacks (whether real or perceived) in your personal and work life drive you back to your old way of eating. In our Success Stories, you've already met nine people like you who confronted their weight and their inner demons. Reread some of their stories, and you'll see that they often struggled not just with their new weight but with their sense of self. It may take some time before you feel completely comfortable with the new you, the permanently slim you.

## TO EXERCISE OR NOT: THAT IS THE QUESTION

If you've reached Lifetime Maintenance, you've already made great strides in achieving a healthy body. If you haven't already done so, now is the time to consider incorporating some enjoyable forms of physical activity into your lifestyle. More often than not, they'll enrich your Atkins experience and offer additional health benefits. Studies indicate that people who are physically active have a better chance of maintaining their weight loss than do sedentary folks.[1] For some of you, the role of exercise in controlling your weight may be small—genetics play a major role—but there are other reasons to consider adopting an exercise routine. For example, bone health and minimizing the risk of osteoporosis are closely linked to activity, especially resistance, or weight-bearing, exercise. Whether you're in your twenties and want to improve your athletic performance or in your eighties and want to maintain normal daily activities, resistance exercises are also the most efficient way to increase your muscle endurance, strength, and power.

Such sustained rhythmic exercises as swimming, cycling, and running are great ways to improve your heart and circulatory and respiratory systems. These endurance forms of exercise also complement many of the metabolic adaptations induced by the Atkins Diet, such as increased fat burning. Do you have to exercise two hours a day to keep your weight under control and maintain appetite control, lack of food cravings, and other benefits? Absolutely not! Remember, if you continue to follow the program's principles you'll have the Atkins Edge, so you don't need to overdo the exercise to control the metabolic bully. But to optimize mental and physical health and well-being, most of us benefit from regularly finding time to exercise.

## THINGS CHANGE

Now that you're getting comfortable with your new lifestyle and feeling that the struggle you've had with your weight is finally history, don't forget this important point. The only constant in life is change. Imagine one or more of these situations:

- You join a swim team and start competing in meets.
- You leave your desk job for one that involves more physical labor.
- You start bicycling three miles to and from work instead of taking the bus.
- You move from the suburbs to the city and walking becomes your usual mode of transportation.

It's possible that any of these changes will increase your daily energy use, enabling you to eat a bit more, either as whole food carbohydrates or as healthy, natural fats, to stay at your goal weight.

Now consider these situations:

- You suffer a ski injury and spend several months in a cast.
- You have a new baby in the house and find yourself stressed and sleep-deprived.
- Your doctor prescribes antidepressants to help you deal with a family crisis.
- A new job requires frequent travel, interfering with your fitness regimen.

Chances are that any of the above will reduce your daily energy use, meaning you'll need to lower your ACE to maintain your weight.

Now let's take a longer view. If you're 40 years old, exercise regularly, and have no health issues, you may be able to continue to manage your weight by staying at your ACE for years to come. As we've discussed before, numerous factors—some in your control and others not (including your genes)—influence your metabolism, which in turn determines your ACE. Aging tends to slow your metabolism, so can certain drugs and hormonal changes. As long as you're attuned to the implications of such changes, you can stay in charge of your weight by either eating fewer carbs, upping your activity level (which works for some people), or both.

## TO ERR IS HUMAN

We know and you know that occasionally, there is the chance that you'll slip up. The following three situations should help you handle smaller and bigger indiscretions.

*Small Stuff.* You find yourself chowing down a cherry Danish, a raisin bagel, or another high-carb food of dubious value. *Recovery tactic:* Once your weight has been stable for several months, it's likely that such an indiscretion won't impact your weight, although it might make you feel sluggish for a day or two. Once you realize what you're doing, stop immediately and get back on track with the healthy way you've been eating.

*A Week of Carb Overindulgence:* You spend a week in Cancún and succumb to the lure of quesadillas and margaritas. Not only do you gain weight, you're also plagued with carb cravings. *Recovery tactic:* Since most of the weight gain from a brief episode of carb overindulgence is water, the best antidote is to reduce your carb intake. As soon as you get home, drop 20 daily grams of Net Carbs below your ACE. If the excess pounds won't budge and you're still experiencing cravings, return to OWL for a week or two until things are back under control.

*Falling off the Wagon:* An event such as a breakup with a significant other, a lost job, or another major disappointment sends you back to your old, unhealthy eating habits. Even a positive event, such as beginning a relationship with someone who doesn't follow the Atkins lifestyle, can trigger a lapse from your new eating habits. After several weeks and several pounds, you're feeling disgusted with yourself. Your pre-Atkins symptoms have returned with a vengeance, and you can't fit into your new clothes. *Recovery tactic:* First of all, don't beat yourself up. Get off the guilt trip, which will just lead to more destructive eating. Instead, go back to OWL until your cravings are under control. Then move to Pre-Maintenance to restore your goal weight and maintain it for a month.

These three examples illustrate several points. First, the longer you wait to take action, the more aggressive your response needs to be. A minor slipup may require no action other than to examine why it happened and plan future defenses. A binge or period during which you depart from your low-carb way of eating demands more proactive measures. Regard any such departure as a learning experience of how thin is the line between your carb threshold and overdoing it. It also clearly demonstrates how a cascading series of events can threaten your long-term weight control program. More important, however, you'll realize that you can reverse the tide. It's as simple as this: You were in control. You fell out of control. Now you know what you have to do to take control again.

At this moment, while you're still new to Lifetime Maintenance, you may honestly believe you'll never backtrack. Maybe you're one of those remarkably strong people who never do, but if you're like many of us, you will occasionally slip up. Just remember that you have all the skills you need to execute a fast reverse and then move forward with the rest of your life full of health and vitality.

## TWO OUTCOMES

Undoubtedly, the question running through your head is "Will I really be able to stay slim and control my eating habits for the rest of my life?" Without claiming to be fortune-tellers, we can predict whether or not you'll succeed in making your goal weight your permanent weight. That's right. We don't even have to meet you. Ask yourself these questions:

1. Are you someone who couldn't wait to reach your goal weight so you could eat all those foods you've been missing?
2. Do you believe that now that you've slimmed down, you'll be able to keep the excess pounds off by eating almost anything in moderation and practicing self-control?
3. Do you want to push your carb intake as high as you possibly can?
4. Do you "get it" that only by permanently changing your way of eating will you avoid repeating the past?
5. Do you understand the role that certain foods play in controlling your appetite?
6. Do you realize that it's better to not push your carb threshold to the max but to settle at a level that you can sustain without cravings?

If you answered yes to any of the first three questions, we predict that your weight will creep (or maybe even lurch) back, along with the attendant health problems. Before you know it, you'll be starting Induction again or trying a new diet. But if you can honestly answer yes to questions 4, 5, and 6—and abide by them—we predict that you'll achieve long-term success. If you're in the second group, you should be able to get on with your life without worrying constantly about your weight and health.

## ADVICE FOR LIFE

If you didn't pass the test above with flying colors, memorize the correct answers to all six questions. For sustained success, also remind yourself frequently of all the things that you've learned in your weight loss journey.

Continue to consume at least 12 to 15 grams of your Net Carbs in the form of foundation vegetables and abide by these twenty tips, and you'll make your goal weight your lifetime weight:

1. *Rely on satisfying foods.* Protein foods keep you feeling pleasantly full and are fundamentally self-limiting. Almost everyone has eaten a couple of dozen cookies in an evening at some time in his or her life, but how many people have eaten as many hard-boiled eggs at one sitting? Other than a contestant at a county fair, probably no one!

2. *Don't skimp on natural fats.* Even though you're now at your goal weight, you're still burning mostly fat for energy, along with a relatively small portion of carbohydrates. Since you're no longer losing weight, it's your dietary fat that's keeping your body warm and your muscles working. Never forget that getting enough fat in your diet keeps your appetite and cravings under control.

3. *Remember the magic number.* Never, ever let yourself gain more than 5 pounds without taking action to restore your goal weight.

4. *Go easy on fruit.* Eating too much fruit pushes up your insulin level and makes you store fat. Even with a relatively high ACE, you should probably confine yourself to no more than two daily servings. With a low ACE, you're better off with at most one serving of berries. Regardless of your carb tolerance, concentrate on those with lower carb counts and more fiber, such as berries, cherries, melon, and that vegetable that pretends it's a fruit: rhubarb.

5. *Keep sipping.* Drink plenty of fluids and take your supplements.

6. *Always read labels.* Be alert to added sugar and other ingredients best avoided in packaged foods.

7. *Steer clear of trigger foods.* You know what they are. Keep them out of the house if at all possible.

8. *Make compromises with excess carbs an increasingly less common behavior.* It's unlikely that the occasional slice of pizza or ice cream cone will never pass your lips. But if you're going to succeed long term, you'll figure out how to recover, return to your ACE, and minimize such lapses in the future.

9. *Keep moving.* Staying active will increase the likelihood that you'll keep your weight under control. Increasing your activity may also help in the event that your weight starts to trend upward. Weight-bearing

and resistance exercise will increase your strength while toning your muscles so you look even better.

10. *Track your numbers.* Weigh and measure yourself weekly or use weight averaging so you can nip in the bud any gains that result from "carb creep."

11. *Eat before you go.* Having a protein-plus-fat snack or even a meal before you go to a foodcentric event will take the edge off your hunger and make you more able to resist inappropriate items on the buffet table.

12. *Take it with you.* For work, on the road, or even a movie, pack snacks such as nuts or cheese so you won't be tempted by the usual sky-high-carb offerings.

13. *Use low-carb specialty foods carefully.* Bars, shakes, and other specialty foods can replace their high-carb analogues, eliminating any sense of deprivation.

14. *Compromise when necessary* (and learn from the experience). When there are no good options, make the best choice available.

15. *Stay in touch.* Continue to share with another Atkins "graduate" and check in with others on the Atkins Community Web site. The challenges don't cease, although they should get easier over time, and you may be able to help others reach their goals.

16. *Get rid of your "fat" wardrobe.* If you have nothing to wear that hides extra pounds, you'll have an early alert system if you start to regain weight and an economic incentive to take immediate action.

17. *Prepare, prepare, prepare.* If you're eating out, check the menu online beforehand. If you're going grocery shopping, make a list and stick to it. Anticipating situations in which temptation might well rear its ugly head is a powerful strategy.

18. *Act quickly.* If you detour from Atkins for a day or more, get back on track ASAP. The longer you're off, the harder it may be to resume.

19. *Remind yourself.* Review your diet journal occasionally, and take a peek at your "before" photo.

20. *Savor your power.* Remind yourself regularly of the tremendous accomplishment you have made and how it impacts not just you but your family and friends. You've made yourself healthier and more attractive and inspired others to do the same.

## THE WAY WE WERE DESIGNED TO EAT

To conclude this portion of the book, we remind you once again that by controlling your carbohydrate intake, you make your body burn primarily body fat and dietary fat for energy. This, in turn, allows you to lose weight and later maintain that new weight, while also improving a host of health indicators. Known as the Atkins Edge, this metabolic adaptation also allows you to enjoy a steady source of energy, making excessive hunger and cravings for carbohydrate foods a thing of the past. With that tool at your disposal, permanent weight control is within your grasp.

After reading part III, "Eating Out, Eating In: Atkins in the Real World," move on to part IV, where we discuss the compelling research that confirms that consuming a high-fat, moderate-protein diet, which describes Atkins, improves a broad range of health indicators that impact heart health, metabolic syndrome, and diabetes.

# EATING OUT, EATING IN:

Atkins in the Real World

# Chapter 11

# LOW-CARB FAST-FOOD AND RESTAURANT MEALS

From fast food to fine cuisine, we've got you covered. Check out our restaurant guides, and then, in chapter 12, move on to our delicious low-carb recipes and meal plans for every phase.

## EATING ON THE RUN

When you're on the road, grabbing lunch between appointments, or taking the family out without breaking the bank, chances are that you'll be patronizing some of the big chain fast-food eateries. Here are some lower-carb options that won't blow your diet. This is not to say that these foods should be your daily fare or that some of them aren't high in calories, have a few grams of added sugar, or contain trans fats.

### ARBY'S/WWW.ARBYS.COM

*Thumbs Up:* Minus the bun: Roast Chicken, Roast Turkey, Roast Ham, Roast Beef, Roast Beef melts, Reuben Corned Beef, and BLT sandwiches and contents of all subs; Chopped Turkey Club Salad with Buttermilk Ranch dressing.
*Thumbs Down:* Popcorn Chicken; Chicken Fillets; most salad dressings and condiments.

### A & W/WWW.AWRESTAURANTS.COM

*Thumbs Up:* Minus the bun: Hot Dog, Cheese Dog, Coney Dog, hamburgers, cheeseburgers, Grilled Chicken sandwich; Ranch dipping sauce.
*Thumbs Down:* Chicken Strips, Crispy Chicken Sandwich, Corn Dog Nuggets, BBQ and Honey-Mustard dipping sauce.

## BLIMPIE/WWW.BLIMPIE.COM

*Thumbs Up:* Minus the bun: Deli Subs, Super Stacked Subs, Hot Philly Cheese Steak and Hot Pastrami subs; also Antipasto, Chef, Grilled Chicken, and Tuna salads; blue cheese, Caesar, and oil and vinegar salad dressings.

*Thumbs Down:* All panini grilled subs, Hot Meatball Sub; Chile Ole and Roast Beef 'n Bleu salads; Blimpie Sauce and Dijon Honey Mustard.

## BURGER KING/WWW.BK.COM

*Thumbs Up:* Minus the bun: All burgers and Whoppers and Tendergrill Chicken Sandwich; Tendergrill Garden Salad (remove the carrots in earlier phases); Ken's Ranch dressing; Ham Omelet Sandwich with/without bacon/ sausage (minus the bun and honey butter sauce); Veggie Burger okay for Phase 3 (minus the bun).

*Thumbs Down:* Tendercrisp Chicken, Tendercrisp Garden Salad, Chicken Tenders; Honey Mustard and Ken's Fat-free Ranch dressings.

## CARL'S JR./WWW.CARLSJR.COM

*Thumbs Up:* Low-Carb Six-Dollar Burger (wrapped in lettuce leaves); minus the bun: Famous Star, Big Carl™, Guacamole Bacon Burger, most other burgers/cheeseburgers, and Charbroiled Chicken Club; Charbroiled Chicken Salad (lose the croutons); house and blue cheese salad dressings; house and Buffalo wing sauces.

*Thumbs Down:* Teriyaki Burger, Parmesan Chicken Sandwich and all other fried chicken and fish dishes; thousand island and low-fat balsamic salad dressings; BBQ, honey mustard, and sweet and sour sauces.

## CHICK-FIL-A/WWW.CHICK-FIL-A.COM

*Thumbs Up:* Minus the biscuit: breakfast egg, cheese, sausage, and bacon dishes; sausage breakfast burrito (unwrap and discard the tortilla); Chargrilled Chicken Club and Chicken Salad sandwiches minus the bread; blue cheese, Caesar, and buttermilk ranch salad dressings; Buffalo and buttermilk ranch sauces.

*Thumbs Down:* All breaded and fried chicken dishes; Chick-fil-A sauce and barbecue, honey mustard, and Polynesian sauces; fat-free honey mustard and other low- or no-fat salad dressings.

## DAIRY QUEEN/WWW.DAIRYQUEEN.COM

*Thumbs Up:* Minus the bun: Grillburgers, hamburgers, cheeseburgers, hot dogs, cheese dogs, grilled chicken and turkey items; side salad (lose the carrots in earlier phases); BBQ, Wild Buffalo, and ranch dipping sauces.

*Thumbs Down:* All crispy chicken items; blue cheese, sweet and sour, honey mustard dipping sauces, all fat-free salad dressings.

## HARDEE'S/WWW.HARDEES.COM

*Thumbs Up:* Hardee's Alternative Options menu: Low-carb Thickburger, low-carb Breakfast Bowl, and Charbroiled Chicken Club "Sandwich" salad.

*Thumbs Down:* All other burgers with buns.

## KFC/WWW.KFC.COM

*Thumbs Up:* Roasted Chicken Caesar or Caesar side salad, both without croutons; roasted chicken BLT salad; Heinz Buttermilk Ranch Dressing; most wing dishes; green beans, KFC Mean Greens.

*Thumbs Down:* All fried, breaded, or crispy dishes and salads; biscuits, most sides.

## MCDONALD'S/WWW.NUTRITION.MCDONALDS.COM

*Thumbs Up:* Minus the bun: Burgers or cheeseburgers; Premium Bacon Ranch or Caesar salad with or without grilled chicken; scrambled eggs and sausage patty minus the bun; Newman's Own Creamy Caesar Dressing.

*Thumbs Down:* Burgers with buns; Chicken McNuggets; all breaded chicken and fish dishes; wraps; all other salad dressings.

## SUBWAY/WWW.SUBWAYFRESHBUZZ.COM

*Thumbs Up:* Any sub can be ordered as a salad (toss any croutons), including cold cut combo, Subway Club, tuna fish, BLT, Black Forest ham, turkey breast, and roast beef; omelets minus the sandwich; vinaigrette dressing.

*Thumbs Down:* Any sub.

## WENDY'S/WWW.WENDYS.COM

*Thumbs Up:* Minus the bun: Any hamburger or cheeseburger; chicken BLT or chicken Caesar salad (omit croutons) with Ultimate Chicken Grill Fillet and Supreme Caesar Dressing.

*Thumbs Down:* Burgers with buns, chicken nuggets, crispy chicken dishes; all wings; Southwest Taco salad; most salad dressings.

# DINING OUT

Whether your tastes run to shish kebab or sashimi, Chicken Piccata or Tandoori Chicken, fajitas or fatoushe, you can eat out with ease in almost any cuisine while complying with your low-carb lifestyle. Here's a peek at what's good to go and what's off the table so you can navigate menus in ten different languages.

## ITALIAN RESTAURANTS

Order dishes that feature chicken, veal, seafood, or pork with the flavorings that mark the cuisine, but without the sides of pasta, rice, or polenta.

*Thumbs Up:* Prosciutto with melon (OWL) or asparagus; Parmigiano Reggiano; antipasto (assorted meat, cheese, and marinated vegetables); caponata (eggplant and caper salad) and most other salads; meat, fish, and poultry entrees, such as Veal Saltimbocca, Chicken Piccata, or Veal Scaloppini (if not breaded, floured, or battered).

*Thumbs Down:* Any pasta or risotto dish; pizza; deep-fried calamari or mozzarella; garlic bread; baked clams; Fettuccine Alfredo; Eggplant (or veal or chicken) Parmesan.

*Tip:* For starters, ask for a bowl of olives instead of the bread basket. To end the meal, order caffè breve, made with half-and-half, instead of cappuccino, made with milk.

## GREEK RESTAURANTS

Olives, olive oil, lemons, eggplant, zucchini, spinach, fennel, grape leaves, yogurt, garlic, mint, dill, rosemary, and tahini (ground sesame seeds) play starring roles in this healthful cuisine.

*Thumbs Up:* Tzatziki (cucumber, yogurt, and garlic dip); Taramosalata (creamy fish-roe spread); Avgolemono soup; feta and other sheep and goat cheeses; roasted, skewered (souvlaki), or grilled or braised lamb, beef, pork, and chicken; gyro platter; grilled shrimp, octopus, or fish.

*Thumbs Down:* Pita bread; rice-stuffed grape leaves; Skordalia (garlic-potato spread); Spanakopita or Tyropita tarts; Moussaka, Pastitsio (lamb with pasta), pilafs, fried calamari, and baklava.

*Tip:* A Greek diner is almost always a good low-carb bet for a Greek salad full of feta cheese, olives, olive oil, lettuce, tomatoes, and fresh basil. Ask for more feta instead of the stuffed grape leaves that are a typical garnish.

## MIDDLE EASTERN RESTAURANTS

Many popular dishes are built around rice, chickpeas, and lentils. Instead, concentrate on lamb and other meat dishes. Eggplant also gets star treatment in this cuisine.

*Thumbs Up:* Babaganoosh (roasted eggplant mixed with garlic and tahini); Loubieh (green beans cooked with tomatoes) and other vegetable dishes; grilled skewered dishes: lamb shish kebab, kofta (ground lamb and onion balls), and Shish Taouk (chicken pieces). In later phases: hummus, labnee (thickened yogurt with mint), tabbouleh, fatoushe, kibbeh.

*Thumbs Down:* Falafel and other chickpea dishes, pita, and baklava.

*Tip:* Instead of using pita bread for dips, ask for celery sticks, green pepper chunks, or cucumber spears.

## MEXICAN RESTAURANTS

There's much more to this cuisine than the tortillas, beans, and rice in Tex-Mex, New Mexico–style, and Cal-Mex restaurants. The primary seasonings of garlic, chilies, cilantro, and cumin can be found in any number of carb-smart dishes.

*Thumbs Up:* Salsa (with no added sugar) or guacamole (with jicama strips for dipping); jicama salad; grilled chicken wings; Sopa de Albondigas (meatball and vegetable soup); "naked fajitas" (minus tortillas and beans); grilled chicken (Pollo Asado) or fish (pescado); Camarones al Ajili (shrimp in garlic sauce); chicken or turkey mole.

*Thumbs Down:* Chips or nachos; any taco, tamale, burrito, tortilla, or enchilada platter or dish; stuffed jalepeño peppers or Chiles Rellenos; quesadillas, chimichangas, or flautas; shrimp enchiladas.

*Tip:* Ask for dishes such as Enchiladas Verdes without the tortilla and with the sauce atop the chicken. Or order a tostada/taco salad with beef or chicken minus the rice and beans and leave the tostada itself, just as you would a plate.

## FRENCH RESTAURANTS

French food is actually a collection of regional specialties and includes everything from bistro fare to haute cuisine. Many French sauces, such as hollandaise, are based on butter or olive oil and thickened with egg yolks rather than flour.

*Thumbs Up:* French onion soup (without bread topping); frisée salad; Coquilles St. Jacques (scallops in cream sauce); Steak au Poivre, Entrecôte or Tournedos Bordelaise; Veal Marengo, Coq au Vin (minus potatoes and carrots); Boeuf Bourguignon; mussels in white wine sauce or Bouillabaisse (skip the bread for dipping); Duck à l'Orange; cheese plate for dessert.

*Thumbs Down:* Alsatian tart, Vichyssoise, Croque Monsieur, pommes frites and any other potato dish, Crêpes Suzette.

## INDIAN RESTAURANTS

India has several distinct cuisines, many based on rice, wheat, or legumes. But there's still plenty of protein and low-carb vegetables on the typical menu, which also offers many options for vegetarians and vegans.

*Thumbs Up:* Tandooris (meats, fish, and vegetables baked in a clay oven); meat and fish curries; grilled shrimp, meat, or chicken kebabs; raita *(yogurt and* cucumbers—after Induction); korma, saag, and paneer (cheese curd) dishes; chicken Shorba soup.

*Thumbs Down:* Naan and other breads; dals, including mulligatawny soup (acceptable in Pre-Maintenance and Lifetime Maintenance); biryani dishes; chutneys made with added sugar; samosas and fritters.

## CHINESE RESTAURANTS

The regional cuisines include Szechuan, Hunan, Cantonese, and Shandong, but rice is a staple of all of them. Order a small portion of brown rice if you can handle whole grains.

*Thumbs Up:* Egg-drop soup (made without cornstarch) or hot-and-sour soup; sizzling shrimp platter, steamed or stir-fried tofu with vegetables; steamed beef with Chinese mushrooms; stir-fried chicken with garlic; Peking Duck and Moo Shu Pork (minus pancakes and plum sauce).

*Thumbs Down:* Any sweet-and-sour dishes; fried wontons, egg rolls, spring rolls; white or fried rice; any breaded or battered or noodle-based dish.

*Tip:* Most Chinese dishes rely on a sauce thickened with cornstarch, as do many soups. Request the sauce on the side; better yet, ask for it prepared without sugar or cornstarch.

## JAPANESE RESTAURANTS

Again, rice is a staple, as are noodles. As an island nation, Japan has many seafood dishes, but a number of other protein sources have found their way into the cuisine.

*Thumbs Up:* Miso soup; sashimi; Shabu-Shabu; grilled fish or squid; Negamaki (scallions/asparagus tips wrapped in sliced beef); steamed and grilled vegetables; pickled vegetables (oshinko), including daikon radish, Japanese eggplant, and seaweed; Sunomono salad (cucumbers, seaweed, crab); edamame (in the later phases).

*Thumbs Down:* Shrimp and vegetable tempura; sushi; gyoza (fried dumplings); seafood noodle dishes; sukiyaki and beef teriyaki (there is sugar in both the sauces).

## THAI RESTAURANTS

A blend of Chinese and Indian culinary traditions, Thai food has its own unique combination of seasonings: coconut milk, lemongrass, tamarind, cilantro, turmeric, cumin, chili paste, dried shrimp, fish sauce, lime juice, and basil. In general, stick to sautéed dishes and avoid noodle-based ones and dipping sauces.

*Thumbs Up:* Tom Yum Goong (shrimp soup) or Gai Tom Kha (chicken and coconut milk soup); Nuuryungnamtok or Yum Plamuk (main-dish salads with sliced steak or squid, respectively); sautéed shrimp, scallion, pork, beef, or vegetable dishes; curries (without potatoes); steamed fish (sauce on the side); green papaya salad.

*Thumbs Down:* Dumplings and spring rolls: fried and white rice; Pad Thai and any other noodle dish; deep-fried fish.

## KOREAN RESTAURANTS

Korean cuisine is a blend of Mongolian, Japanese, and Chinese elements with many dishes ideal for carb-conscious diners.

*Thumbs Up:* Grilled or stewed fish and shellfish; marinated grilled pork, beef, and chicken dishes (omit rice or noodles); ditto for Kalbi Tang (beef-rib stew); any bulgogi (barbecue) (minus the sugary sauce); Shinsollo (hot pots); tofu; kimchi (fermented vegetables with chilies; pickles).

*Thumbs Down:* Noodle-based soups; dumplings; any rice dish; Pa Jon (scallion pancake).

# Chapter 12

# RECIPES AND MEAL PLANS

Many low-carb cookbooks and hundreds of recipes at www.atkins.com and other low-carb Web sites make it easy to produce Atkins-friendly meals. For that reason and because we simply don't have space to include too many recipes in this book, we've taken a different approach: with the exception of the broths, these dishes aren't designed to be eaten alone. Instead, use these delectable sauces, marinades, salad dressings, and flavored butters to complement or enhance meat, poultry, fish, or tofu, as well as salad greens and other vegetables, while complying with your weight management program. Even your family members who aren't on Atkins will enjoy these tasty recipes. In addition to a protein source and vegetables, just make some brown rice, sweet potatoes, or another nutrient-rich starch for them.

Master several of these simple recipes, and you'll be able to:

1. Add flavor and variety to basic meals, so you'll never get bored eating the low-carb way.
2. Find delicious ways to consume all the healthy, natural fats you need to do Atkins properly.
3. Make low-carb alternatives to condiments such as barbecue sauce and cocktail sauce that usually are full of added sugars.

Different noncaloric sweeteners have varying degrees of sweetness. We've left the choice of sucralose, saccharin, xylitol, or stevia up to you in most cases where a recipe for a sauce, salad dressing, or marinade calls for a sweetening agent, unless the recipe calls for 2 or more tablespoons, in which case we've specified xylitol, which is not as sweet as the other three alternatives.

For each recipe, we've provided appropriate phases, nutritional data, the number and size of servings, and the total amount of time it takes to make, as well as the active time. For example, a sauce may need to simmer for an hour to blend flavors but take only 10 minutes to assemble. In the case of specialty ingredients, we've provided sources or alternatives.

So let's get cooking!

# RECIPE INDEX

## SAUCES

## COMPOUND BUTTERS AND OILS

## SALAD DRESSINGS

## MARINADES AND RUBS

## BROTHS

# SAUCES

There are countless sauces and many ways to make them. Sauces that get their rich texture from cream, butter, oil, or puréed ingredients are a boon for people who are watching their carb intake. Mayonnaise, hollandaise, and basil pesto, for example, rely on eggs, cream, or oil to do the thickening. Even sauces that aren't usually low carb, such as barbecue sauce, are easy to adapt, as our recipes demonstrate. Similarly adaptable are pan sauces, which are usually made by thickening the drippings of roast beef, turkey, or another main dish with a roux (a flour-and-fat mixture). Condiments, such as tartar sauce, salsa, aïoli, and other zesty complements to meals, also add zest to meals.

In most recipes, we've relied on oils such as olive oil and canola oil that are primarily monounsaturated. Occasionally, small amounts of the polyunsaturated sesame or peanut oil are specified to remain faithful to a sauce inspired by an Asian cuisine.

Also check out these sauces on www.atkins.com/recipes: Chimichurri Sauce, Béarnaise Sauce, Classic Mint Sauce, Creamy Herb Sauce, Pico de Gallo (tomato salsa), Guacamole, and Simplest Turkey Gravy.

## Velouté Sauce

Don't be intimidated by the French name. This tasty sauce is easy to make. The classic version relies on flour as thickener, but our version makes it a perfect low-carb accompaniment. The specific broth depends on whether you'll be using the sauce with poultry, meat, or fish.

Phases: 1, 2, 3, 4
Makes: 4 (½-cup) servings
Active Time: 5 minutes
Total Time: 15 minutes

2 cups Chicken Broth or Beef Broth (pages 240 or 241), or canned or Tetra Pak chicken, beef, or fish broth
½ teaspoon salt
⅛ teaspoon pepper
1 tablespoon Thick It Up thickener
2 tablespoons unsalted butter

Combine broth, salt, and pepper in a small saucepan over medium-high heat; bring to a boil. Whisk in thickener; simmer, stirring occasionally, until sauce thickens, about 3 minutes. Remove from heat; swirl in butter until melted. Serve warm or refrigerate in an airtight container for up to 5 days.

PER SERVING: Net Carbs: 1 gram; Total Carbs: 3 grams; Fiber: 2 grams; Protein: 3 grams; Fat: 6 grams; Calories: 70

*Tip:* Thick It Up thickener thickens sauces the way cornstarch or flour does, but without the carbs. All its carbs are fiber, so it has 0 grams of Net Carbs per serving. You can order it online from numerous low-carb food Web sites.

## Béchamel Sauce

Béchamel is a mild sauce that can be used in soufflés or simmered with finely chopped vegetables or meats. Traditionally thickened with a mixture of flour and fat, our version uses heavy cream and a low-carb thickener instead.

Phases: 1, 2, 3, 4
Makes: 6 (¼-cup) servings
Active Time: 10 minutes
Total Time: 30 minutes

1 cup heavy cream
1 cup water
½ small onion, coarsely chopped
1 teaspoon salt
¼ teaspoon pepper
Pinch ground nutmeg
1 tablespoon Thick It Up thickener
1 tablespoon butter

1. Combine cream, water, onion, salt, pepper, and nutmeg in a small saucepan over medium heat; bring to a simmer. Remove from heat; let stand 15 minutes.
2. Strain cream mixture; return to saucepan over medium heat. Whisk in thickener; cook until sauce thickens, about 3 minutes. Remove from heat; swirl in butter until melted. Use right away.

PER SERVING: Net Carbs: 2 grams; Total Carbs: 3 grams; Fiber: 1 gram; Protein: 1 gram; Fat: 17 grams; Calories: 160

## Mushroom Gravy

This low-carb gravy gets its rich flavor from sautéed mushrooms rather than pan drippings. For a vegetarian version, replace the chicken broth with vegetable broth.

Phases: 1, 2, 3, 4
Makes: 10 (¼-cup) servings
Active Time: 25 minutes
Total Time: 35 minutes

4 tablespoons (½ stick) butter, divided
1 small onion, finely chopped
¼ teaspoon salt
⅛ teaspoon pepper
1 (10-ounce) package sliced mixed mushrooms
2 garlic cloves, minced
2 teaspoons soy sauce
2 teaspoons red wine vinegar
2 cups Chicken Broth (page 240), or canned or Tetra Pak chicken broth
1½ teaspoons Thick It Up thickener
2 teaspoons fresh chopped thyme

Melt 2 tablespoons of the butter in a nonstick skillet over medium-high heat. Add onion, salt, and pepper and sauté until soft, about 3 minutes. Add mushrooms and sauté until golden brown, about 8 minutes. Add garlic and sauté until fragrant, about 30 seconds. Add soy sauce and vinegar; simmer until evaporated, about 30 seconds. Add broth and boil until mixture is reduced by one-third, about 10 minutes. Stir in thickener and thyme; simmer until sauce thickens, about 2 minutes. Remove from heat; swirl in remaining 2 tablespoons butter until melted. Serve warm.

PER SERVING: Net Carbs: 2 grams; Total Carbs: 3 grams; Fiber: 1 gram; Protein: 2 grams; Fat: 5 grams; Calories: 60

# Mayonnaise

Store-bought mayonnaise may be convenient, but it's usually made with soybean oil and often with added sugar. Homemade mayonnaise is delicious, especially spooned over steamed vegetables. Use it to make tuna, shrimp, or egg salad or as a base for dips or sauces such as Tartar Sauce (page 210–11) and Rémoulade (page 211).

Phases: 1, 2, 3, 4
Makes: 8 (2-tablespoon) servings
Active Time: 10 minutes
Total Time: 10 minutes

1 large egg yolk (see note, opposite)
2 teaspoons fresh lemon juice
1 teaspoon Dijon mustard
½ teaspoon salt
⅛ teaspoon pepper
½ cup olive or canola oil

Combine egg yolk, lemon juice, mustard, salt, and pepper in a medium bowl; add oil in a slow and steady stream, whisking constantly until sauce is very thick. Serve right away, or refrigerate in an airtight container for up to 4 days. If mayonnaise is too thick, stir in 1 to 2 teaspoons water to thin.

PER SERVING: Net Carbs: 0 grams; Total Carbs: 0 grams; Fiber: 0 grams; Protein: 0 grams; Fat: 29 grams; Calories: 260

## VARIATIONS

### Blender Mayonnaise

Assemble ingredients for Mayonnaise, substituting a whole egg for the egg yolk. Combine egg, lemon juice, mustard, salt, and pepper in a blender and pulse to combine. With blender running on low speed, pour in the oil in a thin, steady stream. If the mixture becomes too thick and the oil is no longer incorporating, pulse the blender.

### Herb Mayonnaise

Prepare Mayonnaise according to directions, adding 3 tablespoons chopped fresh herbs, such as parsley, cilantro, thyme, or basil.

### Lime Mayonnaise

Prepare Mayonnaise according to directions, substituting lime juice for the lemon juice and adding 2 teaspoons grated lime zest.

### Chili-Cilantro Mayonnaise

Prepare Mayonnaise according to directions, substituting lime juice for the lemon juice and adding 3 tablespoons chopped fresh cilantro and 2 teaspoons chili powder.

*Note:* The very young and very old, those with compromised immune systems, and pregnant women should avoid consuming raw eggs.

## Aïoli

Delicious atop poached chicken or fish, this garlicky mayonnaise also can be used as a dip for fresh vegetables, making it a perfect low-carb snack food.

Phases: 1, 2, 3, 4
Makes: 8 (2-tablespoon)
   servings
Active Time: 10 minutes
Total Time: 10 minutes

2 garlic cloves, peeled
½ teaspoon salt
2 large egg yolks (see note, above)
1 teaspoon Dijon mustard
½ cup olive oil
½ cup canola oil

Mince garlic on a cutting board and sprinkle with salt. With the blade of a heavy knife, mash the garlic and salt into a paste. Transfer to a medium bowl. Add egg yolks and mustard; mix well. Combine olive oil and canola oil in a glass measuring cup. Slowly whisk in oil a few drops at a time until the mixture begins to thicken. Add oil slightly faster, pouring in a slow steady stream, whisking constantly, until very thick.

PER SERVING: Net Carbs: 0 grams; Total Carbs: 0 grams; Fiber: 0 grams; Protein: 1 gram; Fat: 29 grams; Calories: 270

### VARIATION
### Rouille

Prepare Aïoli according to directions, adding ½ small roasted red pepper that has been mashed into a paste and ⅛ teaspoon cayenne pepper with the egg yolks.

## Dill Sauce

Dill sauce is the classic accompaniment to cold fish (particularly poached salmon), meat, and poultry dishes. Also try it with eggs and vegetables.

| | |
|---|---|
| Phases: 1, 2, 3, 4 | ½ cup Mayonnaise (page 208) |
| Makes: 12 (2-tablespoon) | ½ cup sour cream |
|    servings | ¾ cup chopped fresh dill |
| Active Time: 10 minutes | 1½ tablespoons Dijon mustard |
| Total Time: 40 minutes | 2 tablespoons heavy cream |
| | 1 tablespoon lemon juice |
| | Salt and pepper to taste |

In a small bowl, whisk together mayonnaise, sour cream, dill, mustard, cream, and lemon juice. Stir in salt and pepper. Cover and refrigerate for at least 30 minutes to allow flavors to blend.

PER SERVING: Net Carbs: 1 gram; Total Carbs: 1 gram; Fiber: 0 grams; Protein: 1 gram; Fat: 10 grams; Calories: 100

**VARIATION**

**Caper-Dill Sauce**

Prepare Dill Sauce according to directions, substituting a pinch of cayenne pepper for the black pepper and stirring in 2 tablespoons drained, chopped capers.

## Tartar Sauce

Tartar sauce is a breeze to make, and making it yourself ensures that it will have no added sugar. This American classic is particularly good with crab cakes and other fried seafood, but try it over vegetables, too.

| | |
|---|---|
| Phases: 1, 2, 3, 4 | ½ cup Mayonnaise (page 208) |
| Makes: 8 (generous | ¼ cup finely chopped kosher dill pickle |
|    2-tablespoon) servings | 2 tablespoons finely chopped onion |
| Active Time: 10 minutes | 1 tablespoon drained, chopped capers |
| Total Time: 10 minutes | 2 teaspoons Dijon mustard |
| | ½ teaspoon granular noncaloric sweetener |

Combine mayonnaise, pickle, onion, capers, mustard, and noncaloric sweetener in a small bowl. Serve right away, or refrigerate in an airtight container for up to 5 days.

PER SERVING: Net Carbs: 1 gram; Total Carbs: 1 gram; Fiber: 0 grams; Protein: 0 grams; Fat: 22 grams; Calories: 205

**VARIATION**
**Rémoulade**
Prepare Tartar Sauce according to directions, omitting the onion and adding 1 finely chopped hard-boiled egg, 1 tablespoon minced parsley, and 1 teaspoon minced tarragon. If possible, replace the pickle with 1 tablespoon finely chopped sour gherkin.

## Mustard-Cream Sauce
Serve this savory sauce over chicken, pork, or veal cutlets or poached salmon or chicken breasts.

Phases: 1, 2, 3, 4
Makes: 4 (generous
    2-tablespoon) servings
Active Time: 5 minutes
Total Time: 5 minutes

½ cup heavy cream
1 scallion, chopped
1½ tablespoons coarse-grain mustard
¼ teaspoon pepper
¼ teaspoon salt

Pour cream into a small skillet and bring to boil over high heat. Stir in scallion and cook, stirring frequently, until cream thickens slightly, about 4 minutes. Remove from heat and stir in mustard, pepper, and salt.

PER SERVING: Net Carbs: 1 gram; Total Carbs: 1 gram; Fiber: 0 grams; Protein: 5 grams; Fat: 11 grams; Calories: 110

## Cocktail Sauce

Unlike most commercial cocktail sauces, this easy-to-make recipe contains no added sugars. Use this tangy sauce on shrimp cocktail or raw oysters or your favorite baked or (nonbreaded) fried seafood.

Phases: 1, 2, 3, 4
Makes: 8 (generous
    2-tablespoon) servings
Active Time: 5 minutes
Total Time: 1 hour, 5 minutes

1 cup no-sugar-added ketchup

3 tablespoons prepared horseradish, drained

½ teaspoon grated lemon zest (optional)

1 tablespoon fresh lemon juice

Hot pepper sauce

Combine ketchup, horseradish, lemon zest, and lemon juice in a small bowl; stir in hot sauce to taste. Cover and refrigerate for at least 1 hour to allow flavors to blend.

PER SERVING: Net Carbs: 3 grams; Total Carbs: 5 grams; Fiber: 2 grams; Protein: 0 grams; Fat: 0 grams; Calories: 25

## Barbecue Sauce

Most commercial barbecue sauces are full of sugar or high-fructose corn syrup. Feel free to customize the sauce to your preferences or to the recipe you'll use this sauce with—more or less cayenne pepper, more or less vinegar, and other spice combinations.

Phases: 2, 3, 4
Makes: 10 (scant
    2-tablespoon) servings
Active Time: 25 minutes
Total Time: 25 minutes

1 tablespoon olive oil

1 small onion, finely chopped

2 tablespoons tomato paste

1 teaspoon chili powder

1 teaspoon ground cumin

¾ teaspoon garlic powder

¾ teaspoon powdered mustard

¼ teaspoon ground allspice

⅛ teaspoon cayenne pepper

1½ cups no-sugar-added ketchup

1 tablespoon cider vinegar

2 teaspoons Worcestershire sauce

2 teaspoons noncaloric sweetener

¼ teaspoon instant coffee granules

Heat oil in a medium saucepan over medium-high heat. Add onion and sauté until soft, about 3 minutes. Add tomato paste, chili powder, cumin, garlic powder, mustard, allspice, and cayenne pepper; cook until fragrant, about 1 minute. Stir in ketchup, vinegar, Worcestershire sauce, noncaloric sweetener, and coffee; simmer, stirring occasionally, until very thick, about 8 minutes. Serve warm or at room temperature, or refrigerate in an airtight container for up to 3 days.

PER SERVING: Net Carbs: 4 grams; Total Carbs: 7 grams; Fiber: 3 grams; Protein: 0 grams; Fat: 1.5 grams; Calories: 45

## Peanut Sauce

Peanut sauce is a standard in the cuisines of Southeast Asia, particularly Thailand and Indonesia. Use it as a dip for chicken, lamb, beef, or tofu kebabs or with any grilled meat or poultry. Also try it on raw or steamed vegetables. Be sure to use natural peanut butter without hydrogenated oils and sweeteners. If you don't have fish sauce, substitute soy sauce.

Phases: 3, 4
Makes: 8 (generous
  2-tablespoon) servings
Active Time: 10 minutes
Total Time: 10 minutes

1 tablespoon peanut oil

1 tablespoon minced fresh ginger

2 garlic cloves, minced

¼ teaspoon red pepper flakes

½ cup chunky natural peanut butter

¼ cup water

1 tablespoon unseasoned rice wine vinegar

1 tablespoon fish sauce (*nam pla*)

1 tablespoon noncaloric sweetener

¾ cup unsweetened coconut milk

1. Heat oil in a small saucepan over medium-high heat. Add ginger, garlic, and pepper flakes and sauté until ginger and garlic start to brown, about 1 minute. Add peanut butter, water, vinegar, fish sauce, and noncaloric sweetener; cook, stirring, until smooth, about 1 minute.
2. Remove from heat and stir in coconut milk. Serve right away, or refrigerate in an airtight container for up to 5 days. If sauce is too thick, stir in 1 to 2 tablespoons water.

PER SERVING: Net Carbs: 5 grams; Total Carbs: 6 grams; Fiber: 1 gram; Protein: 4 grams; Fat: 15 grams; Calories: 170

## Raita

Cooling raita is a staple in Indian and Middle Eastern cuisines. It cools hot curries, but it's also great with mild dishes and spiced grilled meats and even as a dip.

Phases: 2, 3, 4
Makes: 8 (¼-cup) servings
Active Time: 15 minutes
Total Time: 1 hour,
    15 minutes

1 medium cucumber, peeled, seeded, grated, and squeezed dry
1½ cups plain whole milk yogurt
2 tablespoons chopped fresh mint
2 tablespoons chopped fresh cilantro
½ teaspoon salt
⅛ teaspoon curry powder

Combine cucumber, yogurt, mint, cilantro, salt, and curry powder in a medium bowl. Cover and refrigerate for 1 hour to allow flavors to blend.

PER SERVING: Net Carbs: 3 grams; Total Carbs: 3 grams; Fiber: 0 grams; Protein: 2 grams; Fat: 1.5 grams; Calories: 35

### VARIATION
### Tzatziki

Prepare Raita according to directions, omitting the mint, cilantro, and curry powder and adding 2 tablespoons extra-virgin olive oil, 1 minced garlic clove, and 2 teaspoons fresh lemon juice. For a more authentic dish, use Greek yogurt, which is thicker and richer—and lower in carbs—than the standard supermarket variety.

## Romesco Sauce

This traditional Spanish sauce gets body and flavor from puréed bell peppers and almonds—a terrific low-carb combination. Use it on grilled meats, vegetables, poultry, and eggs.

Phases: 2, 3, 4
Makes: 12 (generous
    3-tablespoon) servings
Active Time: 25 minutes
Total Time: 45 minutes

3 medium red bell peppers, halved lengthwise
½ cup extra-virgin olive oil
½ cup blanched sliced almonds
2 garlic cloves, crushed
1 small tomato, seeded
2 teaspoons sherry vinegar
2 teaspoons paprika

Salt to taste

Cayenne pepper to taste

1. Place peppers, skin side up, on a broiler pan in a preheated broiler (or on a skewer over a gas burner set on high heat); cook, turning occasionally, until skin is charred, about 8 minutes. Transfer to a large bowl and cover with plastic wrap. Let steam for 20 minutes; peel and seed.
2. Meanwhile, heat oil in a medium skillet over medium heat. Add almonds and garlic and sauté until golden, about 3 minutes.
3. Combine peppers, almonds, tomato, garlic, vinegar, and paprika in a food processor or blender and purée. Season with salt and cayenne pepper to taste. Serve right away, or refrigerate in an airtight container for up to 3 days.

PER SERVING: Net Carbs: 2 grams; Total Carbs: 3 grams; Fiber: 1 gram; Protein: 1 gram; Fat: 11 grams; Calories: 120

## Alfredo Sauce

One of the simplest and best of all pasta sauces, Alfredo sauce is versatile enough to dress up steamed vegetables as well. For the best flavor, buy blocks of Parmesan and Pecorino Romano and grate them yourself.

Phases: 1, 2, 3, 4
Makes: 6 (¼-cup) servings
Active Time: 10 minutes
Total Time: 20 minutes

2 tablespoons unsalted butter

1½ cups heavy cream

½ cup grated Parmesan

¼ cup grated Pecorino Romano

⅛ teaspoon pepper

Pinch ground nutmeg

Melt butter in a medium saucepan over medium heat. Add cream and simmer until reduced to 1 cup, about 10 minutes. Remove from heat; stir in Parmesan, Pecorino Romano, pepper, and nutmeg until the cheeses have melted and sauce is smooth. Serve right away.

PER SERVING: Net Carbs: 2 grams; Total Carbs: 2 grams; Fiber: 0 grams; Protein: 4 grams; Fat: 28 grams; Calories: 280

**VARIATION**

**Vodka Sauce**

Prepare Alfredo Sauce according to directions, adding 3 tablespoons tomato paste and 2 tablespoons vodka to the heavy cream before reducing.

## Basic Tomato Sauce

This versatile sauce is great not just with meatballs or on low-carb or shirataki pasta, but also on sautéed zucchini, onions, or peppers.

Phases: 2, 3, 4

Makes: 6 (½-cup) servings

Active Time: 15 minutes

Total Time: 40 minutes

¼ cup extra-virgin olive oil

1 medium onion, finely chopped

½ medium celery rib, finely chopped

2 garlic cloves, chopped

1 teaspoon dried basil

1 (28-ounce) can crushed tomatoes

Salt and pepper to taste

1. Heat oil in a medium saucepan over medium heat. Add onion, celery, and garlic and sauté until the vegetables are very soft, about 6 minutes. Add basil and cook, stirring, 30 seconds.
2. Stir in tomatoes. Bring to a boil; reduce heat to medium-low and simmer, partially covered, until thickened, about 30 minutes. Season with salt and pepper and serve hot.

PER SERVING: Net Carbs: 9 grams; Total Carbs: 12 grams; Fiber: 3 grams; Protein: 2 grams; Fat: 10 grams; Calories: 140

## Carbonara Sauce

This rich sauce is best for long strands of shirataki (or low-carb in later phases) pasta such as spaghetti or fettuccine. It can also be served over sautéed eggplant, onions, or peppers. Time the cooking so that the pasta or vegetable base is still very hot when you pour the sauce on. This allows the eggs to continue to cook and thicken.

Phases: 1, 2, 3, 4

Makes: 6 (¼-cup) servings

Active Time: 20 minutes

Total Time: 20 minutes

6 slices bacon, cut into ¼-inch pieces

2 garlic cloves, minced

¾ cup heavy cream

½ cup grated Parmesan

⅛ teaspoon pepper
2 large eggs

1. Cook bacon in a medium skillet over medium heat until crisp, about 6 minutes. Transfer bacon to a plate lined with paper towels; set aside. Spoon off all but 2 tablespoons fat; return skillet to heat. Add garlic and sauté until fragrant, about 30 seconds. Add cream, Parmesan, and pepper; simmer until cheese has melted, about 1 minute.
2. Meanwhile, lightly beat eggs in a medium bowl; slowly whisk hot cream mixture into eggs until completely combined. Return mixture to skillet over low heat; simmer, stirring constantly, until it begins to thicken, about 3 minutes. Remove from heat; stir in reserved bacon. Serve right away.

PER SERVING: Net Carbs: 2 grams; Total Carbs: 2 grams; Fiber: 0 grams; Protein: 8 grams; Fat: 17 grams; Calories: 190

## Basil Pesto

Despite its low carb content, this recipe is not coded for Induction because it contains nuts, but it is certainly appropriate after the first two weeks. Toasting the nuts enhances the flavor. Add more garlic if you prefer. Mix pesto with mayonnaise or cream cheese for a quick dip or thick sauce to spoon over fish, chicken, beef, or steamed vegetables. It's also great atop slices of tomato and mozzarella.

Phases: 2, 3, 4
Makes: 4 (¼-cup) servings
Active Time: 10 minutes
Total Time: 10 minutes

3 cups tightly packed fresh basil leaves
⅓ cup pine nuts
⅓ cup grated Parmesan
1 garlic clove, peeled
½ teaspoon salt
⅓ cup extra-virgin olive oil

Combine basil, pine nuts, Parmesan, garlic, and salt in a food processor or blender; pulse until finely chopped. Add oil in a slow and steady stream with machine running; process until fairly smooth but not puréed. Serve right away, or refrigerate in an airtight container for up to 3 days or freeze for up to one month.

PER SERVING: Net Carbs: 1 gram; Total Carbs: 3 grams; Fiber: 2 grams; Protein: 5 grams; Fat: 29 grams; Calories: 280

**VARIATION**
**Arugula-Walnut Pesto**
Prepare Basil Pesto according to directions, substituting arugula for the basil and walnuts for the pine nuts.

## Sun-Dried Tomato Pesto

A tasty twist on the classic Basil Pesto (page 217), this sauce can be mixed with sour cream or cream cheese for a tasty dip. Found near the produce section of the supermarket, dry-packed sun-dried tomatoes are much less expensive and fresher tasting than oil-packed ones.

Phases: 2, 3, 4
Makes: 8 (3-tablespoon)
   servings
Active Time: 10 minutes
Total Time: 15 minutes

¾ cup sun-dried tomatoes (not packed in oil)
2 cups boiling water
¼ cup water
¾ cup extra-virgin olive oil
½ cup basil leaves
¼ cup pine nuts, toasted
3 tablespoons grated Pecorino Romano
1 garlic clove

1. Combine sun-dried tomatoes and boiling water in a bowl; let stand until tomatoes are pliable, about 10 minutes. Drain; squeeze out excess liquid.
2. Combine tomatoes, water, oil, basil, pine nuts, Pecorino Romano, and garlic in a blender; pulse until fairly smooth. Serve right away, or refrigerate in an airtight container for up to 2 days or freeze for up to 1 week.

PER SERVING: Net Carbs: 3 grams; Total Carbs: 4 grams; Fiber: 1 gram; Protein: 2 grams; Fat: 24 grams; Calories: 240

## Salsa Cruda

This uncooked tomato sauce is delicious over vegetables and makes a summery dish when tossed with grilled shrimp or chicken. If your tomatoes are on the acidic side, add ½ teaspoon granulated sucralose.

Phases: 1, 2, 3, 4
Makes: 10 (¼-cup) servings
Active Time: 15 minutes
Total Time: 45 minutes

4 medium tomatoes, seeded and chopped

¼ cup extra-virgin olive oil

3 tablespoons chopped fresh basil

1 tablespoon red wine vinegar

1 garlic clove, minced

½ teaspoon salt

¼ teaspoon pepper

Combine tomatoes, oil, basil, vinegar, garlic, salt, and pepper in a medium bowl. Let stand 30 minutes before serving.

PER SERVING: Net Carbs: 1.5 grams; Total Carbs: 2 grams; Fiber: 0.5 grams; Protein: 0 grams; Fat: 5.5 grams; Calories: 60

*Tip:* It's a good idea to wear gloves to prevent skin irritation when chopping jalapeños. Also, be careful not to rub your eyes after touching the peppers.

## Tomatillo Salsa (Salsa Verde)

Break out of your red salsa rut! This green salsa is tangy and slightly spicy and has a bit of crunch, too. If you haven't experimented with tomatillo, a member of the tomato family that's particularly low in carbs, this is a good first recipe to try.

Phases: 2, 3, 4
Makes: 12 (¼-cup) servings
Active Time: 15 minutes
Total Time: 15 minutes

1 pound tomatillos, husked and chopped

½ small red onion, finely chopped

¾ cup chopped fresh cilantro

2 tablespoons fresh lime juice

2 tablespoons extra-virgin olive oil
1 jalapeño, finely chopped (see note on page 219)
½ teaspoon salt
⅛ teaspoon pepper

Mix tomatillos, onion, cilantro, lime juice, oil, jalapeño, salt, and pepper in a medium bowl. Let stand 30 minutes to allow flavors to blend. Serve chilled or at room temperature. Refrigerate leftovers in an airtight container for up to 3 days.

PER SERVING: Net Carbs: 4 grams; Total Carbs: 6 grams; Fiber: 2 grams; Protein: 1 gram; Fat: 5 grams; Calories: 70

## Hollandaise Sauce

This is the classic sauce for asparagus, broccoli, and Eggs Benedict, but don't overlook it for fish and shellfish. This recipe calls for clarified butter—meaning the milk solids are removed, which makes the sauce more stable. If you prefer, simply melt the butter and add it in step 2 without straining it.

Phases: 1, 2, 3, 4
Makes: 16 (2-tablespoon)
    servings
Active Time: 15 minutes
Total Time: 25 minutes

1½ cups (3 sticks) unsalted butter
3 large egg yolks
3 tablespoons water
1 tablespoon fresh lemon juice
½ teaspoon salt
⅛ teaspoon pepper

1. Line a sieve with a damp paper towel and set over a 2-cup measuring cup. Bring butter to a boil in a small saucepan over medium heat; cook until foam on top falls to the bottom and the butter begins to clear, about 8 minutes. Pour butter through sieve; set aside.
2. Combine egg yolks and water in the top of a double boiler set over (not in) simmering water set over medium-low heat; simmer until mixture has tripled in volume, about 3 minutes. Add butter in a slow and steady stream, whisking constantly until sauce thickens. Whisk in lemon juice, salt, and pepper; serve right away.

PER SERVING: Net Carbs: 0 grams; Total Carbs: 0 grams; Fiber: 0 grams; Protein: 1 gram; Fat: 18 grams; Calories: 160

## Brown Butter Sauce

Butter cooked just until it browns has a lovely nutty flavor and aroma. This simple French classic pairs well with any white fish or scallops, eggs, and vegetables.

Phases: 1, 2, 3, 4
Makes: 4 (2-tablespoon)
    servings
Active Time: 10 minutes
Total Time: 10 minutes

½ cup (1 stick) unsalted butter
1 tablespoon lemon juice
½ teaspoon salt
⅛ teaspoon pepper

Melt butter in a small saucepan over medium heat; cook until butter begins to brown and smell nutty, about 5 minutes. Remove from heat; stir in lemon juice, salt, and pepper. Serve right away.

PER SERVING: Net Carbs: 0 grams; Total Carbs: 0 grams; Fiber: 0 grams; Protein: 0 grams; Fat: 23 grams; Calories: 200

## COMPOUND BUTTERS AND OILS

## Butter-Oil Blend

This mix is high in monounsaturated fats and includes some omega-3 fatty acids. It also has a nice mouthfeel and spreads the way soft margarine does. Serve on vegetables, fish, or meat.

Phases: 1, 2, 3, 4
Makes 32 (1-tablespoon)
    servings
Active Time: 5 minutes
Total Time: 5 minutes

1 cup (2 quarters) salted butter
½ cup light olive oil
½ cup canola oil

Blend butter and both oils in a food processor until smooth. Scrape into a container with a snap top. Keeps in the refrigerator for up to one month.

PER SERVING: Net Carbs: 0 grams; Total Carbs: 0 grams; Fiber: 0 grams; Protein: 0 grams; Fat: 16 grams; Calories: 110

## Herb-Butter Blend

This savory version of the Butter-Oil Blend is delicious on vegetables, fish, and meats.

| Phases 1, 2, 3, 4 | ½ teaspoon salt |
| Makes 32 (1-tablespoon) | 1 teaspoon finely ground black pepper |
|   servings | ½ cup light olive oil |
| Active Time: 7 minutes | 2 cloves garlic, peeled |
| Total Time: 7 minutes | 3 (3-inch) sprigs fresh oregano leaves, stemmed |
|   | 5–10 fresh basil leaves |
|   | 1 cup (2 quarters) salted butter |
|   | ½ cup canola oil |

Place salt, pepper, olive oil, garlic, oregano, and basil in a food processor. Pulse until herbs are finely ground and there are no visible specks of pepper (30–60 seconds total). Add butter and canola oil, blending until smooth. Scrape into a container with a snap top and refrigerate up to 1 month.

PER SERVING: Net Carbs: 0 grams; Total Carbs: 0 grams; Fiber: 0 grams; Protein: 0 grams; Fat: 12.5 grams; Calories: 110

## Parsley Butter

Top vegetables or grilled meats and poultry with this seasoned butter or use it to cook eggs. Substitute a minced clove of garlic and a little onion if shallots aren't available. Feel free to substitute chopped fresh cilantro for the parsley, lime juice for the lemon juice, and a pinch of cayenne pepper for the pepper.

| Phases 1, 2, 3, 4 | 6 tablespoons salted butter, at room temperature |
| Makes: 4 (2-tablespoon) | 1 small shallot (or garlic), minced |
|   servings | 2 tablespoons minced parsley |
| Active Time: 10 minutes | 2 teaspoons fresh lemon juice |
| Total Time: 2 hours, | ¼ teaspoon salt |
|   10 minutes | ⅛ teaspoon pepper |

Combine butter, shallot, parsley, lemon juice, salt, and pepper in a medium bowl; blend well to distribute ingredients thoroughly. Spoon seasoned butter onto waxed paper; roll paper around butter to form a log. Twist ends to secure butter; roll gently across counter to form an even cylinder. Refrigerate until chilled, at least 2 hours and up to 1 week. Slice into small pats and use as desired.

PER SERVING: Net Carbs: 1 gram; Total Carbs: 1 gram; Fiber: 0 grams; Protein: 0 grams; Fat: 17 grams; Calories: 150

## Herb-Flavored Oil
Use herb oils to garnish vegetables, soups, and meats or in salad dressings.

Phases 1, 2, 3, 4
Makes: 16 (1-tablespoon)
   servings
Active Time: 10 minutes
Total Time: 8 hours

1 bunch fresh leafy herbs, such as basil, parsley, or cilantro
1 cup extra-virgin olive oil or canola oil

1. Bring a large pot of salted water to a boil. Have a bowl of cold water ready. Add the herbs (stems and all) to the boiling water and leave until just softened and bright green, about 30 seconds. Drain and plunge into cold water to stop cooking. Drain again and pat dry with paper towels.
2. Combine herbs and oil in a blender. Blend until smooth. Transfer to a glass jar, cover and refrigerate 8 hours or overnight.
3. Strain oil through a fine-mesh sieve. Refrigerate oil in an airtight container for up to 1 week.

PER SERVING: Net Carbs: 0 grams; Total Carbs: 0 grams; Fiber: 0 grams; Protein: 0 grams; Fat: 14 grams; Calories: 130

## SALAD DRESSINGS
To get the most monounsaturated fats and minimize your consumption of polyunsaturates, of which we already get plenty, make salad dressings with olive oil—use the extra-virgin type—and canola oil. A few of our dressings call for another oil to lend a certain flavor. In recipes that call for rice wine vinegar, be sure to use the unseasoned kind with no added sugar. For additional salad dressings, such as Lemon Vinaigrette, Green Goddess Dressing, and Garlic Ranch Dressing, go to www.atkins.com/recipes.

## Caesar Salad Dressing

This is the classic dressing for a Caesar salad made with Romaine, but it enlivens any salad greens. For a real treat, make this dressing with homemade Mayonnaise (page 208).

| | |
|---|---|
| Phases: 1, 2, 3, 4 | ¼ cup mayonnaise |
| Makes: 4 (2-tablespoon) | 3 tablespoons grated Parmesan |
| servings | 1 tablespoon anchovy paste |
| Active Time: 5 minutes | 1 tablespoon fresh lemon juice |
| Total Time: 5 minutes | 2 garlic cloves, finely chopped |
| | 2 teaspoons extra-virgin olive oil |
| | 1 teaspoon Worcestershire sauce |
| | 1 teaspoon Dijon mustard |
| | ½ teaspoon pepper |
| | Hot pepper sauce |

Combine mayonnaise, cheese, anchovy paste, lemon juice, garlic, oil, Worcestershire sauce, mustard, pepper, and hot sauce in a small bowl. Use right away or refrigerate in an airtight container for up to 2 days.

PER SERVING: Net Carbs: 1.5 grams; Total Carbs: 1.5 grams; Fiber: 0 grams; Protein: 2 grams; Fat: 15 grams; Calories: 150

## Greek Vinaigrette

Serve this tangy lemon-garlic dressing on iceberg lettuce with some black olives, red onions, tomatoes, cucumbers, and feta cheese for a Greek salad. Add grilled shrimp to turn it into a hearty salad supper.

| | |
|---|---|
| Phases: 1, 2, 3, 4 | 6 tablespoons extra-virgin olive oil |
| Makes: 4 (2-tablespoon) | 1 garlic clove, finely minced |
| servings | ½ teaspoon dried oregano, crumbled |
| Active Time: 7 minutes | ½ teaspoon salt |
| Total Time: 7 minutes | ¼ teaspoon pepper |
| | 2 tablespoons fresh lemon juice |
| | 1 teaspoon red wine vinegar |

Whisk together oil, garlic, oregano, salt, and pepper in a small bowl; whisk in lemon juice and vinegar. Use right away or refrigerate in an airtight container for up to 2 days.

PER SERVING: Net Carbs: 1 gram; Total Carbs: 1 gram; Fiber: 0 grams; Protein: 0 grams; Fat: 20 grams; Calories: 185

## Hot Bacon Vinaigrette

Perfect for a winter meal, this hot dressing wilts the salad greens. Serve it over spinach, iceberg, tender chicory, or Romaine. Add a few hard-boiled eggs, and/or a little leftover roast chicken to make a filling lunch or a light dinner.

Phases 1, 2, 3, 4
Makes: 6 (2-tablespoon) servings
Active Time: 12 minutes
Total Time: 12 minutes

6 slices thick-cut bacon, cut into ¼-inch strips
¼ cup sherry vinegar
¼ cup extra-virgin olive oil
Salt and pepper

Brown bacon in a skillet over medium heat, stirring occasionally, until crisp, about 10 minutes. Using a slotted spoon, transfer to a paper towel–lined plate to drain; keep bacon fat in skillet. Add vinegar and oil; whisk, scraping up browned bits from bottom of pan. Season with salt and pepper to taste. Pour over greens while still hot.

PER SERVING: Net Carbs: 0 grams; Total Carbs: 0 grams; Fiber: 0 grams; Protein: 3 grams; Fat: 12.5 grams; Calories: 125

*Tip:* Instead of whisking salad dressing ingredients, you can use a blender or place them in a jar with a tight-fitting lid and shake it vigorously.

## Sherry Vinaigrette

Serve this creamy dressing over spinach, watercress, arugula, or other dark leafy greens.

Phases: 1, 2, 3, 4
Makes: 6 (2-tablespoon)
   servings
Active Time: 3 minutes
Total Time: 3 minutes

2 tablespoons sherry vinegar
1 small shallot, minced
1 teaspoon Dijon mustard
½ teaspoon salt
¼ teaspoon pepper
6 tablespoons extra-virgin olive oil

Combine vinegar, shallot, mustard, salt, and pepper in a small bowl. Add oil in a slow, steady stream, whisking until dressing thickens. Use right away or refrigerate in an airtight container for up to 2 days.

PER SERVING: Net Carbs: 0.5 grams; Total Carbs: 0.5 grams; Fiber: 0 grams;
Protein: 0 grams; Fat: 13.5 grams; Calories: 125

## Creamy Coleslaw Dressing

This makes enough dressing for one small green cabbage or two 8-ounce bags of shredded cabbage.

Phases: 1, 2, 3, 4
Makes: 12 (2-tablespoon)
   servings
Active Time: 15 minutes
Total Time: 15 minutes

¾ cup mayonnaise
¼ cup sour cream
2 tablespoons cider vinegar
1 garlic clove, chopped
1 teaspoon caraway seeds
½ teaspoon salt
¼ teaspoon pepper

Combine mayonnaise, sour cream, vinegar, garlic, caraway seeds, salt, and pepper in a small bowl. After adding dressing to cabbage, cover and refrigerate for at least 30 minutes before serving.

PER SERVING: Net Carbs: 0.5 grams; Total Carbs: 0.5 grams; Fiber: 0 grams;
Protein: 0 grams; Fat: 12 grams; Calories: 110

## Fresh Raspberry Vinaigrette

If your berries are tart, you may want to add the noncaloric sweetener, but in-season berries are likely to be fine without it.

Phases: 2, 3, 4
Makes: 8 (2-tablespoon)
    servings
Active Time: 10 minutes
Total Time: 10 minutes

½ cup fresh raspberries

2 tablespoons water

3 tablespoons red wine vinegar

1 teaspoon granular noncaloric sweetener (optional)

1 shallot, minced

¾ teaspoon salt

½ teaspoon pepper

½ cup extra-virgin olive oil

Purée raspberries and water in a blender; strain into a bowl. Stir in vinegar, noncaloric sweetener, shallot, salt, and pepper. Add oil in a slow stream, whisking until dressing thickens. Use right away or refrigerate in an airtight container for up to 2 days.

PER SERVING: Net Carbs: 1 gram; Total Carbs: 0 grams; Fiber: 1 gram; Protein: 0 grams; Fat: 14 grams; Calories: 130

## Blue Cheese Dressing

Drizzle this thick and creamy dressing over iceberg lettuce or other salad greens, or serve as a dip for fresh vegetables or Buffalo chicken wings or atop cold roast beef. If you can, make the dressing a day ahead to let the flavors develop. Homemade Mayonnaise (page 208) produces scrumptious results.

Phases 1, 2, 3, 4
Makes: 14 (2-tablespoon)
    servings
Active Time: 10 minutes
Total Time: 10 minutes

4 ounces blue cheese, crumbled (1 cup)

½ cup mayonnaise

½ cup sour cream

⅓ cup heavy cream

1 tablespoon fresh lemon juice

½ teaspoon Dijon mustard

½ teaspoon pepper

Combine cheese, mayonnaise, sour cream, heavy cream, lemon juice, mustard, and pepper in a medium bowl, mashing with a fork to break up the cheese. Use right away or refrigerate in an airtight container for up to 3 days.

PER SERVING: Net Carbs: 1 gram; Total Carbs: 1 gram; Fiber: 0 grams; Protein: 2 grams; Fat: 12 grams; Calories: 120

## Italian Dressing

This traditional favorite achieves the perfect ratio of oil to vinegar. If you don't have a garlic press, crush the cloves with the flat side of a knife and then mince them very finely.

Phases: 1, 2, 3, 4
Makes: 8 (2-tablespoon) servings
Active Time: 10 minutes
Total Time: 10 minutes

¾ cup extra-virgin olive oil
4 tablespoons red wine vinegar
2 tablespoons fresh lemon juice
2 garlic cloves, pressed
3 tablespoons minced fresh parsley
1 tablespoon minced fresh basil
2 teaspoons dried oregano
½ teaspoon red pepper flakes
¼ teaspoon salt
¼ teaspoon pepper
½ teaspoon granular noncaloric sweetener

Combine oil, vinegar, lemon juice, garlic, parsley, basil, oregano, red pepper flakes, salt, pepper, and sugar substitute in a jar with a tight-fitting lid; shake vigorously. (This can also be done in a blender.) Use right away or refrigerate in an airtight container for up to 3 days.

PER SERVING: Net Carbs: 1 gram; Total Carbs: 1 gram; Fiber: 0 grams; Protein: 0 grams; Fat: 21 grams; Calories: 200

## Roasted Garlic-Basil Dressing

Roasted garlic emulsifies this creamy dressing, keeping it from separating into oil and vinegar. Roasting tames the garlic's pungency, resulting in a paste that's actually sweet. If you have a ceramic garlic roaster, use it instead of aluminum foil.

Phases: 1, 2, 3, 4
Makes: 15 (2-tablespoon)
    servings
Active Time: 10 minutes
Total Time: 90 minutes

1 large garlic bulb
1 cup plus 1 tablespoon extra-virgin olive oil, divided
⅓ cup unseasoned, unsweetened rice wine vinegar
10 fresh basil leaves
1 ounce grated Parmesan (optional)
½ teaspoon salt
1 teaspoon pepper
2 tablespoons xylitol

1. Preheat the oven to 400°F. Trim the top ¼ inch off the garlic bulb to expose the cloves. Place on a large square of aluminum foil, drizzle the top with a tablespoon of olive oil, and close tightly to form a packet. Bake until garlic is very soft, about 45 minutes. Remove from oven and let cool at room temperature for about 25 minutes.
2. Place vinegar, basil, and grated Parmesan in food processor and pulse until very finely ground. Separate garlic into cloves. Squeeze roasted garlic out of skins into food processor and add olive oil, salt, and pepper. Process until smooth, 2 or 3 minutes. Refrigerate in a squeeze bottle or closed container for up to a week.

PER SERVING: Net Carbs: 1 gram; Total Carbs: 1 gram; Fiber: 0 grams; Protein: 0 grams; Fat: 20 grams; Calories: 180

## Ranch Dressing

An all-American favorite, this homemade version of the creamy garlic-and-herb dressing is smooth and satisfying.

| | |
|---|---|
| Phases: 1, 2, 3, 4<br>Makes: 8 (2½-tablespoon)<br>  servings<br>Active Time: 10 minutes<br>Total Time: 10 minutes | ¾ cup mayonnaise<br>½ cup heavy cream<br>2 tablespoons chopped fresh parsley<br>2 tablespoons chopped chives<br>2 teaspoons fresh lemon juice<br>2 teaspoons Dijon mustard<br>1 garlic clove, minced<br>1 teaspoon chopped fresh dill<br>½ teaspoon salt<br>¼ teaspoon pepper |

Whisk mayonnaise, cream, parsley, chives, lemon juice, mustard, garlic, dill, salt, and pepper in a small bowl. Use right away or refrigerate in an airtight container for up to 3 days.

PER SERVING: Net Carbs: 1 gram; Total Carbs: 1 gram; Fiber: 0 grams; Protein: 0 grams; Fat: 22 grams; Calories: 200

## Sweet Mustard Dressing

Use this sweet-and-sour dressing to bring out the best in any salad containing meat or cheese, or to dress up steamed green vegetables.

| | |
|---|---|
| Phases: 1, 2, 3, 4<br>Makes: 10 (2-tablespoon)<br>  servings<br>Active Time: 10 minutes<br>Total Time: 10 minutes | ⅓ cup coarse-grain mustard<br>⅓ cup cider vinegar<br>¼ cup sugar-free pancake syrup<br>½ teaspoon salt<br>¼ teaspoon pepper<br>⅔ cup canola oil |

Combine mustard, vinegar, syrup, salt, and pepper in a small bowl. Add oil in a slow, steady stream, whisking until dressing thickens. Use right away or refrigerate in an airtight container for up to 2 days.

PER SERVING: Net Carbs: 1 gram; Total Carbs: 1 gram; Fiber: 0 grams; Protein: 1 gram; Fat: 15 grams; Calories: 140

## Carrot-Ginger Dressing

This colorful dressing adds exotic flavor to iceberg lettuce, steamed green beans, or chicken, salmon, or low-carb or shirataki noodle salads.

Phases: 3, 4
Makes: 12 (3-tablespoon)
  servings
Active Time: 15 minutes
Total Time: 15 minutes

3 medium carrots, grated

3 tablespoons minced fresh ginger

¼ cup chopped white onion

¼ cup unseasoned, unsweetened rice wine vinegar

¼ cup water

1 tablespoon soy sauce

1 tablespoon dark sesame oil

1 teaspoon salt

½ teaspoon granular noncaloric sweetener

½ cup canola oil

Purée carrots, ginger, onion, vinegar, water, soy sauce, sesame oil, salt, and sugar substitute in a blender. With motor running, add oil in a slow, steady stream until dressing thickens. Use right away or refrigerate in an airtight container for up to 1 day.

PER SERVING: Net Carbs: 1 gram; Total Carbs: 2 grams; Fiber: 1 gram; Protein: 0 grams; Fat: 10 grams; Calories: 100

## Creamy Italian Dressing

This creamy dressing, bold with aged cheese, herbs, and spices, might become your favorite. If you don't have Italian seasoning on hand, use a combination of basil, oregano, and parsley instead.

Phases: 1, 2, 3, 4
Makes: 10 (2-tablespoon)
  servings
Active Time: 10 minutes
Total Time: 15 minutes

½ cup mayonnaise

⅓ cup white wine vinegar

2 tablespoons xylitol

¼ cup grated Parmesan

1 garlic clove, minced

2 teaspoons dried Italian seasoning

¼ teaspoon red pepper flakes

¼ teaspoon salt

¼ teaspoon pepper

2 tablespoons chopped fresh parsley

Whisk mayonnaise, vinegar, and xylitol in a medium bowl. Stir in Parmesan, garlic, Italian seasoning, pepper flakes, salt, pepper, and parsley until well blended. Let stand 5 minutes. Use right away or refrigerate in an airtight container for up to 3 days; stir before using.

PER SERVING: Net Carbs: 2 grams; Total Carbs: 2 grams; Fiber: 0 grams; Protein: 1 gram; Fat: 10 grams; Calories: 100

## Parmesan Peppercorn Dressing

This simple dressing is especially good with shaved fennel or strongly flavored greens and vegetables. To crack whole peppercorns, place them under a heavy-bottomed pan and press down on them, or use a mortar and pestle.

| | |
|---|---|
| Phases: 1, 2, 3, 4 | 3 tablespoons fresh lemon juice |
| Makes: 8 (2-tablespoon) | 3 tablespoons grated Parmesan |
| servings | 1 garlic clove, chopped |
| Active Time: 10 minutes | 1 teaspoon red wine vinegar |
| Total Time: 10 minutes | 1 teaspoon granular noncaloric sweetener |
| | 1 teaspoon cracked black peppercorns |
| | ½ teaspoon salt |
| | ½ cup extra-virgin olive oil |

Combine lemon juice, Parmesan, garlic, vinegar, sugar substitute, peppercorns, and salt in a small bowl. Add oil in a slow, steady stream, whisking until dressing thickens. Use right away or refrigerate in an airtight container for up to 3 days.

PER SERVING: Net Carbs: 1 gram; Total Carbs: 1 gram; Fiber: 0 grams; Protein: 1 gram; Fat: 15 grams; Calories: 140

**VARIATION**
**Lemon-Dill Vinaigrette**
Prepare Parmesan Peppercorn Dressing according to directions, replacing the Parmesan with 1 tablespoon drained capers and 1 tablespoon chopped fresh dill.

## French Dressing

Try this classic sweet-tart American salad dressing with crisp pieces of iceberg lettuce and wedges of sweet ripe tomatoes. If you don't have garlic powder, crush one garlic clove with the flat side of a chef's knife and add it to the dressing; remove and discard the garlic before serving or storing.

Phases: 1, 2, 3, 4
Makes: 10 (2-tablespoon) servings
Active Time: 10 minutes
Total Time: 10 minutes

½ cup low-carb ketchup
½ cup canola oil
¼ cup cider vinegar
1 tablespoon xylitol
½ teaspoon salt
¼ teaspoon garlic powder
Pinch cayenne pepper

Whisk ketchup, oil, vinegar, xylitol, salt, garlic powder, and cayenne pepper in a medium bowl. Use right away, or refrigerate in an airtight container for up to 3 days.

PER SERVING: Net Carbs: 1 gram; Total Carbs: 2 grams; Fiber: 1 gram; Protein: 0 grams; Fat: 11 grams; Calories: 110

## Russian Dressing

Despite its name, this is an American recipe. It's said that at one time it called for caviar as an ingredient, hence the name. You can also spoon it over cold sliced chicken or hard-boiled eggs.

Phases: 1, 2, 3, 4
Makes: 8 (2-tablespoon) servings
Active Time: 10 minutes
Total Time: 10 minutes

¾ cup mayonnaise
¼ cup low-carb ketchup
1 tablespoon finely chopped onion
1 tablespoon chopped fresh parsley
2 teaspoons prepared horseradish
1 teaspoon Worcestershire sauce

Combine mayonnaise, ketchup, onion, parsley, horseradish, and Worcestershire sauce in a bowl, mixing well. Use right away or refrigerate in an airtight container for up to 3 days.

PER SERVING: Net Carbs: 0 grams; Total Carbs: 1 gram; Fiber: 1 gram; Protein: 0 grams; Fat: 17 grams; Calories: 160

*Tip:* Heinz and other manufacturers make ketchup with no added sugar. If your grocery store doesn't carry it, ask the manager to order it or purchase it online.

## MARINADES AND RUBS

Unlike sauces and condiments, marinades and rubs work their magic before cooking. Marinades are liquids that usually contain an acidic ingredient—wine, vinegar, lemon or lime juice, or yogurt—and flavorings. Meat, chicken, fish, and even vegetables are soaked in marinades to heighten their flavors, and enzymes in the acids work to break down fibers. Tough cuts of meat may take several hours (or even days) to become tender when marinated, but delicate fish should be marinated briefly—no more than 20 or 30 minutes—or it may actually "cook" in the acid, giving your finished dish an unpleasant texture. Whether you're marinating fish, tofu, vegetables, poultry, or meat, heed the instructions given in the recipe; if no times are given, err on the side of caution—figure 15 to 20 minutes for fish and tofu, 2 hours for chicken parts or thin steaks, 6 to 8 hours for roasts.

Rubs are dry mixtures of spices and sometimes herbs. As the name suggests, they're rubbed onto cuts of meat or fish and allowed to permeate it before cooking. Ideally, you'll have the time to let the rubbed meat stand overnight, but even a half hour will add flavor.

### Latin Marinade

Garlic and lime, suggesting a Cuban mojo, flavor this marinade. It's particularly good with all cuts of pork and chicken (marinate at least 2 hours and up to 24) and fish and shellfish (marinate no longer than 20 minutes).

Phases: 1, 2, 3, 4
Makes: 8 (2-tablespoon)
   servings (enough for
   1½ to 2 pounds meat,
   fish, or vegetables)
Active Time: 5 minutes
Total Time: 5 minutes

5 garlic cloves, peeled
¼ cup fresh lemon juice
2 tablespoons fresh lime juice
2 tablespoons chopped cilantro leaves
½ small onion, chopped
1½ teaspoons grated orange zest
¾ teaspoon dried oregano

1½ teaspoons salt
¾ cup canola oil

Combine garlic, lemon juice, lime juice, cilantro, onion, orange zest, oregano, and salt in a blender; blend until smooth. Add the oil and pulse to
combine.

PER SERVING: Net Carbs: 2.5 grams; Total Carbs: 3 grams; Fiber: 0.5 gram;
Protein: 0.5 gram; Fat: 21 grams; Calories: 190

*Tip:* Many of the ingredients in marinades and rubs contain carbohydrates, but since you usually discard the marinade, you'll actually consume only negligible amounts.

## Asian Marinade

Try this simple marinade with chicken kebabs, salmon or tuna steaks, pork
chops, or beef tenderloin. Marinate chicken and meat for up to 24 hours,
fish for up to 2 hours.

Phases: 1, 2, 3, 4
Makes: 6 (2-tablespoon)
  servings (enough for 1 to
  1½ pounds meat, fish, or
  vegetables)
Active Time: 5 minutes
Total Time: 5 minutes

½ cup soy sauce
2 tablespoons unseasoned rice wine vinegar
2 tablespoons xylitol
1 tablespoon grated peeled ginger
2 garlic cloves, minced
2 teaspoons dark sesame oil
2 tablespoons canola oil

Combine soy sauce, vinegar, sugar substitute, ginger, garlic, and sesame oil
in a bowl. Slowly whisk in canola oil until combined.

PER SERVING: Net Carbs: 5 grams; Total Carbs: 5 grams; Fiber: 0 grams;
Protein: 1.5 grams; Fat: 4 grams; Calories: 60

*Tip:* Discard marinades after soaking food. Even if you've refrigerated it, the marinade may harbor potentially harmful bacteria. If you want to use the marinade as a basting sauce or to pass it at the table, it's much safer to reserve some before adding the food, or to make a fresh batch.

## Chipotle Marinade

Chipotles en adobo are available in cans in the Mexican food sections of most supermarkets. This pastelike marinade is terrific on bone-in chicken, short ribs, all pork cuts. and boneless, skinless turkey cutlets.

| | |
|---|---|
| Phases: 1, 2, 3, 4 | 6 garlic cloves, minced |
| Makes: 4 (2-tablespoon) | 4 chipotles en adobo, finely chopped |
| servings (enough for | 2 teaspoons granular noncaloric sweetener |
| about 1 pound meat, fish, | 2 tablespoons fresh lime juice |
| or vegetables) | 2 tablespoons extra-virgin olive oil |
| Active Time: 5 minutes | 2 teaspoons ground cumin |
| Total Time: 5 minutes | 1 teaspoon salt |

Combine garlic, chipotles, noncaloric sweetener, lime juice, oil, cumin, and salt in a bowl; mix well.

PER SERVING: Net Carbs: 2 grams; Total Carbs: 3 grams; Fiber: 1 gram; Protein: 1 gram; Fat: 8 grams; Calories: 80

## Mediterranean Marinade

Rosemary, garlic, and lemon are the base of this versatile marinade. It's great on just about anything you grill, broil, sauté, or roast, but particularly chicken, veal chops, eggplant slices, mild-flavored whole fish such as snapper or bass, and sea scallops. Because it's low in acid, even fish and shellfish can be marinated in it for up to 24 hours.

| |
|---|
| Phases: 1, 2, 3, 4 |
| Makes: 4 (2-tablespoon) |
| servings (enough for |
| about 1 pound meat, fish, |
| or vegetables) |
| Active Time: 5 minutes |
| Total Time: 5 minutes |

2 tablespoons Dijon mustard

2 tablespoons fresh chopped rosemary leaves

3 garlic cloves, peeled

1 teaspoon grated lemon zest

½ teaspoon ground fennel

½ teaspoon pepper

1 teaspoon salt

½ cup extra-virgin olive oil

Combine mustard, rosemary, garlic, lemon zest, fennel, pepper, and salt in a blender. With the motor running, slowly drizzle in the oil until incorporated.

PER SERVING: Net Carbs: 1 gram; Total Carbs: 2 grams; Fiber: 1 gram; Protein: 1 gram; Fat: 29 grams; Calories: 270

## Hearty Red Wine Marinade

Steaks, venison, bison or other game, thick onion slices, and summer squash are among the foods that stand up well to this full-flavored marinade. Substitute a small onion for the shallot if you wish.

| |
|---|
| Phases: 1, 2, 3, 4 |
| Makes: 8 (2-tablespoon) |
| servings (enough for 1½ |
| to 2 pounds meat, fish, or |
| vegetables) |
| Active Time: 5 minutes |
| Total Time: 5 minutes |

½ cup dry red wine

¼ cup extra-virgin olive oil

2 tablespoons red wine vinegar

1 medium shallot, chopped

1 garlic clove, minced

2 teaspoons granular noncaloric sweetener

10 juniper berries (optional)

2 teaspoons chopped fresh rosemary leaves

¼ teaspoon coarsely ground black pepper

¾ teaspoon salt

Combine wine, oil, vinegar, shallot, garlic, sugar substitute, juniper berries, rosemary, pepper, and salt in a bowl; mix well.

PER SERVING: Net Carbs: 1 gram; Total Carbs: 1 gram; Fiber: 0 grams; Protein: 0 grams; Fat: 7 grams; Calories: 80

*Tip:* A clean coffee grinder is ideal for grinding whole spices. To clean it, tear up a slice of bread and whirl it in the machine to form crumbs. The bread will absorb the coffee grounds and oils. Repeat after you've ground the spices to absorb their oils.

## BBQ Rub

Use this simple rub to spice up meats before grilling, and for roasting as well. Its flavor pairs beautifully with Barbecue Sauce (page 212). Rub this on ribs before cooking, and then baste the ribs with the sauce during the last 10 to 20 minutes of grilling or cooking.

Phases: 1, 2, 3, 4
Makes: 12 (1-tablespoon)
   servings (enough for 3½
   to 4 pounds meat or fish)
Active Time: 5 minutes
Total Time: 5 minutes

2 tablespoons ground cumin
2 tablespoons garlic powder
2 tablespoons onion powder
2 tablespoons xylitol
1½ tablespoons chili powder
1½ tablespoons pepper
1 tablespoon salt
1 teaspoon powdered mustard
1 teaspoon ground allspice

Combine cumin, garlic powder, onion powder, xylitol, chili powder, pepper, salt, mustard, and allspice in a bowl; mix well.

PER SERVING: Net Carbs: 3 grams; Total Carbs: 4 grams; Fiber: 1 gram; Protein: 1 gram; Fat: 0.5 gram; Calories: 20

*Tip:* You can store extra spice rub mixtures in an airtight container in a cool place for up to two months.

## Moroccan Rub

This exotic mix is a great flavor booster for lamb, shrimp, and chicken.

Phases: 1, 2, 3, 4
Makes: 6 (1-tablespoon)
  servings (enough for
  about 2 pounds meat or
  fish)
Active Time: 5 minutes
Total Time: 5 minutes

2 tablespoons plus 2 teaspoons ground cumin

4 teaspoons ground coriander

4 teaspoons salt

2 teaspoons pepper

2 teaspoons ground ginger

2 teaspoons dried oregano

1½ teaspoons granular noncaloric sweetener

1 teaspoon ground cinnamon

Combine cumin, coriander, salt, pepper, ginger, oregano, sugar substitute, and cinnamon in a bowl; mix well.

PER SERVING: Net Carbs: 1 gram; Total Carbs: 3 grams; Fiber: 2 grams; Protein: 1 gram; Fat: 1 gram; Calories: 25

*Tip:* After food has marinated in a dry rub, remove as much as possible, along with any juices released, before cooking to ensure browning.

## Cajun Rub

This is a classic "blackening" rub for fish steaks such as tuna or swordfish or fillets such as catfish and snapper, but it also works well for poultry or pork chops.

Phases: 1, 2, 3, 4
Makes: 8 (1-tablespoon)
  servings (enough for about
  3 pounds meat or fish)
Active Time: 5 minutes
Total Time: 5 minutes

2 tablespoons plus 2 teaspoons paprika

2 tablespoons dried oregano

1 tablespoon garlic powder

1 tablespoon salt

1 teaspoon dried thyme

1 teaspoon cayenne pepper

Combine paprika, oregano, garlic powder, salt, thyme, and cayenne pepper in a bowl; mix well.

PER SERVING: Net Carbs: 1 gram; Total Carbs: 3 grams; Fiber: 2 grams; Protein: 1 gram; Fat: 0 grams; Calories: 15

# BROTHS

Drinking two cups of broth helps eliminate or minimize side effects such as weakness that may result from the diuretic effects of following a very-low-carb (50 daily grams of Net Carbs or less) diet. Along with fluids, you can lose sodium (salt) and other minerals. These three broths will keep your electrolytes balanced. Plus, they're far more flavorful and nutritious than canned or other packaged versions.

## Chicken Broth

Each cup of this satisfying broth contains 7 grams of protein, providing about an ounce of protein—far more than any store-bought product. The broth is also rich in potassium and magnesium.

Phase 1, 2, 3, 4
Makes: 16 (1-cup) servings
Active Time: 30 minutes
Total Time: 4 hours,
    30 minutes

1 (4-pound) chicken
2 small onions
2 center celery stalks with leaves
2 garlic cloves
2 tablespoons salt
4 quarts (16 cups) water
5 parsley sprigs (optional)
5 thyme sprigs (optional)
2 bay leaves (optional)
10 black peppercorns

1. Combine chicken, onions, celery, garlic, salt, water, optional seasonings, and peppercorns in a large pot over medium heat. Bring just to a boil. Reduce heat to low and simmer, covered, for 2 hours. Stir to break up large pieces of chicken. Add enough water to return to original level and simmer 2 to 4 hours longer. Restore water level again; bring to a boil and remove from heat.
2. After stock has cooled slightly, strain, and discard all solids (including chicken).

3. Chill in the refrigerator until fat congeals. Skim off and discard. Transfer broth to small containers; refrigerate for up to 3 days or freeze for up to 3 months.

PER SERVING: Total Carbs: 1 gram; Fiber: 0 grams; Net Carbs: 1 gram; Protein: 7 grams; Fat: 0 grams; Calories: 28

*Tip:* To ensure a clear broth and optimal flavor, rinse the chicken and the neck, but discard all organs, including the kidney, which is a reddish brown clump against the backbone just inside the cavity. You can use the neck.

## VARIATION
### Beef Broth
Prepare Chicken Broth according to directions above, replacing chicken with 4 pounds chuck or blade roast.

## Vegetable Broth
Canned broths and packaged bouillon cubes can never match the flavor of a homemade stock. In addition, this broth is a good source of potassium, an important mineral during dieting. Use it in place of water or chicken broth in most soup or sauce recipes.

Phase 1, 2, 3, 4
Makes: 16 (1-cup) servings
Active Time: 20 minutes
Total Time: 1 hour, 20 minutes

4 medium leeks, white and light green parts only
2 tablespoons olive oil
2 medium carrots, coarsely chopped
2 celery ribs, coarsely chopped
4 ounces mushrooms, sliced
4 garlic cloves, crushed
4 quarts (16 cups) water
5 parsley sprigs
5 thyme sprigs
2 bay leaves
5 teaspoons table salt

 **2 teaspoons** Morton's Lite Salt (a mix of regular salt and potassium chloride)
**10** peppercorns

1. Cut leeks in half lengthwise and wash in cold water to remove any dirt. Chop coarsely.
2. Heat oil in a large saucepan over medium heat. Add leeks, carrots, celery, mushrooms, and garlic; sauté until vegetables are soft but not browned, about 10 minutes. Add water, parsley, thyme, bay leaves, salt, and pepper. Bring just to a boil. Cover and reduce heat to low and simmer 1 hour, stirring periodically.
3. Remove from heat and strain, pressing on vegetables with a spatula or wooden spoon to release liquid. Discard solids and transfer broth to small containers; refrigerate for up to 3 days or freeze for up to 3 months.

PER SERVING: Net Carbs: 2 grams; Total Carbs: 2 grams; Fiber: 0 grams; Protein: 0 grams; Fat: 2 grams; Calories: 26

# HOW TO USE THE MEAL PLANS

On the following pages, you'll find a wide array of meal plans that should allow you to move at your own pace through the four phases of Atkins. (See Index of Meal Plans on page 245.) They include a week of plans for Phase 1, Induction. Simply repeat this week, with your own variations, as long as you stay in Induction. (Remember, you can add nuts and seeds after two weeks in Induction if you decide to stay there longer.) We include six weeks at progressively higher levels for Phase 2, Ongoing Weight Loss. The five weeks of plans for Phase 3, Pre-Maintenance, are also suitable for Phase 4, Lifetime Maintenance.

Because vegetarians should start Atkins in Ongoing Weight Loss (OWL), our vegetarian plans start at 30 grams of Net Carbs in OWL. We recommend that vegans begin Atkins in OWL at 50 grams of Net Carbs. Once vegans begin to lose weight at this level they can move to higher carb intakes by following the vegetarian meal plans, but substituting plant-based foods for dairy products and eggs.

## TWO TIERS
Most of the plans have two tiers. In OWL, you move up in 5-gram increments, so the first week, you'll stay at the lower level. After a week or more at that level, you can move to the next tier. In Pre-Maintenance, you move up in 10-gram increments, so we've provided similarly incremental versions in the first two meal plans for this phase. (See below for more detail on how to read the incremental plans.)

## FOCUS ON CARBS
While you're welcome to follow these plans to the letter, they're designed to show how to gradually increase your carb intake and, following the carb ladder (see page 120), to add new foods. Feel free to substitute foods with

similar carb counts, swapping asparagus for green beans or cottage cheese for Greek yogurt, for example.

The meal plans focus on carbs; however, we have not indicated carbs from sugar substitutes, cream, drinks with acceptable sweeteners, most condiments, or acceptable desserts. If you add these foods, be sure to make adjustments to remain in the right carb range, so long as you consume at least 12 to 15 grams of Net Carbs as foundation vegetables.

## PROTEIN AND FAT

Intake varies from one person to another, so protein and fat portions aren't usually indicated, although both will make up the majority of your calorie intake. Most people eat roughly 4 to 6 ounces of protein with each meal. Eat enough fat to feel satisfied. We have, however, indicated portions for the few protein foods that also contain carbs, such as Canadian bacon and vegetarian and vegan protein sources. Likewise, we've included serving sizes and carb content for salad dressings and a few sauces. Feel free to add other fats such as butter, olive oil, and sour cream.

You'll follow the same meal plans for Pre-Maintenance and Lifetime Maintenance, but once you've achieved your goal weight, you'll need to consume more fatty foods to offset the body fat that you were burning during weight loss. Check out our recipes for delicious salad dressings and other condiments.

## JUST TO BE CLEAR

We've packed a lot of information into the plans. Here's how to read them:

- Recipes that appear in this book are in boldface. See the recipe index on page 203 for page numbers.
- Meals and snacks show the carb content of each item and a subtotal.
- When a meal or snack includes an incremental food for the higher level of Net Carbs, it appears in bold italics.
- When a meal or snack includes an incremental food the higher level of carb content in the subtotal follows the lower level and is in parentheses.
- The day's total appears at the bottom of each day. In the case of two-tiered plans, the higher level of carb intake appears in parentheses.
- Foundation vegetables are also listed in the day's tally.

Finally, a daily variance at any carb level is natural and fine as long as you don't consistently overshoot your carb tolerance level, as you'll see in the daily totals.

# INDEX OF MEAL PLANS

## Phase 1, Induction

### BREAKFAST

| Day | Food | Grams of Net Carbs |
| --- | --- | --- |
| Day 1 | 2 scrambled eggs | 1 |
| | Sausages | 0 |
| | ½ cup steamed spinach | 2 |
| | **Subtotal** | **3** |
| Day 2 | Ground beef sautéed with | 1 |
| | ¼ cup scallions and | 0 |
| | ½ cup red bell peppers, topped with | 2 |
| | ¼ cup shredded mozzarella cheese | 0.5 |
| | **Subtotal** | **3** |
| Day 3 | ¼ cup shredded mozzarella cheese melted on | 0.5 |
| | 1 medium tomato | 3.5 |
| | Low-carb shake | 3 |
| | **Subtotal** | **4.5** |
| Day 4 | 2 slices Swiss cheese | 0.5 |
| | Roast deli turkey slices wrapped around | 0 |
| | 4 asparagus spears | 2 |
| | **Subtotal** | **5** |
| Day 5 | 2 fried eggs | 1 |
| | 2 Tbsp. no-sugar-added red salsa | 0 |
| | ½ Haas avocado | 2 |
| | **Subtotal** | **2.5** |
| Day 6 | Smoked salmon wrapped around | 1 |
| | 2 Tbsp. cream cheese and | 0.5 |
| | ½ cup sliced cucumber | 2 |
| | **Subtotal** | **3.5** |
| Day 7 | Bacon strips | 0 |
| | 1 slice Swiss cheese | 1 |
| | 1 hard-boiled egg | 0.5 |
| | 3 asparagus spears | 1.5 |
| | **Subtotal** | **3** |

### SNACK

| Day | Food | Grams of Net Carbs |
| --- | --- | --- |
| Day 1 | 1 stick string cheese | 0.5 |
| | ½ Haas avocado | 2 |
| | **Subtotal** | **2.5** |
| Day 2 | 1 hard-boiled egg | 0.5 |
| | 1 celery stalk | 2 |
| | **Subtotal** | **2.5** |
| Day 3 | 6 radishes | 0.5 |
| | 2 slices Muenster cheese | 1 |
| | **Subtotal** | **1.5** |
| Day 4 | Low-carb bar | 0.5 |
| | ½ medium cucumber | 0.5 |
| | **Subtotal** | **1** |
| Day 5 | ½ cup sliced cucumber | 2 |
| | 2 slices Cheddar cheese | 1 |
| | **Subtotal** | **3** |
| Day 6 | 2 celery stalks | 1 |
| | 2 Tbsp. Blue Cheese Dressing | 1 |
| | **Subtotal** | **2** |
| Day 7 | 10 green olives stuffed with | 0 |
| | 2 Tbsp. cream cheese | 1 |
| | **Subtotal** | **1** |

### LUNCH

| Day | Food | Grams of Net Carbs |
| --- | --- | --- |
| Day 1 | Roast beef on | 0 |
| | 4 cups mixed salad greens | 1.5 |
| | ½ cup mung bean sprouts | 2 |
| | 5 black olives | 0.5 |
| | 2 Tbsp. chopped onions | 1.5 |
| | 2 Tbsp. Lemon-Dill Vinaigrette | 1 |
| | **Subtotal** | **6.5** |
| Day 2 | Grilled chicken on | 0 |
| | 4 cups mixed salad greens with | 1.5 |
| | 5 cherry tomatoes | 1.5 |
| | 2 Tbsp. chopped onion | 2 |
| | 2 Tbsp. grated Parmesan cheese | 0.5 |
| | 2 Tbsp. Caesar Dressing | 1.5 |
| | **Subtotal** | **7** |
| Day 3 | Cobb salad: | 0 |
| | 4 cups Romaine lettuce | 1.5 |
| | Grilled chicken | 2 |
| | 1 hard-boiled egg | 0.5 |
| | ¼ cup shredded Cheddar cheese | 1.5 |
| | ½ cup raw mushrooms | 0.5 |
| | 2 Tbsp. Sweet Mustard Dressing | 1 |
| | **Subtotal** | **7** |
| Day 4 | 4 cups mixed salad greens with | 1.5 |
| | canned sardines | 0 |
| | 1 oz. feta cheese | 0.5 |
| | 5 black olives | 0.5 |
| | 5 cherry tomatoes | 0.5 |
| | 2 Tbsp. Greek Vinaigrette | 1 |
| | **Subtotal** | **4.5** |
| Day 5 | 1 can tuna fish on | 0 |
| | 2 cups mixed salad greens | 1.5 |
| | ½ cup cooked broccoli | 0.5 |
| | ¼ cup scallions | 2 |
| | 4 pieces marinated artichoke hearts | 1 |
| | 2 Tbsp. Lemon-Dill Vinaigrette | 1 |
| | **Subtotal** | **6** |
| Day 6 | Grilled chicken on | 0 |
| | 4 cups mixed salad greens with | 1 |
| | ½ Haas avocado | 2 |
| | 10 black olives | 1.5 |
| | ½ cup alfalfa sprouts | 1 |
| | 2 Tbsp. Italian Dressing | 1 |
| | **Subtotal** | **6.5** |
| Day 7 | Sliced roast beef on | 0 |
| | 4 cups mixed salad greens | 1.5 |
| | ¼ cup shredded mozzarella | 0.5 |
| | 6 radishes | 0.5 |
| | ½ cup sliced cucumbers | 1 |
| | 1 Tbsp. Parmesan Peppercorn Dressing | 1 |
| | **Subtotal** | **4.5** |

## Phase 1, Induction

| | Day 1 | Grams of Net Carbs | Day 2 | Grams of Net Carbs | Day 3 | Grams of Net Carbs | Day 4 | Grams of Net Carbs | Day 5 | Grams of Net Carbs | Day 6 | Grams of Net Carbs | Day 7 | Grams of Net Carbs |
|---|---|---|---|---|---|---|---|---|---|---|---|---|---|---|
| **SNACK** | 10 green olives | 0 | ½ Haas avocado | 2 | 2 Tbsp. cream cheese on | 1 | 1 oz. Gouda cheese | 0.5 | Roast deli turkey slices and | 0 | Low-carb bar | 2 | Low-carb bar | 2 |
| | 1 slice Cheddar cheese | 0.5 | 2 slices Muenster cheese | 0.5 | 2 celery stalks | 1.5 | 5 green olives | 0 | 2 Tbsp. **Aïoli** | 0 | 1 slice Cheddar cheese | 0.5 | 1 medium tomato | 3.5 |
| | **Subtotal** | 0.5 | **Subtotal** | 2.5 | **Subtotal** | 2.5 | **Subtotal** | 0.5 | **Subtotal** | 0 | **Subtotal** | 2.5 | **Subtotal** | 5.5 |
| **DINNER** | Baked salmon steak topped with | 0 | Grilled pork chops | 0 | Grilled tuna steak | 0 | Grilled beef tenderloin | 0 | Hamburger patty topped with | 0 | Chef salad: | 0 | Grilled chicken | 0 |
| | 2 Tbsp. **Aïoli** | 0 | ½ cup mashed cauliflower with | 1 | 2 Tbsp. **Herb–Butter Blend** | 0 | ½ cup steamed zucchini | 1 | 2 Tbsp. sautéed onions and | 1.5 | 4 cups Romaine lettuce | 1.5 | 2 Tbsp. **Brown Butter Sauce** | 0 |
| | 6 steamed asparagus spears | 2.5 | ¼ cup shredded Cheddar cheese | 0.5 | ½ cup sautéed zucchini | 1 | 2 cups mixed salad greens with | 1.5 | ¼ cup sautéed mushrooms and | 1 | turkey and ham | 0 | ½ cup steamed spinach | 2 |
| | Salad of 2 cups arugula | 1 | 2 cups mixed salad greens with | 1 | 2 cups mixed salad greens | 1.5 | ¼ cup roasted red peppers | 1 | 2 slices Cheddar cheese | 3.5 | 1 small tomato | 2.5 | 2 cups mixed salad greens | 1 |
| | 5 cherry tomatoes | 2 | 6 radishes | 0.5 | ½ Haas avocado | 2 | 2 Tbsp. chopped onions | 2 | 2 cups mixed salad greens | 1.5 | 2 Tbsp. chopped onions | 1.5 | 1 cup endive | 1 |
| | ½ cup sliced cucumbers | 1 | ½ cup raw string beans | 1 | 2 Tbsp. blue cheese | 0.5 | 2 Tbsp. **Parmesan Peppercorn Dressing** | 1 | 2 Tbsp. **Sweet Mustard Dressing** | 1 | ¼ cup shredded Cheddar cheese | 0.5 | ½ Haas avocado | 2 |
| | 2 Tbsp. **Italian Dressing** | 1 | 2 Tbsp. **Italian Dressing** | 1 | 2 Tbsp. **Parmesan Peppercorn Dressing** | 1 | | | | | 2 Tbsp. **French Dressing** | 1 | 2 Tbsp. **Italian Dressing** | 1 |
| | **Subtotal** | 7.5 | **Subtotal** | 7.5 | **Subtotal** | 6 | **Subtotal** | 7 | **Subtotal** | 8.5 | **Subtotal** | 8 | **Subtotal** | 7 |
| | **Total** | 20 | **Total** | 21.5 | **Total** | 20 | **Total** | 20.5 | **Total** | 20 | **Total** | 20 | **Total** | 21 |
| | **Foundation vegetables** | 16 | **Foundation vegetables** | 16.5 | **Foundation vegetables** | 12.5 | **Foundation vegetables** | 14.5 | **Foundation vegetables** | 15 | **Foundation vegetables** | 13 | **Foundation vegetables** | 14 |

## Phase 2, Ongoing Weight Loss, at 25 and 30 Grams of Net Carbs (30-gram additions in bold italics)

| | Day 1 | Day 2 | Day 3 | Day 4 | Day 5 | Day 6 | Day 7 |
|---|---|---|---|---|---|---|---|
| **BREAKFAST** | 3 pieces Canadian bacon — 1<br>1 cup mashed cauliflower with — 2<br>1/4 cup shredded Cheddar cheese — 0.5<br>***1/4 cup blueberries*** — 4<br>**Subtotal** 3.5 (7.5) | 2-egg omelet with — 1<br>1/4 cup sautéed onion and — 1<br>1/2 cup shredded Cheddar cheese — 4.5<br>***5 large strawberries*** — 5<br>**Subtotal** 6.5 (11.5) | Sliced boiled ham — 0<br>2 slices Swiss cheese — 2<br>1/2 Haas avocado — 2<br>***1/4 cup blueberries*** — 4<br>**Subtotal** 4 (8) | Low-carb shake — 1<br>1 oz. pecans — 1.5<br>***3/4 cup raspberries*** — 5<br>**Subtotal** 2.5 (7.5) | Turkey sausage sautéed with — 0<br>1/4 cup scallions and — 1<br>1 cup shredded green cabbage — 2<br>***1/4 cup blueberries*** — 4<br>**Subtotal** 3 (7) | 2 fried eggs — 1<br>1/2 cup steamed spinach — 1<br>3 bacon strips — 1<br>***4 large strawberries*** — 4<br>**Subtotal** 3 (7) | Low-carb bar — 2<br>1 deviled egg — 0.5<br>***1/4 cup blackberries*** — 2.5<br>**Subtotal** 2.5 (5) |
| **SNACK** | 2 celery stalks — 1.5<br>1 Tbsp. natural peanut butter — 2<br>**Subtotal** 3.5 | 1 oz. almonds — 2.5<br>10 green olives — 0<br>**Subtotal** 2.5 | 1 cup sliced cucumber — 2.5<br>2 oz. walnuts — 2<br>**Subtotal** 4.5 | 1/2 Haas avocado — 2<br>2 oz. Cheddar cheese — 3<br>**Subtotal** 5 | 2 slices Provolone cheese around — 1<br>4 asparagus spears — 2<br>**Subtotal** 3 | 2 celery stalks — 1.5<br>2 Tbsp. natural peanut butter — 5<br>**Subtotal** 6.5 | 5 Brazil nuts — 2<br>5 cherry tomatoes — 2<br>**Subtotal** 4 |
| **LUNCH** | Canned sardines on — 0<br>2 cups spinach and — 0.5<br>2 cups Romaine lettuce — 1<br>1/4 cup roasted red peppers — 1.5<br>1/2 cup raw broccoli — 1<br>1/2 Haas avocado — 2<br>2 Tbsp. **Lemon-Dill Vinaigrette** — 1<br>**Subtotal** 7 | London broil (left over from Day 1) over — 0<br>4 cups mixed salad greens and — 0.5<br>1/4 cup diced celery — 0.5<br>1 small tomato — 2.5<br>1/2 Haas avocado — 1.5<br>2 Tbsp. **Ranch Dressing** — 2<br>**Subtotal** 7 | Canned salmon mixed with — 0<br>1/2 cup diced celery — 0.5<br>2 Tbsp. chopped onions and — 1.5<br>2 Tbsp. **Blender Mayonnaise** over<br>4 cups Romaine lettuce — 1.5<br>5 black olives — 0.5<br>**Subtotal** 4 | Grilled chicken (left over from Day 3) over — 0<br>1 cup watercress and — 0.5<br>3 cups leaf lettuce — 1.5<br>1 small tomato — 2.5<br>1/2 cup raw green beans — 1.5<br>2 Tbsp. **Blue Cheese Dressing** — 1<br>**Subtotal** 7 | Grilled shrimp over — 0<br>4 cups mixed salad greens — 0.5<br>5 black olives — 1.5<br>1 small tomato — 2.5<br>2 oz. goat cheese — 0.5<br>2 Tbsp. **Lemon-Dill Vinaigrette** — 2<br>**Subtotal** 7 | Hamburger — 0<br>1/2 Haas avocado — 2<br>1 slice Cheddar cheese — 0.5<br>1 small tomato — 2.5<br>1 cup loose-leaf lettuce — 0.5<br>2 Tbsp. onions — 0.5<br>**Subtotal** 6 | Grilled chicken (left over from Day 6) over — 0<br>4 cups baby spinach salad with — 1<br>1/4 cup feta cheese — 1.5<br>1 oz. walnuts — 1.5<br>1/2 Haas avocado — 2<br>5 black olives — 0.5<br>2 Tbsp. **Fresh Raspberry Vinaigrette** — 1<br>**Subtotal** 7.5 |

## Phase 2, Ongoing Weight Loss, at 25 and 30 Grams of Net Carbs (30-gram additions in bold italics)

| | Day 1 | Grams of Net Carbs | Day 2 | Grams of Net Carbs | Day 3 | Grams of Net Carbs | Day 4 | Grams of Net Carbs | Day 5 | Grams of Net Carbs | Day 6 | Grams of Net Carbs | Day 7 | Grams of Net Carbs |
|---|---|---|---|---|---|---|---|---|---|---|---|---|---|---|
| **SNACK** | 5 Brazil nuts | 2 | 1 oz. pecans | 1.5 | 1 slice Cheddar cheese | 1.5 | 1 oz. walnuts | 1.5 | 1 oz. pecans | 1.5 | Low-carb bar | 1.5 | ½ cup steamed broccoli | 1.5 |
| | 1 hard-boiled egg | 0.5 | Low-carb shake | 1 | 5 cherry tomatoes | 1 | 4 pieces marinated artichoke hearts | 2 | Low-carb shake | 2 | 1 slice Swiss cheese | 1 | 2 slices Cheddar cheese | 1 |
| | Subtotal | 2.5 | Subtotal | 2.5 | Subtotal | 2.5 | Subtotal | 3.5 | Subtotal | 3.5 | Subtotal | 2.5 | Subtotal | 2.5 |
| **DINNER** | London broil topped with | 0 | Baked cod | 0 | Grilled chicken | 0 | Lamb kebabs cooked with | 0 | Pork tenderloin | 0 | Grilled chicken with | 0 | Rainbow trout | 0 |
| | ¼ cup sautéed shiitake mushrooms | 4.5 | *2 Tbsp. **Herb-Butter Blend*** | 0 | *1 Tbsp. **Barbecue Sauce*** | 0 | 1 cup cubed eggplant and | 2 | *2 Tbsp. **Mustard-Cream Sauce*** | 2 | *¼ cup **Basil Pesto*** | 1 | *2 Tbsp. **Butter-Oil Blend*** | 0 |
| | 2 cups mixed salad greens with | 1 | 1 cup steamed broccoli | 3 | ½ cup steamed spinach | 3 | ¼ cup cubed onions and | 2 | ½ cup cooked green beans topped with | 2 | 1 cup mashed cauliflower with | 1 | 1 steamed medium artichoke | 7 |
| | 1 oz. pine nuts | 1.5 | 2 cups mixed salad greens | 1 | 2 cups arugula topped with | 1 | ½ cup cubed red bell peppers | 1 | 1 oz. slivered almonds | 3 | ¼ cup shredded Cheddar cheese | 0.5 | 2 cups mixed salad greens with | 1 |
| | 2 Tbsp. crumbled blue cheese | 0.5 | ½ cup alfalfa sprouts | 0 | 4 pieces marinated artichoke hearts | 0 | 2 cups mixed salad greens | 2 | 2 cups mixed salad greens with | 1 | 4 cups arugula | 2.5 | ½ cup sliced cucumber | 1 |
| | *2 Tbsp. **Fresh Raspberry Vinaigrette*** | 1 | *2 Tbsp. **Lemon-Dill Vinaigrette*** | 1 | ¼ cup scallions | 1 | *2 Tbsp. **Greek Vinaigrette*** | 1 | ¼ cup roasted red peppers | 0 | *2 Tbsp. **Fresh Raspberry Vinaigrette*** | 1 | *2 Tbsp. **Italian Dressing*** | 1 |
| | | | | | *2 Tbsp. **Blue Cheese Dressing*** | 1 | | | *2 Tbsp. **Lemon-Dill Vinaigrette*** | 1 | | | | |
| | Subtotal | 8.5 | Subtotal | 5 | Subtotal | 5 | Subtotal | 9 | Subtotal | 9 | Subtotal | 6 | Subtotal | 10 |
| | Total | 25 (29) | Total | 24 (29) | Total | 24.5 (28.5) | Total | 25 (30) | Total | 26.5 (30.5) | Total | 26 (30) | Total | 26 (28.5) |
| | Foundation vegetables | 15 | Foundation vegetables | 15 | Foundation vegetables | 16 | Foundation vegetables | 16 | Foundation vegetables | 17 | Foundation vegetables | 14 | Foundation vegetables | 16 |

## Phase 2, Ongoing Weight Loss, at 35 and 40 Grams of Net Carbs (40-gram additions in bold italics)

### BREAKFAST

| | Day 1 | Net Carbs | Day 2 | Net Carbs | Day 3 | Net Carbs | Day 4 | Net Carbs | Day 5 | Net Carbs | Day 6 | Net Carbs | Day 7 | Net Carbs |
|---|---|---|---|---|---|---|---|---|---|---|---|---|---|---|
| | 3 pieces Canadian bacon | 1 | 2-egg omelet with | 1 | Boiled deli ham slices | 0 | Low-carb shake | 1 | Turkey sausage sautéed with | 0 | 2 fried eggs over | 1 | ½ cup cottage cheese | 4 |
| | 1 cup mashed cauliflower with | | ¼ cup sautéed onion and | 4.5 | 2 slices Swiss cheese | 2 | 1 oz. almonds | 2.5 | ¼ cup chopped onions and | 3 | ½ cup steamed spinach | 2 | ¼ cup cantaloupe melon balls | 3.5 |
| | ¼ cup sautéed onion | 2 | ¼ cup sautéed shiitake mushrooms | 4.5 | ½ Haas avocado | 2 | ¼ cup blueberries | 4 | ½ cup red bell peppers | 3 | 3 strips bacon | 0 | ***¼ cup cantaloupe melon balls*** | 3.5 |
| | ¼ cup shredded Cheddar cheese | 0.5 | ¼ cup shredded Cheddar cheese | 0.5 | ½ cup sliced strawberries | 3.5 | ***½ cup cantaloupe melon balls*** | 7 | ¼ cup blackberries | 2.5 | ¼ cup sweet cherries | 4 | 1 oz. hazelnuts | 0.5 |
| | ***¼ cup sweet cherries*** | 4 | | | | | | | | | ***¼ cup sweet cherries*** | 4 | | |
| | **Subtotal** | 3.5 (7.5) | **Subtotal** | 10.5 | **Subtotal** | 7.5 | **Subtotal** | 7.5 (14.5) | **Subtotal** | 8.5 | **Subtotal** | 7 (11) | **Subtotal** | 8 (11.5) |

### SNACK

| | Day 1 | Net Carbs | Day 2 | Net Carbs | Day 3 | Net Carbs | Day 4 | Net Carbs | Day 5 | Net Carbs | Day 6 | Net Carbs | Day 7 | Net Carbs |
|---|---|---|---|---|---|---|---|---|---|---|---|---|---|---|
| | 2 celery stalks | 1.5 | ½ cup ricotta cheese | 4 | 1 cup sliced cucumber | 2 | ½ Haas avocado | 2 | 2 slices Provolone cheese around | 1 | 2 celery stalks | 1.5 | ½ cup raw broccoli | 1 |
| | 2 Tbsp. natural peanut butter | 5 | ¼ cup raspberries | 1.5 | 2 slices Cheddar cheese | 1 | 2 slices Cheddar cheese | 1 | 4 asparagus spears | 2 | 2 Tbsp. natural peanut butter | 5 | 2 Tbsp. **Aïoli** | 0 |
| | **Subtotal** | 6.5 | **Subtotal** | 5.5 | **Subtotal** | 3 | **Subtotal** | 3 | **Subtotal** | 3 | **Subtotal** | 6.5 | **Subtotal** | 1 |

### LUNCH

| | Day 1 | Net Carbs | Day 2 | Net Carbs | Day 3 | Net Carbs | Day 4 | Net Carbs | Day 5 | Net Carbs | Day 6 | Net Carbs | Day 7 | Net Carbs |
|---|---|---|---|---|---|---|---|---|---|---|---|---|---|---|
| | Canned sardines on | 0 | London broil (left over from Day 1) over | 0 | Canned salmon mixed with | 0 | Grilled chicken (left over from Day 3) over | 0 | Grilled shrimp over | 0 | Hamburger patty | 0 | Grilled chicken (left over from Day 6) over | 0 |
| | 2 cups baby spinach and | 0.5 | 4 cups mixed salad greens and | 0.5 | ½ cup diced celery | 0.5 | 1 cup watercress and | 0.5 | 4 cups mixed salad greens | 0 | ½ Haas avocado | 2 | 4 cups baby spinach with | 0 |
| | 2 cups Romaine lettuce | 1 | 1 cup diced celery | 1 | 2 Tbsp. chopped onions and | 1.5 | 3 cups leaf lettuce | 1.5 | 5 black olives | 1.5 | 1 slice Cheddar cheese | 1.5 | 2 oz. feta cheese | 2.5 |
| | ¼ cup roasted red peppers | 3.5 | 1 small tomato | 2.5 | 2 Tbsp. **Blender Mayonnaise** over | 0 | 1 medium tomato | 3.5 | 1 small tomato | 3.5 | 1 small tomato | 1 | 1 oz. walnuts | 1.5 |
| | 4 pieces marinated artichoke hearts | 2 | ½ cup alfalfa sprouts | 0 | 4 cups Romaine lettuce | 1 | 5 black olives | 0.5 | 2 Tbsp. **Lemon-Dill Vinaigrette** | 1 | 1 cup leaf lettuce | 0.5 | 6 radishes | 1 |
| | ½ cup raw broccoli | 1 | 2 Tbsp. **Greek Vinaigrette** | 1 | 5 black olives | 1.5 | 2 Tbsp. **Blue Cheese Dressing** | 0 | ***5 large strawberries*** | 5 | 2 Tbsp. onions | 0.5 | 5 black olives | 1.5 |
| | 2 Tbsp. **Lemon-Dill Vinaigrette** | 1 | | | ***4 oz. tomato juice*** | 4 | | | | | 2 Tbsp. **Aïoli** | 0 | 2 Tbsp. **Fresh Raspberry Vinaigrette** | 1 |
| | **Subtotal** | 9 | **Subtotal** | 5 | **Subtotal** | 4.5 (8.5) | **Subtotal** | 6 | **Subtotal** | 6 (11) | **Subtotal** | 5.5 | **Subtotal** | 7.5 |

## Phase 2, Ongoing Weight Loss, at 35 and 40 Grams of Net Carbs (40-gram additions in bold italics)

### SNACK

| | Day 1 | Day 2 | Day 3 | Day 4 | Day 5 | Day 6 | Day 7 |
|---|---|---|---|---|---|---|---|
| | 4 oz. low-carb yogurt (3) | 2 oz. pistachios (5) | 2 oz. pecans (3) | 1 oz. almonds (2.5) | 2 oz. pine nuts (3.5) | Low-carb bar (3.5) | 4 oz. tomato juice (4) |
| | ¼ cup blueberries (4) | ½ cup jicama sticks (2.5) | ½ cup cottage cheese (3) | 4 oz. low-carb yogurt (3) | ½ cup cottage cheese (3) | ½ cup ricotta cheese (3) | 4 oz. plain whole milk Greek yogurt (3.5) |
| **Subtotal** | 7 | 7.5 | 6 | 5.5 | 6.5 | 6 | 7.5 |

### DINNER

| | Day 1 | Day 2 | Day 3 | Day 4 | Day 5 | Day 6 | Day 7 |
|---|---|---|---|---|---|---|---|
| | London broil topped with (0) | Baked cod (0) | Grilled chicken with (0) | Lamb kebabs broiled with (0) | Pork tenderloin (0) | Grilled chicken with (0) | Rainbow trout (0) |
| | ¼ cup **Mushroom Gravy** (2) | 2 Tbsp. **Herb-Butter Blend** (0) | 2 Tbsp. **Barbecue Sauce** (4) | 1 cup cubed eggplant and (4) | 2 Tbsp. **Mustard-Cream Sauce** (0) | ¼ cup **Basil Pesto** (1) | 2 Tbsp. **Butter-Oil Blend** (1) |
| | ½ steamed medium artichoke (3.5) | 1 cup steamed broccoli (2) | ½ cup steamed Brussels sprouts (3.5) | ¼ cup cubed onions and (3.5) | ½ cup cooked green beans (2) | 1 cup mashed cauliflower with (1) | 1 steamed medium artichoke (2) |
| | 2 cups mixed salad greens with (1) | 2 cups mixed salad greens (3.5) | Salad of 2 cups arugula and (1) | 1 cup cubed red bell peppers (1) | 2 cups mixed salad greens with (3) | ¼ cup shredded Cheddar cheese (2) | 2 cups mixed salad greens with (0.5) |
| | 2 Tbsp. crumbled blue cheese (0.5) | ½ cup sliced cucumber (1) | 4 pieces marinated artichoke hearts and (1) | 2 cups mixed salad greens (2) | ¼ cup roasted red peppers and (6) | 4 cups arugula (0.5) | ½ cup sliced cucumber (1.5) |
| | ¼ cup scallions (1) | 2 Tbsp. **Lemon-Dill Vinaigrette** (1) | 1 small tomato (2.5) | 5 black olives (2.5) | ½ cup sliced cucumber (1) | 1 small tomato (1.5) | ½ Haas avocado (2.5) |
| | 2 Tbsp. **Fresh Raspberry Vinaigrette** (1) | ***¼ cup sweet cherries*** (4) | 2 Tbsp. **Ranch Dressing** (4) | 2 Tbsp. **Greek Vinaigrette** (1) | 2 Tbsp. **Lemon-Dill Vinaigrette** (0.5) | 2 Tbsp. **Fresh Raspberry Vinaigrette** (2.5) | 2 Tbsp. **Italian Dressing** (1) |
| **Subtotal** | 9 | 6.5 (10.5) | 14 | 14 | 12.5 | 8.5 | 8.5 |

| | Day 1 | Day 2 | Day 3 | Day 4 | Day 5 | Day 6 | Day 7 |
|---|---|---|---|---|---|---|---|
| **Total** | 35 (39) | 35 (39) | 35 (39) | 34.5 (41.5) | 34 (39) | 35.5 (39.5) | 35.5 (39) |
| **Foundation vegetables** | 17 | 22 | 17.5 | 20 | 21 | 16.5 | 14 |

## Phase 2, Ongoing Weight Loss, at 45 and 50 Grams of Net Carbs (50-gram additions in bold italics)

### BREAKFAST

| Day | Food | Grams of Net Carbs |
| --- | --- | --- |
| Day 1 | 3 pieces Canadian bacon | 1 |
| | 1 cup mashed cauliflower with | 2 |
| | ¼ cup shredded Cheddar cheese | 0.5 |
| | ¼ cup honeydew melon balls | 7 |
| | **Subtotal** | **10.5** |
| Day 2 | 2-egg omelet with | 1 |
| | ¼ cup sautéed onion and | 4.5 |
| | ¼ cup sautéed shiitake mushrooms | 4.5 |
| | ¼ cup fresh raspberries | 1.5 |
| | **Subtotal** | **10.5** |
| Day 3 | Sliced boiled ham | 0 |
| | 2 slices Swiss cheese and | 2 |
| | ½ Haas avocado | 2 |
| | *4 oz. tomato juice* | 4 |
| | **Subtotal** | **4 (8)** |
| Day 4 | ½ cup creamed cottage cheese | 3 |
| | 1 oz. almonds | 2.5 |
| | ½ cup blueberries | 8 |
| | **Subtotal** | **7.5 (14.5)** |
| Day 5 | Turkey sausage sautéed with | 0 |
| | ¼ cup chopped onion | 3 |
| | 1 cup shredded green cabbage | 2 |
| | ¼ cup shredded Cheddar cheese | 0.5 |
| | **Subtotal** | **5.5** |
| Day 6 | 2 fried eggs | 1 |
| | ½ cup steamed beet greens | 0 |
| | 3 bacon strips | 3.5 |
| | 4 oz. tomato juice | 4 |
| | **Subtotal** | **8.5** |
| Day 7 | **2 Atkins Waffles*** | 6 |
| | ½ cup cottage cheese | 4 |
| | ½ cup cantaloupe melon balls | 7.5 |
| | **Subtotal** | **17.5** |

### SNACK

| Day | Food | Grams of Net Carbs |
| --- | --- | --- |
| Day 1 | 2 celery stalks | 1.5 |
| | 2 Tbsp. natural peanut butter | 5 |
| | **Subtotal** | **6.5** |
| Day 2 | 2 oz. almonds | 1.5 |
| | ½ cup ricotta cheese | 5 |
| | **Subtotal** | **6.5** |
| Day 3 | 1 cup sliced cucumbers | 2 |
| | 2 Tbsp. hummus | 4.5 |
| | **Subtotal** | **6.5** |
| Day 4 | ½ Haas avocado | 2 |
| | 2 slices Cheddar cheese | 1 |
| | **Subtotal** | **3** |
| Day 5 | 2 slices Provolone cheese | 2 |
| | ½ cup honeydew melon | 1 |
| | **Subtotal** | **3** |
| Day 6 | 1 celery stalk | 1 |
| | 2 Tbsp. natural peanut butter | 7 |
| | **Subtotal** | **8** |
| Day 7 | 2 Tbsp. hummus | 4.5 |
| | ½ cup jicama sticks | 2.5 |
| | **Subtotal** | **7** |

### LUNCH

| Day | Food | Grams of Net Carbs |
| --- | --- | --- |
| Day 1 | Canned sardines on | 0 |
| | 2 cups baby spinach and | 0.5 |
| | 2 cups Romaine lettuce | 1 |
| | ¼ cup roasted red peppers | 3.5 |
| | ¼ cup cooked kidney beans | 6.5 |
| | 2 Tbsp. **Lemon-Dill Vinaigrette** | 1 |
| | **Subtotal** | **12.5** |
| Day 2 | London broil (left over from Day 1) over | 0 |
| | 4 cups mixed salad greens and | 0.5 |
| | 1 cup diced celery | 1 |
| | 1 small tomato | 3.5 |
| | ¼ cup cooked chickpeas | 6.5 |
| | 2 Tbsp. **Ranch Dressing** | 1 |
| | *1 low-carb pita* | 3.5 |
| | **Subtotal** | **12.5 (16)** |
| Day 3 | Can of salmon mixed with | 0 |
| | ½ cup diced celery | 0.5 |
| | 2 Tbsp. chopped onions and | 1.5 |
| | 2 Tbsp. **Blender Mayonnaise** | 2.5 |
| | 4 cups Romaine lettuce | 6 |
| | 1 medium tomato | 3.5 |
| | 2 Tbsp. **Blue Cheese Dressing** | 1 |
| | **Subtotal** | **8** |
| Day 4 | Grilled chicken (left over from Day 3) over | 0 |
| | 1 cup watercress and | 0 |
| | 3 cups loose-leaf lettuce | 1.5 |
| | 1 medium tomato | 3.5 |
| | ¼ cup cooked black-eyed peas | 6 |
| | 2 Tbsp. **Lemon-Dill Vinaigrette** | 1 |
| | **Subtotal** | **11** |
| Day 5 | Lamb kebabs (left over from Day 4) over | 0 |
| | 4 cups mixed salad greens | 0 |
| | 5 black olives | 1.5 |
| | 1 small tomato | 2.5 |
| | ¼ cup baby lima beans | 6 |
| | 2 Tbsp. **Lemon-Dill Vinaigrette** | 1 |
| | **Subtotal** | **12.5 (17.5)** |
| Day 6 | Hamburger(s) | 0 |
| | ½ Haas avocado | 2 |
| | 1 slice Cheddar cheese | 0.5 |
| | 1 small tomato | 2.5 |
| | 1 cup loose-leaf lettuce | 1 |
| | 2 Tbsp. chopped onions | 1.5 |
| | *low-carb hamburger bun* | 5 |
| | **Subtotal** | **7.5 (11.5)** |
| Day 7 | Grilled chicken (left over from Day 6) over | 0 |
| | Salad of 4 cups baby spinach with | 1 |
| | ¼ cup feta cheese | 1 |
| | 4 pieces marinated artichoke hearts | 2 |
| | 1 small tomato | 2.5 |
| | 2 Tbsp. **Greek Vinaigrette** | 1 |
| | *1 low-carb pita* | 4 |
| | **Subtotal** | **6.5 (10.5)** |

## Phase 2, Ongoing Weight Loss, at 45 and 50 Grams of Net Carbs (50-gram additions in bold italics)

| | Day 1 | Grams of Net Carbs | Day 2 | Grams of Net Carbs | Day 3 | Grams of Net Carbs | Day 4 | Grams of Net Carbs | Day 5 | Grams of Net Carbs | Day 6 | Grams of Net Carbs | Day 7 | Grams of Net Carbs |
|---|---|---|---|---|---|---|---|---|---|---|---|---|---|---|
| **SNACK** | 5 cherry tomatoes | 2 | 2 slices Cheddar cheese | 1 | 2 oz. roasted pumpkin seeds | 4 | 1 oz. walnuts | 1.5 | ½ cup sliced strawberries | 3.5 | 4 oz. plain whole milk yogurt | 5.5 | Low-carb bar | 2 |
| | 4 oz. low-carb yogurt | 3 | ½ cup jicama sticks | 2.5 | ½ cup blueberries | 8.5 | 5 large strawberries | 5 | ½ cup creamed cottage cheese | 3 | ¼ cup blueberries | 4 | 2 oz. walnuts | 3 |
| | Subtotal | 5 | Subtotal | 3.5 | Subtotal | 12.5 | Subtotal | 6.5 | Subtotal | 6.5 | Subtotal | 9.5 | Subtotal | 5 |
| **DINNER** | London broil topped with | 0 | Baked cod topped with | 0 | Grilled chicken | 0 | Lamb kebabs cooked with | 0 | Pork tenderloin with | 0 | Grilled chicken with | 0 | Rainbow trout | 0 |
| | ¼ cup **Mushroom Gravy** | | 2 Tbsp. **Herb-Butter Blend** | | 2 Tbsp. **Barbecue Sauce** | | 1 cup cubed eggplant and | 4 | 2 Tbsp. **Mustard-Cream Sauce** | 0 | ¼ cup **Basil Pesto** | 1 | 2 Tbsp. **Butter-Oil Blend** | 0 |
| | 1 cup steamed green beans | 2 | 1 cup steamed broccoli | 3.5 | 1 cup steamed Brussels sprouts | 3.5 | ¼ cup cubed onion and | 7 | 1 cup cooked green beans topped with | 2 | 1 cup mashed cauliflower with | 2 | 1 steamed medium artichoke | 7 |
| | 2 cups mixed salad greens with | 6 | 2 cups mixed salad greens | 6 | Salad of 2 cups arugula topped with | 1 | ½ cup cubed red bell peppers | 1 | 1 oz. slivered almonds | 3 | ¼ cup shredded Cheddar cheese | 0.5 | 2 cups mixed salad greens with | 1 |
| | ½ cup mung bean sprouts | 1 | ½ cup mung bean sprouts | 1 | 4 pieces marinated artichoke hearts | 2 | 2 cups mixed salad greens | 2 | 2 cups mixed salad greens with | 3 | 4 cups arugula | 1.5 | 5 black olives | 0.5 |
| | 2 Tbsp. crumbled blue cheese | 0.5 | 4 pieces marinated artichoke hearts | 0.5 | ¼ cup scallions | 2 | *¼ cup cooked lentils* | 1 | ¼ cup roasted red peppers and | 6 | 1 small tomato | 2.5 | ½ cup sliced cucumber | 1 |
| | *1 low-carb roll* | 4 | 2 Tbsp. **Lemon-Dill Vinaigrette** | 1 | 2 Tbsp. **Lemon-Dill Vinaigrette** | 1 | 2 Tbsp. **Greek Vinaigrette** | 1 | 2 Tbsp. **Greek Vinaigrette** | 0 | ¼ cup cooked lentils | 6 | 2 Tbsp. **Fresh Raspberry Vinaigrette** | 1 |
| | 1 Tbsp. **Fresh Raspberry Vinaigrette** | 0.5 | | | | | | | | | 2 Tbsp. **Italian Dressing** | 1 | | |
| | Subtotal | 10 (14) | Subtotal | 9.5 | Subtotal | 9.5 | Subtotal | 16 | Subtotal | 10.5 (16.5) | Subtotal | 14.5 | Subtotal | 10.5 |
| | Total | 44.5 (48.5) | Total | 45.5 (49.5) | Total | 47 (51) | Total | 32 (39) | Total | 46.5 (51.5) | Total | 46 (50) | Total | 46.5 (50.5) |
| | Foundation vegetables | 17.5 | Foundation vegetables | 25 | Foundation vegetables | 22 | Foundation vegetables | 20 | Foundation vegetables | 20 | Foundation vegetables | 17.5 | Foundation vegetables | 17.5 |

*www.atkins.com/Recipes/ShowRecipe884/Atkins-Cuisine-Waffles.aspx.

## Phase 3, Pre-Maintenance, and Phase 4, Lifetime Maintenance, at 55 and 65 Grams of Net Carbs (65-gram additions in bold italics)

| | Day 1 | Grams of Net Carbs | Day 2 | Grams of Net Carbs | Day 3 | Grams of Net Carbs | Day 4 | Grams of Net Carbs | Day 5 | Grams of Net Carbs | Day 6 | Grams of Net Carbs | Day 7 | Grams of Net Carbs |
|---|---|---|---|---|---|---|---|---|---|---|---|---|---|---|
| **BREAKFAST** | 2-egg omelet | 1 | **1 Atkins Waffle\*** | 6 | Smoothie: ½ cup plain unsweetened almond milk | 0.5 | 4 oz. plain whole milk yogurt | 5.5 | 4 oz. plain whole milk Greek yogurt | 3.5 | 2 scrambled eggs | 1 | **2 Atkins Pancakes\*\*** | 6 |
| | ¼ cup sautéed shiitake mushrooms | 4.5 | ¼ cup ricotta cheese | 2 | 4 oz. plain whole milk yogurt | 5.5 | Low-carb bar | 2 | ¼ cup blueberries | 4 | ¼ cup sautéed onions | 4.5 | 4 oz. ricotta cheese | 4 |
| | ½ cup shredded Cheddar cheese | 1 | ½ cup blueberries | 8 | ½ cup raspberries | 3 | ½ cup mango | 12.5 | 2 oz. almonds | 4.5 | ½ cup shredded Cheddar cheese | 1 | ½ cup blueberries | 4 |
| | | | 1 oz. slivered almonds | 2.5 | 1 oz. almonds | 2.5 | | | | | 4 oz. tomato juice | 4 | | |
| | **Subtotal** | 6.5 | **Subtotal** | 18.5 | **Subtotal** | 11.5 | **Subtotal** | 20 | **Subtotal** | 12 | **Subtotal** | 10.5 | **Subtotal** | 14 |
| **SNACK** | 2 oz. pine nuts | 3.5 | 2 slices Swiss cheese around | 2 | 2 slices Swiss cheese | 2 | 2 slices Swiss cheese around | 2 | ½ Haas avocado | 2 | Low-carb bar | 2 | ½ Haas avocado | 2 |
| | ½ cup blackberries | 5.5 | 4 asparagus spears | 2 | ½ cup edamame | 2 | 4 spears asparagus | 6 | ½ cup mango | 12.5 | ½ cup blackberries | 5.5 | *1 medium carrot stick* | 5.5 |
| | | | 1 tsp. Dijon mustard | 0.5 | | | | | | | | | | |
| | **Subtotal** | 9 | **Subtotal** | 4.5 | **Subtotal** | 4 | **Subtotal** | 8 | **Subtotal** | 14.5 | **Subtotal** | 7.5 | **Subtotal** | 2 (7.5) |
| **LUNCH** | Grilled chicken with | 0 | Lamb kebabs (left over from Day 1) | 0 | Sliced turkey (left over from Day 2) on | 0 | 2 deviled eggs made with | 0 | Shrimp (left over from Day 4) topped with | 0 | Grilled chicken over | 0 | Ham (left over from Day 5) and | 0 |
| | **2 Tbsp. Peanut Sauce** | 5 | 2 Tbsp. hummus | 4.5 | 4 cups mixed salad greens and | 1.5 | **2 Tbsp. Blender Mayonnaise** | 0 | **2 Tbsp. Blender Mayonnaise** and | 0 | 4 cups mixed salad greens | 1.5 | 2 slices Swiss cheese on | 1.5 |
| | 4 cups mixed salad greens | 1.5 | 2 cups mixed salad greens | 1.5 | ¼ cup roasted red peppers | 3.5 | 1 low-carb pita with | 4 | 1 dill pickle, chopped | 2 | ½ cup pickled okra | 1.5 | Low-carb bagel with | 5.5 |
| | ½ cup green bell peppers | 2 | 1 medium tomato | 3.5 | ½ Haas avocado | 2 | 2 Tbsp. hummus | 4.5 | 1 low-carb bagel | 5 | ¼ cup roasted red peppers | 2 | 1 tsp. Dijon mustard | 0.5 |
| | ½ cup chopped jicama | 2.5 | ½ Haas avocado | 2 | 1 small tomato | 2.5 | 2 cups mixed salad greens | 2 | 4 cups Romaine lettuce | 2 | ½ cup snow peas | 5 | ½ cup loose-leaf lettuce | 0.5 |
| | 1 small tomato | 2.5 | **2 Tbsp. Greek Vinaigrette** | 1 | **2 Tbsp. Italian Dressing** | 1 | 1 small tomato | 2.5 | ¼ cup cooked lentils | 6 | **2 Tbsp. Parmesan Peppercorn Dressing** | 2 | 1 small tomato | 2.5 |
| | **2 Tbsp. Creamy Italian Dressing** | 2 | | | | | **2 Tbsp. Parmesan Peppercorn Dressing** | 1 | **2 Tbsp. Italian Dressing** | 1 | | | 2 Tbsp. hummus | 4.5 |
| | **Subtotal** | 15.5 | **Subtotal** | 12.5 | **Subtotal** | 10.5 | **Subtotal** | 14 | **Subtotal** | 16 | **Subtotal** | 12 | **Subtotal** | 15 |

## Phase 3, Pre-Maintenance, and Phase 4, Lifetime Maintenance, at 55 and 65 Grams of Net Carbs (65-gram additions in bold italics)

| | Day 1 | Grams of Net Carbs | Day 2 | Grams of Net Carbs | Day 3 | Grams of Net Carbs | Day 4 | Grams of Net Carbs | Day 5 | Grams of Net Carbs | Day 6 | Grams of Net Carbs | Day 7 | Grams of Net Carbs |
|---|---|---|---|---|---|---|---|---|---|---|---|---|---|---|
| **SNACK** | ½ cup plain whole milk yogurt<br>½ medium apple<br>**Subtotal** | 5.5<br>8.5<br>**14** | 1 oz. almonds<br>½ white grapefruit<br>**Subtotal** | 2.5<br>8.5<br>**11** | 1 oz. almonds<br>½ cup pineapple<br>**Subtotal** | 2.5<br>8.5<br>**11** | ¼ cup sweet cherries<br>2 oz. almonds<br>**Subtotal** | 4<br>4.5<br>**8.5** | 4 oz. tomato juice<br>2 oz. goat cheese<br>**Subtotal** | 4<br>0.5<br>**4.5** | ½ cup pineapple<br>1 oz. macadamias<br>**Subtotal** | 8.5<br>2<br>**10.5** | 2 oz. almonds<br>½ medium apple<br>**Subtotal** | 4.5<br>8.5<br>**13** |
| **DINNER** | Lamb kebabs<br>½ ***baked sweet potato***<br>2 cups mixed salad greens<br>¼ cup cooked chickpeas<br>5 black olives<br>1 oz. blue cheese<br>2 Tbsp. **Greek Vinaigrette**<br>**Subtotal** | 0<br>12<br>1<br>6.5<br>0.5<br>0.5<br>1<br>**9.5 (21.5)** | Roast turkey<br>½ cup **Velouté Sauce**<br>½ ***baked potato***<br>1 cup grilled eggplant<br>2 cups mixed salad greens<br>6 radishes<br>2 Tbsp. **Greek Vinaigrette**<br>**Subtotal** | 0<br>1<br>12.5<br>4<br>1<br>0.5<br>1<br>**7.5 (20)** | Fajitas: broiled sliced skirt steak with<br>¼ cup sautéed onions and<br>1 cup sautéed green bell peppers<br>¼ cup **Salsa Cruda**<br>½ ***ear corn on the cob***<br>2 cups mixed salad greens<br>2 Tbsp. **Parmesan Peppercorn Dressing**<br>**Subtotal** | 0<br>2.5<br>8<br>1.5<br>8.5<br>1<br>1<br>**14 (22.5)** | Sautéed shrimp on<br>½ cup steamed leeks<br>¼ cup **Alfredo Sauce**<br>2 cups baby spinach salad<br>1 small tomato<br>½ ***cup pickled beets***<br>2 Tbsp. **Creamy Italian Dressing**<br>**Subtotal** | 0<br>3.5<br>2<br>0.5<br>2.5<br>7<br>2<br>**10.5 (17.5)** | Baked ham<br>¼ cup **Mushroom Gravy**<br>½ ***cup mashed butternut squash***<br>Salad of 1 cup chopped raw fennel and<br>½ cup chopped jicama<br>2 Tbsp. **Blue Cheese Dressing**<br>**Subtotal** | 0<br>2<br>7<br>3.5<br>2.5<br>1<br>**9 (16)** | Flank steak<br>¼ cup cooked baby lima beans<br>½ ***cup corn kernels***<br>2 cups mixed salad greens<br>½ cup chopped cucumber<br>1 small tomato<br>2 Tbsp. **Creamy Italian Dressing**<br>**Subtotal** | 0<br>7<br>12.5<br>1<br>1<br>2.5<br>2<br>**13.5 (26)** | Salmon steak over<br>1 cup roasted fennel and<br>¼ cup roasted onions<br>¼ cup **Raita**<br>Salad of 2 cups arugula<br>4 pieces marinated artichoke hearts<br>2 Tbsp. **Fresh Raspberry Vinaigrette**<br>**Subtotal** | 0<br>3<br>4.5<br>3<br>0.5<br>2<br>1<br>**14** |
| | **Total<br>Foundation vegetables** | **54.5 (66.5)**<br>14.5 | **Total<br>Foundation vegetables** | **54 (66.5)**<br>14.5 | **Total<br>Foundation vegetables** | **55 (63.5)**<br>24.5 | **Total<br>Foundation vegetables** | **57 (64)**<br>12 | **Total<br>Foundation vegetables** | **56 (63)**<br>12 | **Total<br>Foundation vegetables** | **54 (66.5)**<br>20 | **Total<br>Foundation vegetables** | **58 (63.5)**<br>15 |

*www.atkins.com/Recipes/ShowRecipe884/Atkins-Cuisine-Waffles.aspx, **www.atkins.com/Recipes/ShowRecipe883/Atkins-Cuisine-Pancakes.aspx, ***www.atkins.com/Recipes/Atkins-Cuisine-Pancakes.aspx.

## Phases 3, Pre-Maintenance, and 4, Lifetime Maintenance, at 75 and 85 Grams of Net Carbs (85-gram additions in bold italics)

### BREAKFAST

| Day | Food | Grams of Net Carbs |
| --- | --- | --- |
| **Day 1** | 2-egg omelet | 1 |
|  | 1/4 cup sautéed shiitake mushrooms | 4.5 |
|  | 1/2 cup shredded Cheddar cheese | 1 |
|  | 4 oz. tomato juice | 4 |
|  | **Subtotal** | **10.5** |
| **Day 2** | 1 Atkins Waffle* | 6 |
|  | 1/2 cup ricotta cheese | 4 |
|  | 1/2 cup pineapple | 8.5 |
|  | 1 oz. slivered almonds | 2.5 |
|  | **Subtotal** | **21** |
| **Day 3** | Smoothie: 1/2 cup plain unsweetened almond milk with | 0.5 |
|  | 4 oz. plain whole milk yogurt and | 5.5 |
|  | 1/2 cup pineapple and | 8.5 |
|  | 1 oz. almonds | 2.5 |
|  | **Subtotal** | **17** |
| **Day 4** | 2 deviled eggs made with | 1 |
|  | 1 Tbsp. **Blender Mayonnaise** | 0 |
|  | 1 low-carb pita with | 4 |
|  | 3 Tbsp. **Sun-Dried Tomato Pesto** | 3 |
|  | **Subtotal** | **8** |
| **Day 5** | 4 oz. plain whole milk yogurt | 5.5 |
|  | 1 medium orange | 13 |
|  | 1 oz. cashews | 4.5 |
|  | **Subtotal** | **23** |
| **Day 6** | 2 scrambled eggs | 1 |
|  | 1/4 cup refried beans | 6.5 |
|  | 1/2 cup shredded Cheddar cheese | 1 |
|  | 4 oz. tomato juice | 4 |
|  | **Subtotal** | **12.5** |
| **Day 7** | 2 Atkins Pancakes** | 6 |
|  | 4 oz. ricotta | 4 |
|  | 1/2 cup honeydew melon balls | 7 |
|  | **Subtotal** | **17** |

### SNACK

| Day | Food | Grams of Net Carbs |
| --- | --- | --- |
| **Day 1** | 2 oz. almonds | 5 |
|  | 1/2 cup cantaloupe melon balls | 7.5 |
|  | **Subtotal** | **12.5** |
| **Day 2** | 2 slices Swiss cheese | 2 |
|  | 1 medium carrot | 5.5 |
|  | **Subtotal** | **7.5** |
| **Day 3** | 1 oz. macadamias | 2 |
|  | 4 oz. tomato juice | 4 |
|  | **Subtotal** | **6** |
| **Day 4** | 1/2 medium apple | 2 |
|  | 2 oz. pecans | 4 |
|  | **Subtotal** | **6** |
| **Day 5** | 1/2 Haas avocado | 8.5 |
|  | 4 oz. tomato juice | 3 |
|  | **Subtotal** | **11.5** |
| **Day 6** | Low-carb bar | 2 |
|  | 1/2 cup blackberries | 4 |
|  | **Subtotal** | **6** |
| **Day 7** | 1/2 Haas avocado | 2 |
|  | 1 small tomato | 2.5 |
|  | **Subtotal** | **4.5** |

### LUNCH

| Day | Food | Grams of Net Carbs |
| --- | --- | --- |
| **Day 1** | Grilled chicken with | 0 |
|  | 2 Tbsp. **Peanut Sauce** | 5 |
|  | 2 cups mixed salad greens | 1 |
|  | 1/2 cup green bell peppers | 2 |
|  | 1/2 cup chopped jicama | 2.5 |
|  | 2 medium carrots, grated | 11 |
|  | ***1/2 cup corn kernels*** | 12.5 |
|  | 2 Tbsp. **Italian Dressing** | 1 |
|  | **Subtotal** | **22.5 (35)** |
| **Day 2** | Lamb kebabs (left over from Day 1) | 0 |
|  | 2 cups salad greens | 1.5 |
|  | 1/4 cup cooked lentils | 6 |
|  | 1 medium tomato | 3.5 |
|  | 1/2 Haas avocado | 2 |
|  | 2 Tbsp. **Creamy Italian Dressing** | 2.5 |
|  | 1 low-carb pita |  |
|  | **Subtotal** | **19** |
| **Day 3** | Sliced turkey (left over from Day 2) on | 0 |
|  | 4 cups mixed salad greens and | 1.5 |
|  | 1/4 cup roasted red peppers | 3.5 |
|  | 1/2 Haas avocado | 2 |
|  | 2 small tomatoes | 2 |
|  | ***1/2 cup corn kernels*** | 12.5 |
|  | 2 1/2 Tbsp. **Ranch Dressing** | 4 |
|  | **Subtotal** | **13 (25.5)** |
| **Day 4** | Beef burger and |  |
|  | 2 slices Swiss cheese and | 2.5 |
|  | 1 small tomato and | 1.5 |
|  | 1/4 cup hummus wrapped in | 3.5 |
|  | 1/2 cup loose-leaf lettuce | 5 |
|  | Coleslaw: 1 cup shredded cabbage and | 5.5 |
|  | 1 medium carrot, grated and | 1 |
|  | 2 Tbsp. **Creamy Coleslaw Dressing** | 2 |
|  | **Subtotal** | **22.5** |
| **Day 5** | Shrimp (left over from Day 4) with | 0 |
|  | 2 Tbsp. **Cocktail Sauce** | 2 |
|  | 4 cups Romaine lettuce | 2 |
|  | 1/2 cup pickled beets | 9 |
|  | ***1/4 cup cooked wild rice*** | 8 |
|  | 2 Tbsp. **Italian Dressing** |  |
|  | **Subtotal** | **13 (21)** |
| **Day 6** | Grilled chicken over | 0 |
|  | 4 cups mixed salad greens | 1.5 |
|  | 2 slices Swiss cheese on | 2.5 |
|  | 1/2 cup pickled okra | 3 |
|  | 1/2 cup roasted red peppers | 2.5 |
|  | ***1/2 cup corn kernels*** | 12.5 |
|  | 1/2 cup snow peas | 2 |
|  | 2 Tbsp. **Parmesan Peppercorn Dressing** | 1 |
|  | **Subtotal** | **12.5 (25)** |
| **Day 7** | Ham (left over from Day 5) and | 0 |
|  | 2 slices Swiss cheese on | 1.5 |
|  | Low-carb bagel with | 9 |
|  | 1 tsp. Dijon mustard | 0.5 |
|  | 1/2 cup loose-leaf lettuce | 0.5 |
|  | 1/2 cup sliced cucumber | 1 |
|  | 1/4 cup hummus | 5.5 |
|  | **Subtotal** | **18** |

**Phases 3, Pre-Maintenance, and 4, Lifetime Maintenance, at 75 and 85 Grams of Net Carbs (85-gram additions in bold italics)**

| Day 1 | Grams of Net Carbs | Day 2 | Grams of Net Carbs | Day 3 | Grams of Net Carbs | Day 4 | Grams of Net Carbs | Day 5 | Grams of Net Carbs | Day 6 | Grams of Net Carbs | Day 7 | Grams of Net Carbs |
|---|---|---|---|---|---|---|---|---|---|---|---|---|---|
| **SNACK** | | | | | | | | | | | | | |
| 1 medium apricot | 3 | 1 oz. cashews | 4.5 | 2 oz. goat cheese | 0.5 | ½ cup sweet cherries | 8 | ½ cup honeydew melon balls | 7 | ½ medium apple | 8.5 | 2 oz. almonds | 4.5 |
| 4 oz. plain whole milk yogurt | 5.5 | ½ medium apple | 8.5 | ½ cup blueberries | 8 | ½ cup cottage cheese | 4 | 2 oz. goat cheese | 0.5 | 2 oz. macadamias | 4 | 1 medium orange | 13 |
| **Subtotal** | 8.5 | **Subtotal** | 13 | **Subtotal** | 8.5 | **Subtotal** | 12 | **Subtotal** | 7.5 | **Subtotal** | 12.5 | **Subtotal** | 17.5 |
| **DINNER** | | | | | | | | | | | | | |
| Lamb kebabs | 0 | Grilled turkey breast | 0 | Fajitas: broiled sliced skirt steak with | 0 | Sautéed shrimp | 0 | Baked ham with | 0 | Flank steak | 0 | Salmon steak over | 0 |
| ½ cup cooked chickpeas | 13 | 2 Tbsp. **Barbecue Sauce** | 13 | ½ cup sautéed onions and | 4 | ***¼ cup cooked brown rice*** | 10 | ¼ cup **Mushroom Gravy** | 2 | ½ baked potato | 10.5 | 1 cup roasted fennel and | 3 |
| 2 cups mixed salad greens | 1 | ***½ cup cooked bulgur*** | 13 | ½ cup sautéed green peppers | 3 | 1 cup steamed leeks with | 9 | ***½ cup baked acorn squash*** | 10 | 4 cups mixed salad greens | 2 | ***¼ cup cooked brown rice*** | 10.5 |
| 4 pieces marinated artichoke hearts | 2 | 2 cups mixed salad greens | 1 | ***½ cup refried beans*** | 13 | ¼ cup **Alfredo Sauce** | 3.5 | Salad of 2 cups chopped raw fennel and | 7 | ½ cup cooked chickpeas | 13 | ½ cup roasted onions | 9 |
| 1 oz. blue cheese | 0.5 | ½ cup chopped fennel | 0.5 | ¼ cup **Salsa Cruda** | 2 | 2 cups baby spinach salad with | 1.5 | ½ cup chopped jicama | 7 | 2 Tbsp. **Fresh Raspberry Vinaigrette** | 1 | ¼ cup **Raita** | 3 |
| 5 black olives | 0.5 | 1 medium tomato | 2.5 | 2 cups mixed salad greens | 3.5 | 1 small tomato | 1.5 | 1 small tomato | 2.5 | | | Salad of 2 cups arugula | 0.5 |
| 1 small tomato | 2.5 | 2 oz. feta cheese | 2.5 | 2 Tbsp. **Parmesan Peppercorn Dressing** | 1 | ½ cup pickled beets | 2.5 | 2 Tbsp. **Blue Cheese Dressing** | 2 | | | 2 Tbsp. **Creamy Italian Dressing** | 2 |
| 2 Tbsp. **Greek Vinaigrette** | 1 | 2 Tbsp. **Greek Vinaigrette** | 1 | | | 2 Tbsp. **Creamy Italian Dressing** | 1 | | | | | | |
| **Subtotal** | 20.5 | **Subtotal** | 20.5 | **Subtotal** | 13.5 (26.5) | **Subtotal** | 19 (29) | **Subtotal** | 21 (31) | **Subtotal** | 26.5 | **Subtotal** | 17.5 (28) |
| **Total** | 74.5 (87) | **Total** | 74 (87) | **Total** | 73.5 (86) | **Total** | 75 (85) | **Total** | 75 (83) | **Total** | 71 (83.5) | **Total** | 74.5 (85) |
| **Foundation vegetables** | 16 | **Foundation vegetables** | 16 | **Foundation vegetables** | 13.5 | **Foundation vegetables** | 25.5 | **Foundation vegetables** | 15 | **Foundation vegetables** | 16.5 | **Foundation vegetables** | 18.5 |

*www.atkins.com/Recipes/ShowRecipe884/Atkins-Cuisine-Waffles.aspx, **www.atkins.com/Recipes/ShowRecipe883/Atkins-Cuisine-Pancakes.aspx.

## Phases 3, Pre-Maintenance, and 4, Lifetime Maintenance, at 95 Grams of Net Carbs

*(Each day lists food items followed by Grams of Net Carbs.)*

### BREAKFAST

**Day 1** (Subtotal 15)
- 2-egg omelet — 1
- ½ cup shredded Cheddar cheese — 1
- 1 medium orange — 13

**Day 2** (Subtotal 14.5)
- 1 Atkins Waffle* — 6
- ½ cup ricotta cheese — 4
- ¼ cup sliced strawberries — 2
- 1 oz. slivered almonds — 2.5

**Day 3** (Subtotal 14.5)
- ½ cup cooked rolled oats — 6
- 2 oz. whole milk — 4
- ¼ cup blueberries — 2
- 1 oz. almonds — 2.5

**Day 4** (Subtotal 28.5)
- ½ cup cottage cheese — 4
- ½ cup mango — 19
- 2 oz. almonds — 5.5

**Day 5** (Subtotal 25.5)
- ½ cup plain whole milk yogurt — 5.5
- ¼ cup cooked wheat berries — 7
- ¼ cup blueberries — 4
- 2 oz. cashews — 9

**Day 6** (Subtotal 14.5)
- 2 scrambled eggs — 1
- ¼ cup sauteed onions — 4.5
- ¼ cup shredded Cheddar cheese — 0.5
- ½ white grapefruit — 8.5

**Day 7** (Subtotal 18)
- 2 Atkins Pancakes*** — 6
- 4 oz. ricotta cheese — 4
- ½ red grapefruit — 8

### SNACK

**Day 1** (Subtotal 7.5)
- 2 oz. pine nuts — 3.5
- 4 oz. tomato juice — 4

**Day 2** (Subtotal 4.5)
- 2 slices Swiss cheese around 4 asparagus spears — 2 / 2
- 1 tsp. Dijon mustard — 0.5

**Day 3** (Subtotal 4.5)
- 1 oz. walnuts — 2
- 4 oz. tomato juice — 2
- 1 tsp. Dijon mustard — 0.5

**Day 4** (Subtotal 5.5)
- 2 slices of Swiss cheese — 1.5
- 1 medium carrot — 4

**Day 5** (Subtotal 7.5)
- ½ Haas avocado — 2
- 4 oz. tomato juice — 5.5

**Day 6** (Subtotal 7.5)
- Low-carb bar — 2
- ½ cup blackberries — 5.5

**Day 7** (Subtotal 4.5)
- ½ Haas avocado — 2
- 1 small tomato — 2.5

### LUNCH

**Day 1** (Subtotal 20)
- Grilled chicken with 2 Tbsp. Peanut Sauce — 5
- 2 cups mixed salad greens — 2
- ½ cup green bell peppers — 1
- ¼ cup roasted red peppers — 2
- 2 small tomatoes — 3.5
- ¼ cup chickpeas — 6.5
- 2 Tbsp. Creamy Italian Dressing — 2

**Day 2** (Subtotal 24)
- Lamb kebabs (left over from Day 1) on — 0
- 2 Tbsp. hummus on — 5
- 2 pieces fiber crisp bread — 1
- 4 cups mixed salad greens — 2
- 2 small tomatoes — 1.5
- ¼ cup roasted red peppers — 5
- ¼ cup chickpeas — 6.5
- 2 Tbsp. Greek Vinaigrette — 2

**Day 3** (Subtotal 30)
- Sliced turkey (left over from Day 2) on — 0
- 1 slice 100% whole grain bread — 4.5
- 4 cups mixed salad greens and — 1.5
- ¼ cup roasted red peppers — 5
- ½ cup cooked lentils — 12
- 2 Tbsp. Fresh Raspberry Vinaigrette — 2

**Day 4** (Subtotal 30)
- 2 deviled eggs topped with — 0
- 1 Tbsp. Blender Mayonnaise — 0
- 2 cups mixed salad greens topped with — 1
- ½ cup cooked wheat berries and — 14
- ¼ cup red bell peppers — 12
- 2 Tbsp. Parmesan Peppercorn Dressing — 1

**Day 5** (Subtotal 22.5)
- Tuna fish salad made with 2 Tbsp. Blender Mayonnaise and — 1
- ½ cup chopped celery and — 0
- 2 Tbsp. chopped onion on — 1.5
- 1 slice 100% whole wheat bread — 12
- 4 cups Romaine lettuce — 2
- 1 medium carrot, grated — 5.5
- 2 Tbsp. Italian Dressing — 0.5

**Day 6** (Subtotal 33.5)
- Grilled chicken over — 0
- 2 cups mixed salad greens — 1
- ½ cup corn kernels — 12.5
- 1 cup red peppers — 6
- ½ cup black beans — 13
- 2 Tbsp. Parmesan Peppercorn Dressing — 1

**Day 7** (Subtotal 27.5)
- Ham (left over from Day 5) and — 0
- 2 slices Swiss cheese on — 2
- 1 slice 100% whole wheat bread with — 12
- 1 tsp. Dijon mustard — 0.5
- ½ cup loose-leaf lettuce — 0.5
- 1 medium tomato — 3.5
- ¼ cup hummus — 9

## Phases 3, Pre-Maintenance, and 4, Lifetime Maintenance, at 95 Grams of Net Carbs

| | Day 1 | Grams of Net Carbs | Day 2 | Grams of Net Carbs | Day 3 | Grams of Net Carbs | Day 4 | Grams of Net Carbs | Day 5 | Grams of Net Carbs | Day 6 | Grams of Net Carbs | Day 7 | Grams of Net Carbs |
|---|---|---|---|---|---|---|---|---|---|---|---|---|---|---|
| SNACK | ½ cup cantaloupe melon balls | 7.5 | 1 oz. cashews | 4.5 | 2 slices Swiss cheese | 2 | 2 Tbsp. hummus | 4.5 | ½ cup red grapes | 13.5 | 1 medium carrot | 5.5 | 2 oz. almonds | 4.5 |
| | ½ cup cottage cheese | 4 | ¼ pomegranate | 6.5 | ½ medium apple | 8.5 | 6 spears asparagus | 2.5 | 2 oz. goat cheese | 0.5 | 2 oz. walnuts | 3 | ½ cup sliced strawberries | 3.5 |
| | **Subtotal** | 11.5 | **Subtotal** | 11 | **Subtotal** | 10.5 | **Subtotal** | 7 | **Subtotal** | 14 | **Subtotal** | 8.5 | **Subtotal** | 8 |
| DINNER | Lamb kebabs with | 0 | Roast turkey | 0 | Fajitas: broiled sliced skirt steak with | 0 | Sautéed shrimp | 0 | Baked ham | 0 | Flank steak | 0 | Salmon steak over | 0 |
| | ¼ cup **Raita** | 3 | ½ cup **Velouté Sauce** | 1 | ¼ cup sautéed onions and | 4.5 | 1 cup sautéed leeks with | 3.5 | ¼ cup **Mushroom Gravy** | 2 | ¼ cup **Mushroom Gravy** | 2 | 1 cup sautéed spinach | 4.5 |
| | 1 cup cooked low-carb penne pasta** | 19 | ½ cup cooked brown rice | 20.5 | ¼ cup sautéed green peppers | 2 | ¼ cup **Alfredo Sauce** | 2 | 1 cup steamed acorn squash | 15 | ½ cup mashed potato | 16.5 | topped with ¼ cup **Raita** | 3 |
| | 1 cup Brussels sprouts | 9.5 | 1 steamed medium artichoke | 7 | ¼ cup refried beans | 6.5 | ½ cup cooked wild rice | 16 | Salad of 1 cup chopped raw fennel and | 3.5 | 2 cups mixed salad greens | 1 | 1 cup cooked low-carb penne pasta** | 19 |
| | 2 cups mixed salad greens | 1 | 2 cups mixed salad greens topped with | 1 | ¼ cup **Salsa Cruda** | 1.5 | 2 cups baby spinach salad with | 0.5 | ½ cup chopped jicama | 2.5 | 1 oz. goat cheese | 0.5 | Salad of 2 cups arugula | 0.5 |
| | 1 medium carrot, grated | 5.5 | ¼ cup roasted red peppers | 3.5 | 2 cups mixed salad greens | 1 | ½ Haas avocado | 2 | 1 small tomato | 2.5 | ½ cup snow peas | 3.5 | 4 pieces marinated artichoke hearts | 2 |
| | ¼ cup shredded jicama | 1.5 | 1 medium carrot, grated | 5.5 | ½ Haas avocado | 2 | ½ cup corn kernels | 12.5 | 2 Tbsp. **Blue Cheese Dressing** | 1 | ½ cup pickled beets | 7 | 1 medium carrot, grated | 5.5 |
| | 2 Tbsp. **Greek Vinaigrette** | 1 | 2 Tbsp. **Greek Vinaigrette** | 1 | 2 Tbsp. **Parmesan Peppercorn Dressing** | 1 | 2 Tbsp. **Creamy Italian Dressing** | 2 | | | 2 Tbsp. **Fresh Raspberry Vinaigrette** | 1 | 2 Tbsp. **Creamy Italian Dressing** | 2 |
| | **Subtotal** | 40.5 | **Subtotal** | 39.5 | **Subtotal** | 18.5 | **Subtotal** | 38.5 | **Subtotal** | 26.5 | **Subtotal** | 31.5 | **Subtotal** | 36.5 |
| | **Total** | 94.5 | **Total** | 93.5 | **Total** | 93 | **Total** | 94 | **Total** | 94.5 | **Total** | 95.5 | **Total** | 94.5 |
| | **Foundation vegetables** | 18.5 | **Foundation vegetables** | 20 | **Foundation vegetables** | 16 | **Foundation vegetables** | 12.5 | **Foundation vegetables** | 14 | **Foundation vegetables** | 16 | **Foundation vegetables** | 15.5 |

*www.atkins.com/Recipes/ShowRecipe884/Atkins-Cuisine-Waffles.aspx, **www.atkins.com/Products/productdetail.aspx?productID=36, ***www.atkins.com/Recipes/ShowRecipe883/Atkins-Cuisine-Pancakes.aspx.

## Phase 2, Ongoing Weight Loss, Vegetarian, at 30 and 35 Grams of Net Carbs (35-gram additions in bold italics)

### BREAKFAST

| Day 1 | Net Carbs | Day 2 | Net Carbs | Day 3 | Net Carbs | Day 4 | Net Carbs | Day 5 | Net Carbs | Day 6 | Net Carbs | Day 7 | Net Carbs |
|---|---|---|---|---|---|---|---|---|---|---|---|---|---|
| 2-egg omelet | 1 | 3 slices tofu Canadian "bacon" | 1.5 | 1 veggie burger | 2 | Low-carb shake | 2 | Smoothie: 1 cup plain unsweetened almond milk and | 1 | 2 fried eggs | 1 | 4 oz. tofu "sausage" patties | 8 |
| 2 cups Swiss chard sautéed with | 1.5 | ½ cup mashed cauliflower with | 1 | 2 slices Swiss cheese | 2 | 2 oz. pecans | 2 | 3 oz. silken soft tofu and | 3 | ½ cup sautéed okra | 2.5 | 2 slices Cheddar cheese | 1 |
| ¼ cup chopped onion | 3 | ¼ cup shredded Cheddar cheese and | 0.5 | ½ Haas avocado | 2 | *½ cup blackberries* | 5 | 2 Tbsp. low-carb strawberry syrup and | 0 | 2 tofu "bacon" strips | 2 | ½ Haas avocado | 2 |
| ¼ cup shredded Cheddar cheese | 0.5 | 2 Tbsp. sautéed onion | 2.5 | *5 large strawberries* | 5 | | | 1 oz. almonds | 2.5 | | | | |
| *¼ cup blueberries* | 4 | *¼ cup blueberries* | 4 | | | | | | | | | | |
| **Subtotal** | 6 (10) | **Subtotal** | 5.5 (9.5) | **Subtotal** | 6 (11) | **Subtotal** | 4 (9) | **Subtotal** | 6.5 | **Subtotal** | 5.5 | **Subtotal** | 11 |

### SNACK

| Day 1 | Net Carbs | Day 2 | Net Carbs | Day 3 | Net Carbs | Day 4 | Net Carbs | Day 5 | Net Carbs | Day 6 | Net Carbs | Day 7 | Net Carbs |
|---|---|---|---|---|---|---|---|---|---|---|---|---|---|
| 1 celery stalk | 1 | 1 oz. almonds | 2.5 | 2 celery stalks | 2.5 | ½ Haas avocado | 1.5 | 8 asparagus spears | 2 | 1 small tomato | 3 | 2 oz. walnuts | 3 |
| 1 Tbsp. natural peanut butter | 2.5 | Low-carb shake | 1 | 2 Tbsp. **Aioli** | 1 | 2 slices Cheddar cheese | 0 | 2 Tbsp. **Aioli** | 1 | 1 oz. roasted pumpkin seeds | 0 | *¼ cup cantaloupe melon balls* | 3.5 |
| **Subtotal** | 3.5 | **Subtotal** | 3.5 | **Subtotal** | 3.5 | **Subtotal** | 1.5 | **Subtotal** | 3 | **Subtotal** | 3 | **Subtotal** | 3 (6.5) |

### LUNCH

| Day 1 | Net Carbs | Day 2 | Net Carbs | Day 3 | Net Carbs | Day 4 | Net Carbs | Day 5 | Net Carbs | Day 6 | Net Carbs | Day 7 | Net Carbs |
|---|---|---|---|---|---|---|---|---|---|---|---|---|---|
| 4 oz. firm tofu sautéed with | 1 | 2 deviled eggs on | 1 | 4 oz. sautéed seitan on | 1 | 2-egg omelet | 1 | 4 slices "turkey"-style cold cuts | 1 | 2 veggie burgers | 3 | 2-egg salad made with | 1 |
| 4 cups mixed salad greens | 2.5 | 4 cups mixed salad greens | 2.5 | 4 cups Romaine lettuce with | 1.5 | ½ cup sautéed spinach | 3.5 | 2 slices Provolone cheese | 1 | ½ Haas avocado | 2 | ½ cup diced celery and | 0.5 |
| 2 cups spinach | 0.5 | ½ cup pickled okra | 1.5 | 10 black olives | 2 | 4 cups mixed salad greens | 2.5 | 1 tsp. Dijon mustard | 0 | 2 slices Cheddar cheese | 1 | 1 Tbsp. **Blender Mayonnaise** | 0 |
| 1 Tbsp. soy sauce | 1 | 6 radishes | 0.5 | ½ cup sliced daikon | 0.5 | ½ cup alfalfa sprouts | 1.5 | 4 cups mixed salad greens | 1 | 1 cup loose-leaf lettuce | 0.5 | Salad of 4 cups baby spinach with | 1 |
| 2 cups Romaine lettuce | 0.5 | 5 black olives | 0.5 | 2 Tbsp. **Caesar Dressing** | 0 | 2 Tbsp. **Blue Cheese Dressing** | 1 | 10 black olives | 1 | 2 Tbsp. chopped onions | 0.5 | 1 small tomato | 2.5 |
| ¼ cup alfalfa sprouts | 0 | 2 Tbsp. **Russian Dressing** | 0 | 2 Tbsp. grated Parmesan cheese | 1 | | | 2 Tbsp. **Italian Dressing** | 0.5 | 2 Tbsp. **Aioli** | 1.5 | 2 Tbsp. **Sweet Mustard Dressing** | 1 |
| 10 black olives | 1 | | | | | | | | | | | | |
| 2 Tbsp. **Fresh Raspberry Vinaigrette** | 1 | | | | | | | | | | | | |
| **Subtotal** | 7.5 | **Subtotal** | 6 | **Subtotal** | 6 | **Subtotal** | 9.5 | **Subtotal** | 4.5 | **Subtotal** | 8.5 | **Subtotal** | 6 |

## Phase 2, Ongoing Weight Loss, Vegetarian, at 30 and 35 Grams of Net Carbs (35-gram additions in bold italics)

| | Day 1 | Grams of Net Carbs | Day 2 | Grams of Net Carbs | Day 3 | Grams of Net Carbs | Day 4 | Grams of Net Carbs | Day 5 | Grams of Net Carbs | Day 6 | Grams of Net Carbs | Day 7 | Grams of Net Carbs |
|---|---|---|---|---|---|---|---|---|---|---|---|---|---|---|
| **SNACK** | 1 oz. pecans | 1.5 | 2 sticks string cheese | 1 | 1 dill pickle | 2 | 1 oz. goat cheese | 0.5 | 1 oz. hazelnuts | 0.5 | 1 oz. walnuts | 1.5 | ½ cup sliced daikon | 1 |
| | 2 oz. goat cheese | 1 | 1 oz. walnuts | 1.5 | 1 oz. peanuts | 1.5 | 10 green olives | 0 | *¼ cup blueberries* | 4 | 2 Tbsp. blue cheese | 0.5 | 2 Tbsp. **Aioli** | 0 |
| | Subtotal | 2.5 | Subtotal | 2.5 | Subtotal | 3.5 | Subtotal | 0.5 | Subtotal | 0.5 (4.5) | Subtotal | 2 | Subtotal | 1 |
| **DINNER** | 5 veggie "meatballs" sautéed with | 4 | 4 oz. Quorn roast with | 4 | 4 oz. firm tofu baked with | 2.5 | ⅔ cup veggie crumbles sautéed with | 4 | ½ cup tempeh sautéed with | 3.5 | 4 oz. baked firm tofu and | 2.5 | 2 tofu "hot dogs" | 4 |
| | ½ cup shirataki soy noodles topped with | 1 | ¼ cup **Mushroom Gravy** | 2 | 2 Tbsp. **Barbecue Sauce** | 2 | 1 cup raw shredded green cabbage topped with | 2 | ½ cup green peppers served over | 2 | 3 Tbsp. **Sun-Dried Tomato Pesto** over | 3 | 1 cup sauerkraut | 2 |
| | 3 Tbsp. **Romesco Sauce** | 2 | ½ cup steamed green beans | 3 | ¼ cup steamed Brussels sprouts | 2 | 2 Tbsp. **Peanut Sauce** | 5 | 1 cup raw shredded green cabbage topped with | 2 | ½ cup cooked spaghetti squash | 4 | ½ cup mashed cauliflower and | 1 |
| | 2 cups mixed salad greens with | 1 | 2 cups mixed salad greens | 1 | Salad of 2 cups arugula and | 1 | 2 cups mixed salad greens | 1 | 3 Tbsp. **Romesco Sauce** and | 2 | Salad of 2 cups mesclun and | 1 | ¼ cup shredded Cheddar cheese | 0.5 |
| | 1 small tomato | 2.5 | 4 pieces marinated artichoke hearts | 2 | 1 oz. walnuts | 1.5 | 8 asparagus spears | 3 | 1 oz. grated Parmesan cheese | 3 | ½ cup alfalfa sprouts | 0 | Salad of 2 cups mixed salad greens | 1 |
| | 2 Tbsp. **Sweet Mustard Dressing** | 1 | 2 Tbsp. **Blue Cheese Dressing** | 1 | 2 Tbsp. **Italian Dressing** | 1 | 1 cup sliced cucumber | 2 | ½ Haas avocado | 2 | *½ cup raspberries* | 3 | ½ cup sliced cucumber | 1 |
| | | | | | | | 2 Tbsp. **Sweet Mustard Dressing** | 1 | | | 2 Tbsp. **Fresh Raspberry Vinaigrette** | 1 | 2 Tbsp. **Italian Dressing** | 1 |
| | Subtotal | 11.5 | Subtotal | 13 | Subtotal | 10 | Subtotal | 18 | Subtotal | 12.5 | Subtotal | 11.5 (14.5) | Subtotal | 10.5 |
| | **Total** | 31 (35) | **Total** | 30.5 (34.5) | **Total** | 30.5 (35) | **Total** | 30 (35) | **Total** | 30 (34) | **Total** | 33 (36) | **Total** | 31.5 (35) |
| | **Foundation vegetables** | 12 | **Foundation vegetables** | 14.5 | **Foundation vegetables** | 12.5 | **Foundation vegetables** | 12.5 | **Foundation vegetables** | 12 | **Foundation vegetables** | 12 | **Foundation vegetables** | 12 |

## Phase 2, Ongoing Weight Loss, Vegetarian, at 40 and 45 Grams of Net Carbs (45-gram additions in bold italics)

*Each food item is followed by its Grams of Net Carbs.*

| | Day 1 | Day 2 | Day 3 | Day 4 | Day 5 | Day 6 | Day 7 |
|---|---|---|---|---|---|---|---|
| **BREAKFAST** | 2-egg omelet with — 1; 2 cups Swiss chard sautéed with — 1.5; ¼ cup chopped onion — 3; ¼ cup shredded Cheddar cheese — 0.5. **Subtotal 6** | 3 slices tofu Canadian "bacon" — 1.5; 1 cup mashed cauliflower with — 1; ½ cup shredded Cheddar cheese and — 0.5; ¼ cup sautéed onion — 1.5. **Subtotal 4.5** | 1 veggie burger — 2; 2 slices Cheddar cheese — 1.5; ½ Haas avocado — 2; ¼ cup blueberries — 4. **Subtotal 9** | Low-carb shake — 2; 1 oz. pecans — 1; ½ cup raspberries — 4. **Subtotal 9** | Smoothie: 1 cup plain unsweetened almond milk with — 1; 1 oz. pecans — 1.5; 3 oz. silken soft tofu and — 3; ½ cup frozen strawberries and — 5; 1 oz. walnuts — 1.5. **Subtotal 10.5** | 2 fried eggs — 1; 2 tofu "bacon" strips — 2; ½ Haas avocado — 2; ¼ cup **Tomatillo Salsa** — 4. **Subtotal 9** | 4 oz. tofu "sausage" patties — 8; ½ cup baked chayote squash — 2; 2 slices Cheddar cheese — 1; ½ Haas avocado — 2. **Subtotal 13** |
| **SNACK** | ½ cup blueberries — 8; 1 oz. goat cheese — 0.5. **Subtotal 8.5** | 1 oz. almonds — 2.5; ¼ cup sliced strawberries — 2. **Subtotal 4.5** | 2 celery sticks — 1.5; 2 oz. walnuts — 3. **Subtotal 4.5** | ½ Haas avocado — 2; *½ cup cottage cheese* — 3. **Subtotal 2 (6)** | *½ cup cottage cheese* — 2; low-carb bar — 4. **Subtotal 2 (6)** | 1 oz. almonds — 2.5; ¼ cup blackberries — 3. **Subtotal 5.5** | 2 oz. hazelnuts — 1; *4 oz. plain whole milk Greek yogurt* — 3.5. **Subtotal 1 (4.5)** |
| **LUNCH** | 4 oz. firm tofu sautéed with — 2.5; 2 cups spinach and — 0.5; 1 Tbsp. soy sauce — 1; Salad of 2 cups Romaine lettuce and — 2.5; 1 small tomato — 2.5; ½ cup chopped celery — 0.5; 2 Tbsp. **Fresh Raspberry Vinaigrette** — 1. **Subtotal 9** | 2 deviled eggs on — 2.5; 4 cups mixed salad greens — 0.5; 1 cup steamed green beans — 1; 1 small tomato — 2.5; 2 Tbsp. **Russian Dressing** — 0.5. **Subtotal 9** | 4 oz. sautéed seitan on — 1; Salad of 4 cups Romaine lettuce — 1.5; 5 black olives — 2.5; ½ cup sliced daikon — 2.5; 2 Tbsp. **Caesar Dressing** — 6; 2 Tbsp. grated Parmesan cheese — 0. **Subtotal 12.5** | 2-egg omelet with — 1; ½ cup chopped watercress and — 3.5; 2 oz. Cheddar cheese — 1.5; 4 cups mixed salad greens — 0.5; 1 small tomato — 2.5; 2 Tbsp. **Blue Cheese Dressing** — 1. **Subtotal 8.5** | 4 slices "turkey"-style cold cuts — 3; 2 slices Provolone cheese — 0; 1 tsp. Dijon mustard — 1; 4 cups mixed salad greens — 1.5; 10 black olives — 2.5; 2 Tbsp. **Italian Dressing** — 1. **Subtotal 8.5** | 2 veggie burgers — 4; 1 small tomato — 2.5; 2 Tbsp. hummus — 4.5; 2 slices Cheddar cheese — 0; 1 cup loose-leaf lettuce — 1; 2 Tbsp. **Aïoli** — 0. **Subtotal 13** | 2-egg salad made with — 1; ½ cup diced celery and — 1; 2 Tbsp. **Blender Mayonnaise** over — 0; 4 cups baby spinach with — 1; ¼ cup cooked chickpeas — 6.5; 2 Tbsp. **Sweet Mustard Dressing** — 1. **Subtotal 10.5** |

## Phase 2, Ongoing Weight Loss, Vegetarian, at 40 and 45 Grams of Net Carbs (45-gram additions in bold italics)

| Day 1 | Grams of Net Carbs | Day 2 | Grams of Net Carbs | Day 3 | Grams of Net Carbs | Day 4 | Grams of Net Carbs | Day 5 | Grams of Net Carbs | Day 6 | Grams of Net Carbs | Day 7 | Grams of Net Carbs |
|---|---|---|---|---|---|---|---|---|---|---|---|---|---|
| **SNACK** | | | | | | | | | | | | | |
| 2 oz. almonds | 5 | 1 oz. almonds | 2.5 | 1 dill pickle | 2 | 1 oz. walnuts | 1.5 | 1 oz. walnuts | 1.5 | 1 oz. walnuts | 1.5 | ¼ cup blueberries | 4 |
| *½ cup cottage cheese* | 4 | *4 oz. plain whole milk yogurt* | 5.5 | *4 oz. plain whole milk Greek yogurt* | 3.5 | ¼ cup roasted red peppers | 3.5 | ½ cup raw green beans | 2 | *½ cup ricotta cheese* | 4 | 2 sticks string cheese | 1 |
| Subtotal | 5 (9) | Subtotal | 2.5 (8) | Subtotal | 2 (5.5) | Subtotal | 5 | Subtotal | 3.5 | Subtotal | 1.5 (5.5) | Subtotal | 5 |
| **DINNER** | | | | | | | | | | | | | |
| 5 veggie "meatballs" sautéed with | 5 | 4 oz. Quorn roast with | 4 | 4 oz. firm tofu grilled and topped with | 4 | ⅔ cup veggie crumbles sautéed with | 4 | ½ cup tempeh sautéed with | 3.5 | 4 oz. baked firm tofu and | | 2 tofu "hot dogs" | |
| ¼ cup **Mushroom Gravy** | 4 | ¼ cup **Mushroom Gravy** | 2 | 2 Tbsp. **Barbecue Sauce** | 2.5 | 1 cup shirataki soy noodles topped with | 2 | 1 cup green peppers over | 4.5 | 3 Tbsp. **Sun-Dried Tomato Pesto** over | 3 | ½ cup sauerkraut | 2.5 |
| ½ cup shirataki soy noodles topped with | 1 | ½ cup sautéed red peppers | 3.5 | 1 cup sautéed kale | 4 | 2 Tbsp. **Peanut Sauce** | 5 | 1 cup raw shredded green cabbage topped with | 2 | ½ cup cooked spaghetti squash | 4 | 1 cup mashed cauliflower and | 3 |
| 3 Tbsp. **Romesco Sauce** | | 2 cups mixed salad greens | 2 | Salad of 2 cups arugula | 1 | 1 cup steamed Brussels sprouts | 7 | 3 Tbsp. **Romesco Sauce** and | | Salad of 2 cups arugula | 2 | ¼ cup Cheddar cheese | 0.5 |
| 2 cups mixed salad greens | 2 | ½ cup sliced cucumber | 1 | 1 small tomato | 2.5 | 2 cups mixed salad greens | 2.5 | 1 oz. grated Parmesan | 1 | ½ cup sliced cucumber | 0.5 | 2 cups mixed salad greens | 2 |
| ½ cup sliced cucumber | 1 | 2 Tbsp. **Blue Cheese Dressing** | 1 | 2 Tbsp. **Italian Dressing** | 1 | 2 Tbsp. **Sweet Mustard Dressing** | 1 | ½ Haas avocado | 1 | 2 Tbsp. **Fresh Raspberry Vinaigrette** | 2 | 4 pieces marinated artichoke hearts | 2 |
| 5 asparagus spears | 2.5 | | | | | | | | | | | 2 Tbsp. **Italian Dressing** | 1 |
| 2 Tbsp. **Sweet Mustard Dressing** | 1 | | | | | | | | | | | | |
| Subtotal | 11.5 | Subtotal | 12.5 | Subtotal | 12.5 | Subtotal | 16 | Subtotal | 15 | Subtotal | 12 | Subtotal | 11.5 |
| Total | 40 (44) | Total | 41 (46.5) | Total | 40 (43.5) | Total | 39.5 (43.5) | Total | 39.5 (43.5) | Total | 41 (45) | Total | 41 (44.5) |
| Foundation vegetables | 12.5 | Foundation vegetables | 23.5 | Foundation vegetables | 17 | Foundation vegetables | 17.5 | Foundation vegetables | 13.5 | Foundation vegetables | 15 | Foundation vegetables | 12 |

## Phase 2, Ongoing Weight Loss, Vegetarian, at 50 and 55 Grams of Net Carbs (55-gram additions in bold italics)

**BREAKFAST**

| Day 1 | Grams of Net Carbs | Day 2 | Grams of Net Carbs | Day 3 | Grams of Net Carbs | Day 4 | Grams of Net Carbs | Day 5 | Grams of Net Carbs | Day 6 | Grams of Net Carbs | Day 7 | Grams of Net Carbs |
|---|---|---|---|---|---|---|---|---|---|---|---|---|---|
| 2-egg omelet | 1 | 3 slices tofu Canadian "bacon" | 1.5 | 1 veggie burger | 2 | Low-carb shake | 1 | Smoothie: 1 cup plain unsweetened almond milk and | 1 | 2 fried eggs | 1 | 4 oz. tofu "sausage" patties | 8 |
| 1 cup sautéed Swiss chard and | 3.5 | 1/4 cup refried beans | 6.5 | 1 slice Cheddar cheese | 0.5 | 2 oz. pecans | 3 | 3 oz. silken soft tofu and | 3 | 1/2 cup sautéed okra | 2.5 | 1/2 cup baked chayote squash | 2 |
| 2 Tbsp. sautéed onion and | 2.5 | 1/4 cup shredded Cheddar cheese | 0.5 | 1/2 Haas avocado | 2 | 1/2 cup cantaloupe melon balls | 7.5 | 3/4 cup frozen strawberries | 7 | 2 tofu "bacon" strips | 1 | 2 slices Cheddar cheese | 1 |
| 1/4 cup shredded Cheddar cheese | 1 | ***4 oz. tomato juice*** | 4 | 1/2 cup blueberries | 8 |  |  | 1 oz. almonds | 2.5 | 1/4 cup **Tomatillo Salsa** | 4 | 1/2 Haas avocado | 2 |
| 1/4 cup cantaloupe melon balls | 3.5 |  |  |  |  |  |  |  |  |  |  |  |  |
| **Subtotal** | 11.5 | **Subtotal** | 8.5 (12.5) | **Subtotal** | 12.5 | **Subtotal** | 11.5 | **Subtotal** | 13.5 | **Subtotal** | 9.5 | **Subtotal** | 13 |

**SNACK**

| Day 1 | Grams of Net Carbs | Day 2 | Grams of Net Carbs | Day 3 | Grams of Net Carbs | Day 4 | Grams of Net Carbs | Day 5 | Grams of Net Carbs | Day 6 | Grams of Net Carbs | Day 7 | Grams of Net Carbs |
|---|---|---|---|---|---|---|---|---|---|---|---|---|---|
| ***4 oz. tomato juice*** | 5 | 5 large strawberries | 4 | 1/2 cup cottage cheese | 5 | 1/2 Haas avocado | 2 | 1/2 cup cottage cheese | 4 | 4 oz. plain whole-milk Greek yogurt | 4 | 2 oz. hazelnuts | 1 |
| 1/2 cup cottage cheese | 4 | 1/2 cup low-carb yogurt | 4 | 1 small tomato | 3 | ***1/4 cup edamame*** | 3 | 8 asparagus spears | 3 | 1 small tomato | 3 | 1/4 cup blackberries | 3 |
| **Subtotal** | 4 (8) | **Subtotal** | 8 | **Subtotal** | 8 | **Subtotal** | 2 (5) | **Subtotal** | 7 | **Subtotal** | 7 | **Subtotal** | 4 |

**LUNCH**

| Day 1 | Grams of Net Carbs | Day 2 | Grams of Net Carbs | Day 3 | Grams of Net Carbs | Day 4 | Grams of Net Carbs | Day 5 | Grams of Net Carbs | Day 6 | Grams of Net Carbs | Day 7 | Grams of Net Carbs |
|---|---|---|---|---|---|---|---|---|---|---|---|---|---|
| 4 oz. firm tofu sautéed with | 2.5 | 2 deviled eggs on | 2.5 | 4 oz. sautéed seitan on | 1 | 2-egg omelet with | 1 | 4 slices "turkey"-style cold cuts | 1 | 2 veggie burgers | 4 | 2-egg salad made with | 1 |
| 1 cup green bell peppers and | 4.5 | 4 cups mixed salad greens | 1.5 | 4 cups Romaine lettuce | 1.5 | 1/2 cup sautéed red bell peppers and | 3.5 | 2 slices Swiss cheese | 2 | 1/2 Haas avocado | 2 | 1/2 cup diced celery and | 0.5 |
| 1/2 cup scallions | 2.5 | 1/2 cup pickled okra | 2.5 | 10 black olives | 2.5 | 2 oz. feta cheese | 1.5 | 1 tsp. Dijon mustard | 0.5 | ***3 Tbsp. hummus*** | 7 | 2 Tbsp. **Blender Mayonnaise** over | 0 |
| 1 Tbsp. soy sauce | 1 | 1 small tomato | 2.5 | 1/2 cup sliced daikon | 2.5 | 2 cups mixed salad greens | 1.5 | 4 cups mesclun greens | 2 | 1/2 cup shredded Cheddar cheese | 0.5 | 4 cups baby spinach with | 1 |
| 2 cups Romaine lettuce | 1 | 4 pieces marinated artichoke hearts | 1 | 2 Tbsp. **Caesar Dressing** | 2 | 1 small tomato | 1 | 1 small tomato | 2.5 | 1 cup loose-leaf lettuce | 1 | 1 small tomato | 2.5 |
| 2 Tbsp. **Fresh Raspberry Vinaigrette** | 1 | 2 cups Romaine lettuce | 1 | 2 Tbsp. grated Parmesan cheese | 0 | ***2 Tbsp. Sweet Mustard Dressing*** | 2.5 | 10 black olives | 2.5 | 2 Tbsp. chopped onions | 1.5 | 1/4 cup cooked chickpeas | 6.5 |
|  |  | 2 Tbsp. **Russian Dressing** | 1 |  |  |  |  | 2 Tbsp. **Italian Dressing** | 2 | 1 Tbsp. **Caesar Dressing** | 1 | ***2 Tbsp. Sweet Mustard Dressing*** | 1 |
| **Subtotal** | 12.5 | **Subtotal** | 12.5 | **Subtotal** | 9.5 | **Subtotal** | 9.5 (11.5) | **Subtotal** | 12.5 | **Subtotal** | 10 (17) | **Subtotal** | 11.5 (12.5) |

## Phase 2, Ongoing Weight Loss, Vegetarian, at 50 and 55 Grams of Net Carbs (55-gram additions in bold italics)

**Day 1**

| Item | Grams of Net Carbs |
|---|---|
| SNACK | |
| ¼ cup edamame | 3 |
| 2 oz. cashews | 9 |
| Subtotal | 12 |
| DINNER | |
| 5 veggie "meatballs" sautéed with | 4 |
| 1 cup shirataki soy noodles topped with | 2 |
| 3 Tbsp. Romesco Sauce | 2 |
| 2 cups mixed salad greens | 2 |
| ½ cup sliced cucumber | 1 |
| 2 Tbsp. Sweet Mustard Dressing | 1 |
| Subtotal | 11 |
| Total | 51 (55) |
| Foundation vegetables | 16 |

**Day 2**

| Item | Grams of Net Carbs |
|---|---|
| SNACK | |
| 1 stick string cheese | 0.5 |
| 2 oz. macadamias | 4 |
| Subtotal | 4.5 |
| DINNER | |
| 4 oz. Quorn roast with | 4 |
| ¼ cup Mushroom Gravy | 2 |
| 1 cup sautéed green bell pepper | 7.5 |
| ¼ cup sautéed onion | 4.5 |
| 2 cups mixed salad greens | 1 |
| 2 Tbsp. Blue Cheese Dressing | 1 |
| Subtotal | 20 |
| Total | 50.5 (54.5) |
| Foundation vegetables | 21.5 |

**Day 3**

| Item | Grams of Net Carbs |
|---|---|
| SNACK | |
| *4 oz. tomato juice* | 4 |
| 2 oz. walnuts | 3 |
| Subtotal | 3 (7) |
| DINNER | |
| 4 oz. firm tofu baked with | 2.5 |
| 2 Tbsp. **Barbecue Sauce** | 4 |
| 2 cups mixed salad greens | 1 |
| ½ cup steamed green beans | 1 |
| ¼ cup cooked chickpeas | 6.5 |
| 2 Tbsp. Italian Dressing | 1 |
| Subtotal | 18 |
| Total | 49.5 (53.5) |
| Foundation vegetables | 12.5 |

**Day 4**

| Item | Grams of Net Carbs |
|---|---|
| SNACK | |
| ½ cup red bell peppers | 3 |
| 2 Tbsp. hummus | 4.5 |
| Subtotal | 7.5 |
| DINNER | |
| ⅔ cup veggie crumbles sautéed with | 4 |
| 1 cup shirataki soy noodles topped with | 2 |
| 2 Tbsp. **Peanut Sauce** | 5 |
| ¾ cup steamed Brussels sprouts | 3 |
| 2 cups mixed salad greens | 1 |
| 2 Tbsp. **Blue Cheese Dressing** | 6.5 |
| Subtotal | 18.5 |
| Total | 51 (54) |
| Foundation vegetables | 18.5 |

**Day 5**

| Item | Grams of Net Carbs |
|---|---|
| SNACK | |
| 1 oz. macadamias | 2 |
| ¼ cup Crenshaw melon balls | 2.5 |
| Subtotal | 4.5 |
| DINNER | |
| ½ cup tempeh sautéed with | 3.5 |
| 1 cup green bell peppers topped with | 4 |
| 3 Tbsp. **Romesco Sauce** and | 2 |
| 1 oz. grated Parmesan cheese | 5.5 |
| 2 cups watercress salad | 1 |
| *¼ cup black beans* | 6.5 |
| 2 Tbsp. **Sweet Mustard Dressing** | 1 |
| Subtotal | 12 (18.5) |
| Total | 49.5 (56) |
| Foundation vegetables | 13.5 |

**Day 6**

| Item | Grams of Net Carbs |
|---|---|
| SNACK | |
| 2 oz. pecans | 3 |
| ¼ cup cantaloupe melon balls | 7.5 |
| Subtotal | 10.5 |
| DINNER | |
| 4 oz. baked firm tofu and | 2.5 |
| ¼ cup cooked lentils topped with | 6 |
| 3 Tbsp. **Sun-Dried Tomato Pesto** | 3 |
| 2 cups salad greens | 1 |
| 6 radishes | 0.5 |
| 2 Tbsp. **Fresh Raspberry Vinaigrette** | 6.5 |
| Subtotal | 14 |
| Total | 50 (57) |
| Foundation vegetables | 15 |

**Day 7**

| Item | Grams of Net Carbs |
|---|---|
| SNACK | |
| *4 oz. tomato juice* | 4 |
| ½ cup cottage cheese | 4 |
| Subtotal | 4 (8) |
| DINNER | |
| 2 tofu "hot dogs" | 4 |
| ½ cup sauerkraut | 1 |
| 1 cup mashed turnip and | 6.5 |
| ½ cup shredded Cheddar cheese | 1 |
| 2 cups salad greens | 1 |
| 4 pieces marinated artichoke hearts | 2 |
| 2 Tbsp. Italian Dressing | 1 |
| Subtotal | 16.5 |
| Total | 50 (54) |
| Foundation vegetables | 18.5 |

## Phase 3, Pre-Maintenance, and Phase 4, Lifetime Maintenance, Vegetarian, at 60 and 70 Grams of Net Carbs (70-gram additions in bold italics)

| | Day 1 | Day 2 | Day 3 | Day 4 | Day 5 | Day 6 | Day 7 |
|---|---|---|---|---|---|---|---|
| **BREAKFAST** | ½ cup cottage cheese (4)<br>1 oz. almonds (2.5)<br>½ cup blueberries (8)<br>**Subtotal 14.5** | **2 Atkins Pancakes\*** (6)<br>½ cup ricotta cheese (4)<br>½ cup raspberries (3)<br>**Subtotal 13** | Smoothie: ½ cup plain unsweetened almond milk (0.5)<br>4 oz. low-carb yogurt (3)<br>¼ cup frozen blackberries (4)<br>1 Tbsp. almond butter (2.5)<br>**Subtotal 10** | 2-egg omelet (1)<br>½ cup sautéed leeks (3.5)<br>1 oz. feta cheese (1)<br>½ cup cantaloupe melon balls (7)<br>**Subtotal 12.5** | **1 Atkins Waffle\*\*** (1)<br>¼ cup ricotta cheese (3.5)<br>¼ cup sliced strawberries (1)<br>1 oz. slivered almonds (7)<br>**Subtotal 12.5** | 4 oz. plain whole milk (6)<br>Greek yogurt (2)<br>½ cup honeydew melon balls (2)<br>2 oz. pecans (2.5)<br>**Subtotal 12.5** | 2 scrambled eggs (1)<br>½ cup sautéed okra (2.5)<br>¼ cup **Salsa Cruda** (1.5)<br>¼ cup shredded Cheddar cheese (0.5)<br>**Subtotal 5.5** |
| **SNACK** | 2 Tbsp. natural peanut butter (5)<br>2 celery stalks (1.5)<br>**Subtotal 6.5** | 2 oz. walnuts (3)<br>1 medium carrot (5.5)<br>**Subtotal 8.5** | 2 slices of Swiss cheese around (2)<br>4 asparagus spears (2)<br>1 tsp. Dijon mustard (0.5)<br>**Subtotal 4.5** | ½ cup red bell peppers (3)<br>2 oz. almonds (4.5)<br>**Subtotal 7.5** | 1 celery stalk (1)<br>1 Tbsp. natural peanut butter (2.5)<br>**Subtotal 3.5** | ½ cup marinated Jerusalem artichoke (12)<br>2 slices Cheddar cheese (2)<br>**Subtotal 14** | 2 oz. macadamias (4)<br>6 large strawberries (6)<br>**Subtotal 10** |
| **LUNCH** | 4 oz. seitan, sautéed, over (3.5)<br>1 cup mesclun greens (0.5)<br>1 oz. feta cheese (1)<br>¼ cup roasted red peppers (3.5)<br>10 black olives (1.5)<br>¼ cup cooked lentils (6)<br>2 Tbsp. **Italian Dressing** (1)<br>**Subtotal 17** | 2 hard-boiled eggs and (1)<br>2 tofu "bacon" strips (2)<br>½ Haas avocado (2)<br>1 small tomato (2.5)<br>¼ cup scallions on (1)<br>4 cups mixed salad greens (1.5)<br>2 Tbsp. **Blue Cheese Dressing** (1)<br>**Subtotal 11** | 2 veggie burgers on (1)<br>1 low-carb hamburger bun (2)<br>½ Haas avocado (2.5)<br>1 small tomato (1)<br>2 cups mixed salad greens (2.5)<br>4 pieces marinated artichoke hearts (4)<br>5 black olives (1)<br>2 Tbsp. **Italian Dressing** (2)<br>**Subtotal 16** | 4 oz. firm tofu simmered with (4)<br>2 Tbsp. **Barbecue Sauce** (4)<br>½ Haas avocado (2)<br>4 cups mixed salad greens with (2.5)<br>¼ cup edamame (1)<br>½ cup pickled beets (3)<br>2 oz. goat cheese (0.5)<br>2 Tbsp. **Greek Vinaigrette** (1)<br>**Subtotal 17** | 2-egg, egg salad made with (2.5)<br>2 Tbsp. **Blender Mayonnaise** and (2)<br>2 Tbsp. chopped onions and (0)<br>½ cup diced celery on (1.5)<br>1 low-carb pita (3)<br>2 cups mixed salad greens (0.5)<br>¼ cup cooked lentils (6)<br>2 Tbsp. **Parmesan Peppercorn Dressing** (1)<br>**Subtotal 19.5** | ⅓ cup veggie crumbles sautéed and topped with (1)<br>¼ cup shredded mozzarella cheese (0.5)<br>¼ cup refried beans (6.5)<br>1 cup shredded mixed greens (0.5)<br>¼ cup **Salsa Cruda** (1.5)<br>1 low-carb tortilla (1)<br>½ Haas avocado (2)<br>**Subtotal 15** | 3 slices tofu "Canadian bacon" (1.5)<br>2 slices Swiss cheese on (2)<br>1 low-carb bagel (5)<br>1 tsp. Dijon mustard (0.5)<br>½ cup loose-leaf lettuce (0.5)<br>1 cup sliced cucumber (2)<br>¼ cup hummus (9)<br>**Subtotal 20.5** |

## Phase 3, Pre-Maintenance, and Phase 4, Lifetime Maintenance, Vegetarian, at 60 and 70 Grams of Net Carbs (70-gram additions in bold italics)

### SNACK

| Day 1 | Grams of Net Carbs | Day 2 | Grams of Net Carbs | Day 3 | Grams of Net Carbs | Day 4 | Grams of Net Carbs | Day 5 | Grams of Net Carbs | Day 6 | Grams of Net Carbs | Day 7 | Grams of Net Carbs |
|---|---|---|---|---|---|---|---|---|---|---|---|---|---|
| 2 oz. goat cheese | 0.5 | 2 slices Swiss cheese | 2 | Low-carb bar | 2 | ¼ cup sweet cherries | 4 | 4 oz. plain whole milk Greek yogurt | 3.5 | ½ cup jicama sticks | 2.5 | ½ cup red bell pepper | 3 |
| ½ cup blueberries | 8 | ½ cup edamame | 6 | ¼ cup honeydew melon balls | 3.5 | ½ cup cottage cheese | 4 | ¼ cup blueberries | 4 | 2 Tbsp. Parmesan Peppercorn Dressing | 1 | 1 slice Swiss cheese | 1 |
| Subtotal | 8.5 | Subtotal | 8 | Subtotal | 5.5 | Subtotal | 8 | Subtotal | 7.5 | Subtotal | 3.5 | Subtotal | 4 |

### DINNER

| Day 1 | Grams of Net Carbs | Day 2 | Grams of Net Carbs | Day 3 | Grams of Net Carbs | Day 4 | Grams of Net Carbs | Day 5 | Grams of Net Carbs | Day 6 | Grams of Net Carbs | Day 7 | Grams of Net Carbs |
|---|---|---|---|---|---|---|---|---|---|---|---|---|---|
| Stuffed pepper: 1 cup sautéed tempeh in | 3.5 | 5 oz. tofu "sausage" sautéed with | 3.5 | 4 oz. sautéed seitan on | 3.5 | ⅔ cup veggie crumbles sautéed with | 4 | 4 oz. firm tofu sautéed with | 2.5 | 2 tofu "hot dogs" | 5 | 2 Quorn unbreaded cutlets | 6 |
| 2 red bell pepper halves and | 4.5 | ¼ cup onions and | 3 | ½ cup baked acorn squash | 10.5 | 1 cup raw shredded cabbage and | 2 | ¼ cup onions | 3 | ½ cup mashed pumpkin | 5 | 2 Tbsp. **Barbecue Sauce** | 4 |
| 1 Tbsp. soy sauce and topped with | 1 | ½ cup green bell peppers over | 2.5 | 4 cups mixed salad greens | 2 | ¼ cup onions | 3 | ½ cup parsnips | 8.5 | 2 cups mixed salad greens | 1 | 6 asparagus spears | 2.5 |
| ¼ cup shredded Cheddar cheese and baked | 0.5 | ½ cup steamed butternut squash | 7 | ¼ cup cooked chickpeas | 7 | *¼ cup cooked bulgur* | 6.5 | 2 cups mixed salad greens | 1.5 | 2 cups watercress | 0.5 | *½ cup cooked brown rice* | 10.5 |
| 2 cups mixed salad greens | 1 | 2 cups mixed salad greens | 2 | ½ cup jicama | 1 | ½ Haas avocado and | 2 | 2 small tomatoes | 5 | 5 black olives | 0.5 | Salad of 1 cup shredded cabbage and | 2 |
| *1 medium carrot, grated* | 5.5 | *¼ cup cooked wild rice* | 8 | *¼ cup cooked brown rice* | 8 | 1 small tomato | 2.5 | *¼ cup cooked millet* | 10 | 2 Tbsp. **Sweet Mustard Dressing** | 1 | 1 medium carrot, shredded | 5.5 |
| 1 medium tomato | 3.5 | 2 Tbsp. Parmesan Peppercorn Dressing | 1 | 2 Tbsp. Russian Dressing | 0 | 1 Tbsp. Russian Dressing | 0 | 2 Tbsp. Parmesan Peppercorn Dressing | 1 | *¼ cup cooked wild rice* | 8 | 2 Tbsp. **Creamy Coleslaw Dressing** | 0.5 |
| 2 Tbsp. Italian Dressing | 1 | | | | | | | | | | | | |
| Subtotal | 15 (20.5) | Subtotal | 19 (27) | Subtotal | 24.5 (35) | Subtotal | 13.5 (20) | Subtotal | 21.5 (31.5) | Subtotal | 13 (21) | Subtotal | 20 (30.5) |
| Total | 61.5 (67) | Total | 59.5 (67.5) | Total | 61.5 (72) | Total | 61 (67.5) | Total | 60 (70) | Total | 61 (69) | Total | 60.5 (71) |
| Foundation vegetables | 16 | Foundation vegetables | 13 | Foundation vegetables | 14 | Foundation vegetables | 17.5 | Foundation vegetables | 13.5 | Foundation vegetables | 13.5 | Foundation vegetables | 14 |

*www.atkins.com/Recipes/ShowRecipe883/Atkins-Cuisine-Pancakes.aspx, **www.atkins.com/Recipes/ShowRecipe884/Atkins-Cuisine-Waffles.aspx

**Phase 3, Pre-Maintenance, and Phase 4, Lifetime Maintenance, Vegetarian, at 80 and 90 Grams of Net Carbs (90-gram additions in bold italics)**

| | Day 1 | Grams of Net Carbs | Day 2 | Grams of Net Carbs | Day 3 | Grams of Net Carbs | Day 4 | Grams of Net Carbs | Day 5 | Grams of Net Carbs | Day 6 | Grams of Net Carbs | Day 7 | Grams of Net Carbs |
|---|---|---|---|---|---|---|---|---|---|---|---|---|---|---|
| BREAKFAST | ½ cup cottage cheese | 4 | 2 **Atkins Pancakes*** | 6 | Smoothie: ½ cup plain unsweetened almond milk | 0.5 | 2-egg omelet | 1 | 1 **Atkins Waffle**** | 6 | Atkins muesli: 3 Tbsp. oat bran and | 9 | 2 scrambled eggs | 1 |
| | ½ cup blueberries | 8 | ½ cup ricotta cheese | 4 | ½ cup plain whole milk yogurt | 5.5 | ½ cup cooked spinach | 2 | ¼ cup ricotta cheese | 2 | 2 oz. pecans and | 3 | ½ cup sautéed okra | 2.5 |
| | 1 slice low-carb bread | 6 | 1 cup sliced strawberries | 7 | ¼ cup frozen blackberries | 4 | 1 oz. feta cheese | 1 | ¼ cup blueberries | 4 | 2 Tbsp. dried unsweetened coconut | 2 | ¼ cup **Salsa Cruda** | 1 |
| | 1 Tbsp. almond butter | 2.5 | | | 1 oz. almonds | 2.5 | ½ cup cantaloupe melon balls | 7 | 1 oz. slivered almonds | 2.5 | ¼ cup raspberries | 1.5 | ½ cup shredded Cheddar cheese | 1 |
| | | | | | | | | | | | ½ cup plain whole milk yogurt | 5.5 | 1 low-carb tortilla | 4 |
| | **Subtotal** | 20.5 | **Subtotal** | 17 | **Subtotal** | 12.5 | **Subtotal** | 11 | **Subtotal** | 14.5 | **Subtotal** | 21 | **Subtotal** | 9.5 |
| SNACK | 1 oz. pistachios | 2.5 | 2 oz. walnuts | 3 | 2 slices Swiss cheese | 2 | ¼ cup sweet cherries | 4 | 1 celery stalk | 1 | ½ Haas avocado | 2 | 2 oz. macadamias | 4 |
| | 1 medium carrot | 5.5 | ½ cup Crenshaw melon balls | 4.5 | 1 medium carrot | 5.5 | ½ cup cottage cheese | 4 | 1 Tbsp. natural peanut butter | 2.5 | ½ cup Crenshaw melon balls | 4.5 | 6 large strawberries | 6 |
| | | | | | 1 tsp. Dijon mustard | 0.5 | | | | | | | | |
| | **Subtotal** | 8 | **Subtotal** | 7.5 | **Subtotal** | 8 | **Subtotal** | 8 | **Subtotal** | 3.5 | **Subtotal** | 6.5 | **Subtotal** | 10 |
| LUNCH | 4 oz. seitan, sautéed, over | 3.5 | Cobb salad: 2 hard-boiled eggs and | 1 | 2 veggie burgers on | 4 | 4 oz. firm tofu simmered with | 2.5 | 2 deviled eggs | 1 | ⅓ cup veggie crumbles sautéed and topped with | 2 | 3 slices tofu "Canadian bacon" | 1.5 |
| | 1 cup mesclun greens | 0.5 | 2 tofu "bacon" strips on | 2 | 1 low-carb hamburger bun | 4 | 2 Tbsp. **Barbecue Sauce** over | 4 | 2 Tbsp. chopped onion and | 1.5 | ¼ cup shredded mozzarella cheese | 0.5 | 2 slices Swiss cheese on | 2 |
| | ¼ cup hummus | 9 | 4 cups mixed greens with | 1.5 | 2 cups mixed salad greens | 1 | ¼ cup brown rice | 10.5 | ½ cup diced celery in | 0.5 | ¼ cup refried beans | 6.5 | 1 slice 100% whole grain bread | 12 |
| | 1 oz. feta cheese | 1 | ½ Haas avocado | 2 | 4 pieces marinated artichoke hearts | 2 | 4 cups mixed salad greens with | 1.5 | 1 low-carb pita | 4 | 1 cup shredded mixed greens | 0.5 | 1 tsp. Dijon mustard | 0.5 |
| | ½ cup red bell peppers | 3 | 1 small tomato | 2.5 | ½ cup jicama | 2.5 | ¼ cup cooked chickpeas | 6.5 | 2 cups mixed salad greens | 1 | ½ cup corn kernels | 12.5 | ½ cup loose-leaf lettuce | 0.5 |
| | 5 black olives | 0.5 | ¼ cup scallions | 1 | ½ Haas avocado | 2 | ***½ cup pickled beets*** | 7 | ½ cup cooked lentils | 12 | ¼ cup **Salsa Cruda** | 1 | 2 small tomatoes | 5 |
| | 1 medium tomato | 3.5 | ½ cup corn kernels | 12.5 | 1 medium tomato | 3.5 | 2 oz. goat cheese | 0.5 | ***¼ cup cooked wild rice*** | 8 | 1 low-carb tortilla | 4 | ***¼ cup hummus*** | 9 |
| | 2 Tbsp. **Greek Vinaigrette** | 1 | 2 Tbsp. **Blue Cheese Dressing** | 1 | 2 Tbsp. **Italian Dressing** | 1 | 2 Tbsp. **Greek Vinaigrette** | 1 | 2 Tbsp. **Parmesan Peppercorn Dressing** | 1 | | | | |
| | **Subtotal** | 22 | **Subtotal** | 23.5 | **Subtotal** | 20 | **Subtotal** | 26.5 (33.5) | **Subtotal** | 21 (29) | **Subtotal** | 27 | **Subtotal** | 21.5 (30.5) |

## Phase 3, Pre-Maintenance, and Phase 4, Lifetime Maintenance, Vegetarian, at 80 and 90 Grams of Net Carbs (90-gram additions in bold italics)

### Day 1

| | Grams of Net Carbs |
|---|---|
| **SNACK** | |
| 2 oz. goat cheese | 0.5 |
| ½ cup sweet cherries | 8.5 |
| Subtotal | 9 |
| **DINNER** | |
| Stuffed pepper: 1 cup sautéed tempeh and | |
| ¼ cup cooked brown rice with | 3.5 |
| 1 Tbsp. soy sauce baked in | 10 |
| 2 green bell pepper halves topped with | 1 |
| ¼ cup shredded Cheddar cheese | 3.5 |
| *½ cup baked butternut squash* | 0.5 |
| 2 Tbsp. Parmesan Peppercorn Dressing | 7 |
| 2 cups mixed salad greens | 1 |
| 6 radishes | 1 |
| 2 Tbsp. Italian Dressing | 0.5 |
| | 1 |
| Subtotal | 21 (28) |
| Total | 80 (87.5) |
| Foundation vegetables | 12.5 |

### Day 2

| | Grams of Net Carbs |
|---|---|
| **SNACK** | |
| 2 slices Swiss cheese | 2 |
| ½ cup edamame | 6 |
| Subtotal | 8 |
| **DINNER** | |
| 5 oz. tofu "sausage" sautéed with | 5 |
| ¼ cup onions and | 3 |
| ½ cup green bell peppers over | 2 |
| ½ cup steamed butternut squash | 1 |
| 2 cups mixed salad greens | 3.5 |
| 1 medium carrot, grated | 0.5 |
| *¼ cup cooked wild rice* | 7 |
| 2 Tbsp. Parmesan Peppercorn Dressing | 1 |
| Subtotal | 24.5 (32.5) |
| Total | 80.5 (88.5) |
| Foundation vegetables | 13 |

### Day 3

| | Grams of Net Carbs |
|---|---|
| **SNACK** | |
| Low-carb bar | 2 |
| 1 small fig | 6 |
| Subtotal | 8 |
| **DINNER** | |
| 4 oz. sautéed seitan on | 5 |
| ½ cup baked acorn squash | 3 |
| 4 cups mixed salad greens | 2 |
| ½ cup cooked green beans | 7 |
| ½ cup cooked chickpeas | 1 |
| *¼ cup cooked wheat berries* | 5.5 |
| 2 Tbsp. Russian Dressing | 8 |
| Subtotal | 31.5 (38.5) |
| Total | 80.5 (87.5) |
| Foundation vegetables | 15.5 |

### Day 4

| | Grams of Net Carbs |
|---|---|
| **SNACK** | |
| ¼ cup roasted red peppers | 3.5 |
| 2 oz. walnuts | 3 |
| Subtotal | 6.5 |
| **DINNER** | |
| ⅔ cup veggie crumbles sautéed with | 4 |
| ¼ cup onions | 3 |
| 1 cup raw shredded cabbage | 2 |
| ½ cup cooked brown rice | 10.5 |
| Chopped salad of ½ Haas avocado | 3 |
| 1 small tomato | 2.5 |
| ¼ cup corn kernels | 13 |
| 2 Tbsp. Parmesan Peppercorn Dressing | 7 |
| | 0 |
| Subtotal | 31 |
| Total | 83 (90) |
| Foundation vegetables | 16.5 |

### Day 5

| | Grams of Net Carbs |
|---|---|
| **SNACK** | |
| ½ cup plain whole milk yogurt | 5.5 |
| ½ cup Crenshaw melon balls | 4.5 |
| Subtotal | 10 |
| **DINNER** | |
| 4 oz. firm tofu sautéed with | 2.5 |
| ½ cup onions and | 6 |
| 1 cup eggplant | 2 |
| ½ baked sweet potato | 12 |
| 2 cups mixed salad greens | 1.5 |
| 1 small tomato | 2.5 |
| 1 medium carrot, grated | 6 |
| 2 Tbsp. **Carrot-Ginger Dressing** | |
| Subtotal | 33 |
| Total | 82 (90) |
| Foundation vegetables | 15 |

### Day 6

| | Grams of Net Carbs |
|---|---|
| **SNACK** | |
| 1 cup jicama sticks | 5 |
| 2 slices Cheddar cheese | 1 |
| Subtotal | 6 |
| **DINNER** | |
| 2 tofu "hot dogs" | 5 |
| 1 cup sauerkraut | 2.5 |
| *½ baked potato* | 10.5 |
| 2 cups mixed salad greens | 2 |
| 2 cups watercress | 0.5 |
| 5 black olives | 0.5 |
| ¼ cup cooked wild rice | 1.5 |
| 2 Tbsp. **Sweet Mustard Dressing** | 8 |
| | 1 |
| Subtotal | 18.5 (29) |
| Total | 79 (89.5) |
| Foundation vegetables | 13 |

### Day 7

| | Grams of Net Carbs |
|---|---|
| **SNACK** | |
| ½ cup red bell peppers | 3 |
| 2 slices Cheddar cheese | 1 |
| Subtotal | 4 |
| **DINNER** | |
| 2 Quorn unbreaded cutlets | 6 |
| 2 Tbsp. **Barbecue Sauce** | 4 |
| 6 asparagus spears | 2.5 |
| ½ baked sweet potato | 12 |
| Salad of 1 cup shredded cabbage and | 2 |
| 1 medium carrot, grated | 5.5 |
| 2 Tbsp. **Creamy Coleslaw Dressing** | 0.5 |
| Subtotal | 32.5 |
| Total | 77.5 (86.5) |
| Foundation vegetables | 16.5 |

**Phase 3, Pre-Maintenance and Phase 4, Lifetime Maintenance, Vegetarian, at 100 Grams of Net Carbs**

### BREAKFAST

| Day | Food | Grams of Net Carbs |
|---|---|---|
| **Day 1** | ½ cup cottage cheese | 4 |
| | ½ cup blueberries | 8 |
| | 1 slice low-carb bread | 6 |
| | 2 Tbsp. almond butter | 5 |
| | **Subtotal** | **23** |
| **Day 2** | 2 Atkins Pancakes* | 6 |
| | ½ cup ricotta cheese | 4 |
| | 1 cup sliced strawberries | 7 |
| | **Subtotal** | **17** |
| **Day 3** | Smoothie: ½ cup plain unsweetened almond milk | 0.5 |
| | ½ cup plain whole milk yogurt | 5.5 |
| | ¼ cup frozen blackberries | 4 |
| | 1 oz. almonds | 2.5 |
| | **Subtotal** | **12.5** |
| **Day 4** | 2-egg omelet | 1 |
| | ½ cup cooked spinach | 2 |
| | 1 oz. feta cheese | 1 |
| | 1 medium nectarine | 14 |
| | **Subtotal** | **18** |
| **Day 5** | 1 Atkins Waffle** | 6 |
| | ¼ cup ricotta cheese | 2 |
| | 1 orange | 13 |
| | 1 oz. slivered almonds | 2.5 |
| | **Subtotal** | **23.5** |
| **Day 6** | Atkins muesli: 3 Tbsp. oat bran and | 9 |
| | 2 oz. pecans and | 3 |
| | 2 Tbsp. dried unsweetened coconut | 2 |
| | ½ cup raspberries | 3 |
| | ½ cup plain whole milk yogurt | 5.5 |
| | **Subtotal** | **22.5** |
| **Day 7** | 2 scrambled eggs | 1 |
| | ½ cup sautéed okra | 2.5 |
| | ¼ cup Salsa Cruda | 1 |
| | ½ cup shredded Cheddar cheese | 1 |
| | 1 low-carb tortilla | 4 |
| | **Subtotal** | **9.5** |

### SNACK

| Day | Food | Grams of Net Carbs |
|---|---|---|
| **Day 1** | 1 oz. pistachios | 2.5 |
| | 1 medium carrot | 5.5 |
| | **Subtotal** | **8** |
| **Day 2** | 2 oz. walnuts | 2.5 |
| | ½ cup Crenshaw melon balls | 5.5 |
| | **Subtotal** | **8** |
| **Day 3** | 2 slices Swiss cheese | 3 |
| | 1 medium carrot | 4 |
| | 1 tsp. Dijon mustard | 0.5 |
| | **Subtotal** | **7.5** |
| **Day 4** | ¼ cup sweet cherries | 4 |
| | ½ cup cottage cheese | 4 |
| | **Subtotal** | **8** |
| **Day 5** | 1 celery stalk | 1 |
| | 1 Tbsp. natural peanut butter | 2.5 |
| | **Subtotal** | **3.5** |
| **Day 6** | ½ Haas avocado | 2 |
| | 2 small figs | 13 |
| | **Subtotal** | **15** |
| **Day 7** | 2 oz. macadamias | 4 |
| | 1 medium nectarine | 14 |
| | **Subtotal** | **18** |

### LUNCH

| Day | Food | Grams of Net Carbs |
|---|---|---|
| **Day 1** | 4 oz. seitan, sautéed, over | 3.5 |
| | 1 cup mesclun greens | 0.5 |
| | ¼ cup hummus | 9 |
| | 1 oz. feta cheese | 1 |
| | ½ cup red bell peppers | 3 |
| | 5 black olives | 0.5 |
| | 1 medium tomato | 3.5 |
| | 2 Tbsp. Greek Vinaigrette | 1 |
| | **Subtotal** | **22** |
| **Day 2** | Cobb salad: 2 hard-boiled eggs and | 1 |
| | 2 tofu "bacon" strips on | 2 |
| | 4 cups mixed greens with | 2 |
| | ½ Haas avocado | 2 |
| | 1 small tomato | 2.5 |
| | ¼ cup scallions | 0.5 |
| | ¼ cup corn kernels | 12.5 |
| | 2 Tbsp. Blue Cheese Dressing | 1 |
| | **Subtotal** | **23.5** |
| **Day 3** | 2 veggie burgers on | 3.5 |
| | 1 low-carb hamburger bun | 5 |
| | ½ Haas avocado | 2 |
| | 1 medium tomato | 1.5 |
| | 2 cups mixed salad greens | 2 |
| | 4 pieces marinated artichoke hearts | 2.5 |
| | 5 black olives | 0.5 |
| | 2 Tbsp. Italian Dressing | 1 |
| | **Subtotal** | **18** |
| **Day 4** | 4 oz. firm tofu simmered with | 4 |
| | 2 Tbsp. Barbecue Sauce over | 5.5 |
| | ¼ cup brown rice | 10.5 |
| | 4 cups mixed salad greens with | 3.5 |
| | ¼ cup cooked chickpeas | 6.5 |
| | ½ cup pickled beets | 2 |
| | 2 oz. goat cheese | 0.5 |
| | 2 Tbsp. Greek Vinaigrette | 1 |
| | **Subtotal** | **33.5** |
| **Day 5** | 2-egg salad made with | 1 |
| | Blender Mayonnaise and | 0 |
| | 2 Tbsp. chopped onions and | 1.5 |
| | ½ cup diced celery on | 0.5 |
| | 1 low-carb pita | 4 |
| | 2 cups mixed salad greens | 1 |
| | ½ cup cooked lentils | 12 |
| | ¼ cup cooked wild rice | 8 |
| | 2 Tbsp. Parmesan Peppercorn Dressing | 1 |
| | **Subtotal** | **29** |
| **Day 6** | ⅓ cup veggie crumbles sautéed and topped with | 1 |
| | ¼ cup shredded mozzarella cheese | 1.5 |
| | ¼ cup refried beans | 6.5 |
| | 1 cup shredded mixed greens | 0.5 |
| | ¼ cup corn kernels | 12.5 |
| | ¼ cup Salsa Cruda | 1.5 |
| | 1 low-carb tortilla | 4 |
| | **Subtotal** | **27.5** |
| **Day 7** | 3 slices tofu "Canadian bacon" | 1.5 |
| | 2 slices Swiss cheese or | 2 |
| | 1 slice 100% whole grain bread | 12 |
| | 1 tsp. Dijon mustard | 0.5 |
| | ¼ cup loose-leaf lettuce | 0.5 |
| | 2 small tomatoes | 5 |
| | ¼ cup hummus | 9 |
| | **Subtotal** | **30.5** |

**Phase 3, Pre-Maintenance and Phase 4, Lifetime Maintenance, Vegetarian, at 100 Grams of Net Carbs**

| | Day 1 | Grams of Net Carbs | Day 2 | Grams of Net Carbs | Day 3 | Grams of Net Carbs | Day 4 | Grams of Net Carbs | Day 5 | Grams of Net Carbs | Day 6 | Grams of Net Carbs | Day 7 | Grams of Net Carbs |
|---|---|---|---|---|---|---|---|---|---|---|---|---|---|---|
| SNACK | 2 oz. goat cheese | 0.5 | 2 slices Swiss cheese | 2 | Low-carb bar | 2 | ¼ cup roasted red peppers | 3.5 | ½ cup plain whole milk yogurt | 5.5 | 1 cup jicama sticks | 5 | 1 cup red bell peppers | 6 |
| | ½ medium apple | 8.5 | ½ cup red grapes | 13.5 | 1 small Bosc pear | 17.5 | 2 oz. walnuts | 3 | ½ cup Crenshaw melon balls | 4.5 | 2 slices Cheddar cheese | 1 | 2 slices Cheddar cheese | 1 |
| | **Subtotal** | 9 | **Subtotal** | 15.5 | **Subtotal** | 19.5 | **Subtotal** | 6.5 | **Subtotal** | 10 | **Subtotal** | 6 | **Subtotal** | 7 |
| DINNER | Stuffed pepper: 1 cup sautéed tempeh and | 3.5 | 5 oz. tofu "sausage" sautéed with | 5 | 4 oz. sautéed seitan on | 3.5 | ⅔ cup veggie crumbles sautéed with | 4 | 4 oz. firm tofu sautéed with | 2.5 | 2 tofu "hot dogs" | 5 | 2 Quorn unbreaded cutlets | 6 |
| | ½ cup cooked brown rice baked with | 20 | ¼ cup onions and | 3 | ½ cup baked acorn squash | 7 | ¼ cup chopped onions | 3 | ½ cup onions and | 6 | 1 cup sauerkraut | 2.5 | 2 Tbsp. **Barbecue Sauce** | 4 |
| | 1 Tbsp. soy sauce in | 1 | ½ cup green bell peppers over | 3 | 4 cups mixed salad greens | 1.5 | 1 cup raw shredded cabbage | 2 | 1 cup eggplant | 2 | ½ baked potato | 10.5 | 6 asparagus spears | 2.5 |
| | 2 green bell pepper halves topped with | 3.5 | ¾ cup steamed butternut squash | 10.5 | ½ cup cooked green beans | 3 | ½ cup cooked brown rice | 10.5 | ½ baked sweet potato | 12 | 2 cups mixed salad greens | 1 | ½ baked sweet potato | 12 |
| | ¼ cup shredded Cheddar cheese | 0.5 | 2 cups mixed salad greens | 1 | ½ cup cooked cannellini beans | 17 | Chopped salad of ½ Haas avocado | 2 | 2 cups mixed salad greens | 1.5 | 2 cups watercress | 0.5 | Salad of 1 cup shredded cabbage and | 2 |
| | ½ cup baked butternut squash | 7 | 1 medium carrot, grated | 5.5 | ½ cup jicama | 2.5 | 2 small tomatoes | 5 | 1 small tomato | 2.5 | 5 black olives | 0.5 | 1 medium carrot, grated | 5.5 |
| | 2 cups mixed salad greens | 1 | ¼ cup cooked wild rice | 8 | ¼ cup cooked wheat berries | 7 | ¼ cup corn kernels | 6 | 1 medium carrot, grated | 5.5 | ¼ cup cooked wild rice | 8 | 2 Tbsp. **Creamy Coleslaw Dressing** | 0.5 |
| | 6 radishes | 0.5 | 2 Tbsp. **Parmesan Peppercorn Dressing** | 1 | 2 Tbsp. **Russian Dressing** | 0 | 2 Tbsp. **Parmesan Peppercorn Dressing** | 1 | 2 Tbsp. **Carrot-Ginger Dressing** | 1 | 2 Tbsp. **Sweet Mustard Dressing** | 1 | | |
| | 2 Tbsp. **Italian Dressing** | 1 | | | | | | | | | | | | |
| | **Subtotal** | 38 | **Subtotal** | 37 | **Subtotal** | 41.5 | **Subtotal** | 33.5 | **Subtotal** | 33 | **Subtotal** | 29 | **Subtotal** | 32.5 |
| | **Total** | 100 | **Total** | 100.5 | **Total** | 99.5 | **Total** | 99.5 | **Total** | 99 | **Total** | 100 | **Total** | 97.5 |
| | **Foundation vegetables** | 12.5 | **Foundation vegetables** | 14 | **Foundation vegetables** | 16 | **Foundation vegetables** | 19 | **Foundation vegetables** | 16 | **Foundation vegetables** | 13.5 | **Foundation vegetables** | 19 |

*www.atkins.com/Recipes/ShowRecipe883/Atkins-Cuisine-Pancakes.aspx, **www.atkins.com/Recipes/ShowRecipe884/Atkins-Cuisine-Waffles.aspx

## Phase 2, Ongoing Weight Loss, Vegan, at 50 Grams of Net Carbs

| Day 1 | Grams of Net Carbs | Day 2 | Grams of Net Carbs | Day 3 | Grams of Net Carbs | Day 4 | Grams of Net Carbs | Day 5 | Grams of Net Carbs | Day 6 | Grams of Net Carbs | Day 7 | Grams of Net Carbs |
|---|---|---|---|---|---|---|---|---|---|---|---|---|---|
| **BREAKFAST** | | | | | | | | | | | | | |
| 4 oz. tofu "scrambled eggs" | 2 | 3 slices tofu Canadian "bacon" | 2 | 1 vegan burger | 2 | 3 tofu "link sausages" | 6 | 4 oz. tofu "scrambled eggs" | 4 | 2 tofu "bacon" strips | 2 | Smoothie: 1 cup plain unsweetened almond milk and | 2 |
| 2 cups Swiss chard sautéed with | 1 | 1/4 cup refried beans | 6.5 | 1 slice vegan "cheese" | 6 | 1/2 cup baked chayote squash | 6 | 1 small tomato | 2 | 1/2 cup sautéed okra | 2.5 | 3 oz. silken soft tofu and | 1.5 |
| 1/4 cup chopped onion | 1.5 | 1/4 cup vegan "Cheddar cheese" | 1.5 | 1/2 Haas avocado | 2 | 8 oz. unsweetened almond milk | 2 | 1/2 Haas avocado | 2 | 1 slice vegan "cheese" | 6 | 1/4 cup frozen strawberries | 3 |
| 2 Tbsp. grated vegan "Parmesan cheese" | 3 | | | 1/4 cup blueberries | 4 | | | 1 Tbsp. grated vegan "Parmesan cheese" | 1 | | | | |
| Subtotal | 7.5 | Subtotal | 10 | Subtotal | 14 | Subtotal | 14 | Subtotal | 9 | Subtotal | 10.5 | Subtotal | 6.5 |
| **SNACK** | | | | | | | | | | | | | |
| 1/4 cup edamame | 3 | 2 Tbsp. vegan "cream cheese" | 2 | 8 oz. unsweetened almond milk | 2 | 1/4 cup boysenberries | 3 | 10 green olives, stuffed with | 2 | 1 small tomato | 2 | 2 celery stalks | 2.5 |
| 2 slices vegan "cheese" | 12 | 1/2 cup cucumber sliced | 1 | 2 oz. pecans | 1 | 2 oz. hazelnuts | 1 | 2 Tbsp. vegan "cream cheese" | 2 | 10 black olives | 0 | 1/4 cup guacamole | 1.5 |
| Subtotal | 15 | Subtotal | 3 | Subtotal | 3 | Subtotal | 4 | Subtotal | 4 | Subtotal | 2 | Subtotal | 4 |
| **LUNCH** | | | | | | | | | | | | | |
| 4 oz. firm tofu sautéed with | 2.5 | 2/3 cup veggie crumbles sautéed and topped with | 3.5 | 1/2 cup tempeh sautéed with | 6.5 | 2 slices vegan deli "ham" over | 2 | 2 slices vegan deli "turkey" and | 6 | 2 vegan burgers | 4 | 2 tofu "hot dogs" with | 4 |
| 1/2 cup green bell peppers and | 2 | 1/4 cup Salsa Cruda | 1.5 | 1/4 cup chopped onion and | 3 | 4 cups mixed salad greens and | 3 | 1 slice vegan "Swiss cheese" with | 1 | 1/2 Haas avocado | 6 | 1/4 cup sautéed onions | 2 |
| 1/2 cup scallions and | 2.5 | 4 cups mixed salad greens with | 1.5 | 1/2 cup chopped celery | 0.5 | 1/2 cup red bell peppers and | 0.5 | 1/4 cup Basil Pesto on | 3 | 2 Tbsp. hummus | 4.5 | 2 cups mixed salad greens | 4.5 |
| 1 Tbsp. soy sauce | 1 | 1/2 cup pickled okra and | 2.5 | 2 cups mixed salad greens | 1.5 | 1/4 cup cooked black beans | 6.5 | 1 low-carb pita | 6.5 | 1 cup loose-leaf lettuce | 1 | 1 small tomato | 1 |
| 2 cups Romaine lettuce | 1 | 4 pieces marinated artichoke hearts | 2 | 1/4 cup cooked lentils and | 2.5 | 1 small tomato | 1 | 2 cups mixed salad greens | 2.5 | 2 Tbsp. chopped onions | 4 | 1/4 cup cooked chickpeas | 6.5 |
| 2 Tbsp. Fresh Raspberry Vinaigrette | 1 | 5 black olives | 0.5 | 6 radishes | 1 | 2 Tbsp. Sweet Mustard Dressing | 0.5 | 5 black olives | 0.5 | 1 Tbsp. Italian Dressing | 0.5 | 2 Tbsp. Sweet Mustard Dressing | 1 |
| | | 2 Tbsp. Russian Dressing | 0.5 | 2 Tbsp. Sweet Mustard Dressing | 0.5 | | | 2 Tbsp. Italian Dressing | 1 | | | | |
| Subtotal | 10 | Subtotal | 12 | Subtotal | 15.5 | Subtotal | 13.5 | Subtotal | 20.5 | Subtotal | 19.5 | Subtotal | 20 |

## Phase 2, Ongoing Weight Loss, Vegan, at 50 Grams of Net Carbs

### Day 1

| | Grams of Net Carbs |
|---|---|
| **SNACK** | |
| 10 green olives | 0 |
| 2 oz. almonds | 4.5 |
| **Subtotal** | **4.5** |
| **DINNER** | |
| 5 veggie "meatballs" sautéed with | 4 |
| 1 cup shirataki soy noodles topped with | 2 |
| 3 Tbsp. **Romesco Sauce** | 2 |
| ½ cup steamed green beans | 2 |
| 2 cups mixed salad greens and | 1 |
| ½ cup sliced cucumber | 1 |
| 1 small tomato | 2.5 |
| 2 Tbsp. **Sweet Mustard Dressing** | 1 |
| **Subtotal** | **13.5** |
| **Total** | **50.5** |
| **Foundation vegetables** | **14.5** |

### Day 2

| | Grams of Net Carbs |
|---|---|
| **SNACK** | |
| 2 oz. walnuts | 3 |
| ¼ cup Crenshaw melon balls | 2.5 |
| **Subtotal** | **5.5** |
| **DINNER** | |
| 4 oz. firm tofu baked with | 2.5 |
| 1 Tbsp. **Barbecue Sauce** | 2 |
| ½ cup steamed green beans | 3 |
| 2 cups mixed salad greens and | 1 |
| 1 small tomato | 1 |
| ¼ cup cooked chickpeas | 6.5 |
| 2 Tbsp. **Italian Dressing** | 1 |
| **Subtotal** | **16** |
| **Total** | **50.5** |
| **Foundation vegetables** | **13** |

### Day 3

| | Grams of Net Carbs |
|---|---|
| **SNACK** | |
| 10 green olives | 0 |
| 1 slice vegan "cheese" | 5 |
| **Subtotal** | **5** |
| **DINNER** | |
| 4 oz. baked tofu and | 2.5 |
| 1 cup shirataki soy noodles topped with | 2 |
| ¼ cup **Basil Pesto** | 2 |
| 1 cup braised fennel | 3 |
| 2 cups mixed salad greens and | 1 |
| 1 small tomato | 1 |
| 2 Tbsp. **Sweet Mustard Dressing** | 6.5 |
| **Subtotal** | **16** |
| **Total** | **51.5** |
| **Foundation vegetables** | **13.5** |

### Day 4

| | Grams of Net Carbs |
|---|---|
| **SNACK** | |
| ½ cup jicama sticks | 2.5 |
| 2 Tbsp. hummus | 4.5 |
| **Subtotal** | **7** |
| **DINNER** | |
| ½ cup tempeh sautéed with | 3.5 |
| ½ cup okra and | 2 |
| ½ cup button mushrooms and | 3 |
| 2 Tbsp. chopped onions | 1.5 |
| 2 cups mixed salad greens | 1 |
| ½ Haas avocado | 2.5 |
| 2 Tbsp. **Russian Dressing** | 0 |
| **Subtotal** | **13** |
| **Total** | **52** |
| **Foundation vegetables** | **19.5** |

### Day 5

| | Grams of Net Carbs |
|---|---|
| **SNACK** | |
| 2 oz. hazelnuts | 1 |
| 6 radishes | 0.5 |
| **Subtotal** | **1.5** |
| **DINNER** | |
| 4 pieces sautéed seitan | 8 |
| ½ cup steamed string beans | 3 |
| ½ cup mashed pumpkin | 5 |
| 2 cups mixed salad greens | 1 |
| 6 radishes | 0.5 |
| ¼ cup edamame | 3 |
| 2 Tbsp. **Russian Dressing** | 0 |
| **Subtotal** | **20.5** |
| **Total** | **50** |
| **Foundation vegetables** | **16** |

### Day 6

| | Grams of Net Carbs |
|---|---|
| **SNACK** | |
| 1 oz. almonds | 2.5 |
| ¼ cup raspberries | 1.5 |
| **Subtotal** | **4** |
| **DINNER** | |
| ⅔ cup veggie crumbles sautéed with | 4 |
| 2 cups bok choy | 1 |
| ½ cup red bell peppers | 3 |
| ¼ cup cooked chickpeas | 6.5 |
| Salad of 1 cup shredded green cabbage with | 2 |
| 1 oz. chopped peanuts and | 1.5 |
| 2 Tbsp. **Coleslaw Dressing** | 0.5 |
| **Subtotal** | **19** |
| **Total** | **50.5** |
| **Foundation vegetables** | **17** |

### Day 7

| | Grams of Net Carbs |
|---|---|
| **SNACK** | |
| 2 oz. walnuts | 3 |
| 1 slice vegan "Cheddar cheese" | 5 |
| **Subtotal** | **8** |
| **DINNER** | |
| 4 veggie "meatballs" and | 4 |
| 3 Tbsp. **Romesco Sauce** over | 2 |
| ½ cup spaghetti squash | 4 |
| ½ cup steamed broccoli | 1.5 |
| 2 cups mixed salad greens | 1 |
| 10 black olives | 1.5 |
| 2 Tbsp. **Russian Dressing** | 0 |
| **Subtotal** | **14** |
| **Total** | **51.5** |
| **Foundation vegetables** | **19.5** |

# Part IV

# A DIET FOR LIFE:

The Science of Good Health

# Chapter 13

# METABOLIC SYNDROME AND CARDIOVASCULAR HEALTH

The words *healthy* and *low fat* seem inextricably linked, but the rationale for a low-fat diet is based on two overly simplistic ideas that we now understand to be incorrect.

In this and the following chapter, we'll highlight how carbohydrate-restricted approaches can address cardiovascular disease (and metabolic syndrome) and diabetes and look at the impressive body of research in both these areas. (You may want to share these chapters with your health care professional.)

One in four deaths in the United States stems from heart disease, making it the leading cause of death for both women and men. Heart disease develops over decades, and a poor diet can aggravate and accelerate its progression. Whether you have a strong family history of heart disease or you're blessed with cardioprotective genes, you can improve your quality of life by adopting a healthy diet that targets some of the known modifiable risk factors.

Although the majority of the medical establishment has focused on LDL cholesterol, an increased understanding of the progression of heart disease has directed attention and appreciation toward other risk factors. For example did you know that LDL cholesterol is actually a family of particles of various sizes and that the smallest particles are the most dangerous ones? The Atkins Diet eradicates small LDL particles like a strategic missile defense system. You'll soon understand the significance of this fact for both cardiovascular disease and metabolic syndrome.

Before we go any further, two brief definitions are in order. In simple terms, metabolic syndrome is a collection of markers that amplifies your risk for heart disease, including high blood triglyceride level, low HDL cholesterol level, and elevated glucose and insulin levels. Likewise, in simple terms, inflammation is a catchall word that encompasses the processes by which your body protects you from unfamiliar and potentially damaging substances. As part of your body's natural defense system, a certain amount of inflammation is healthy, especially when it responds to infection, irritation, or injury. But once the battle has been fought, inflammation should return to normal levels. Unchecked inflammation, which can be detected during the early phases of heart disease by elevated levels of C-reactive protein (CRP), is now understood to be one of the best predictors of future heart problems. Levels of triglycerides, HDL cholesterol, glucose, and insulin are also important markers that provide a complete picture of your overall risk status. We'll explore both conditions in detail below.

This chapter will explore the ascendancy of scientific studies supporting the effectiveness of diets low in carbohydrate as a way to achieve cardiovascular heath. This is true even though you'll be eating plenty of fat. If you've read the rest of this book, we can assume that you've put aside any fear of fat. In case you still have any lingering anxiety, however, the following pages will convince you otherwise. First, however, let's consider the rationale for a low-fat diet and issue a report card.

## ARE LOW-FAT DIETS A MAJOR SUCCESS OR A SERIOUS DISTRACTION?

Most of you know that for the last few decades, the government agencies concerned with health care have beamed forth a strong and unwavering message: reduce your total fat, saturated fat, and cholesterol intake to achieve a healthy weight and decrease heart disease. The message has been so unrelenting that the terms "healthy" and "low fat" seem inextricably linked, but the rationale for a low-fat diet is based on two overly simplistic ideas that we now understand to be incorrect.

First, fat contains 9 Calories per gram, more than twice the 4 Calories per gram of both protein and carbohydrate. Since fat is more calorically dense, reducing intake of it should be the easiest way to promote weight loss, while still allowing you to eat a greater total volume of food and thus feel satisfied. This logic is expressed in the axiom "You are what you eat." In other words, if you eat fat, you must get fat. The corollary is that if you eat less fat, then you'll easily lose body fat. Many Americans have embraced this seemingly intuitive strategy hook, line, and sinker, only to find themselves drowning in disappointment.

As a nation, our consumption of total fat and saturated fat has remained relatively steady and even trended slightly downward over the last two decades. So why are we experiencing frightening twin epidemics of obesity and diabetes? And why has metabolic syndrome become a significant health threat to tens of millions of Americans? Not because we failed to pay attention to dietary recommendations focused on lowering fat. Rather, we replaced fat calories with an abundance of carbohydrate calories, without understanding that many people have a metabolism that cannot process the additional carbohydrate. Basically, the low-fat approach has backfired.

A second reason for the major emphasis on reducing dietary fat, saturated fat, and cholesterol is based on the belief that consumption of fatty foods will lead to increased blood cholesterol levels, which, in turn, will increase the incidence of heart disease. This belief system, often called the "diet-heart hypothesis," has shaped nutrition policy in this country for the last forty years. Despite decades of research and billions of taxpayer dollars earmarked to prove this hypothesis, there's little evidence to support its basic premise.

The largest and most expensive study on the role of fat in the diet was the Women's Health Initiative, a randomized, controlled trial in which almost 50,000 postmenopausal women aged 50 to 79 were tracked for an average of eight years. Researchers assigned participants either to a low-fat diet that reduced total fat intake and increased the intake of vegetables, fruits, and grains, or to a control group who could eat whatever they wanted. Multiple research papers reported on the results of this colossal experiment, which can be summarized as nothing short of a major public health disappointment. A low-fat eating pattern revealed no significant effect on weight loss or the incidence of heart disease, diabetes, or cancer.[1] You can see why the low-fat dietary approach to weight control gets a failing grade.

## METABOLIC SYNDROME

As waistlines expand, so does the epidemic of metabolic syndrome. It's estimated that nearly one of every four American adults has this condition,[2] which puts them on the fast track to developing type 2 diabetes and triples their risk for developing heart disease. The identification of metabolic syndrome two decades ago[3] is now recognized as a turning point in our understanding of metabolism as it plays out in the clinical states of obesity, diabetes, and cardiovascular disease. As a theory, metabolic syndrome represents an alternative and conflicting paradigm to the diet-heart hypothesis because elevated LDL cholesterol is typically not a problem in metabolic syndrome. More important, the most effective treatment for metabolic syndrome is restriction of carbohydrate, not fat. Restricting dietary fat and replacing it with carbohydrate actually exacerbates many of the problems of metabolic syndrome. The metabolic syndrome paradigm has therefore caused a great deal of distress—and pushback—among those advocating low-fat diets.

Metabolic syndrome involves a cluster of markers that predispose people to diabetes and heart disease. Because metabolic syndrome includes the presence of more than one of several potential markers, the public health community has struggled with the decision of how best to define, diagnose, and treat it. Obesity is a common characteristic, particularly excessive fat in the waist and stomach area, which makes a person look "apple-shaped." Problems with fat metabolism manifest as high plasma levels of triglycerides, and although a patient's LDL cholesterol is usually within the normal range, the *size* of the LDL particles tends to be the small, more dangerous type. High blood pressure is another common marker, as is elevated blood glucose. Additional markers include chronically elevated inflammation and abnormal blood vessel function (see the sidebar "Do You Have Metabolic Syndrome?").

## DO YOU HAVE METABOLIC SYNDROME?

A person is defined as having metabolic syndrome if he or she has three or more of the following markers.[4]

|  | Men | Women |
|---|---|---|
| Waist Circumference | ≥ 40 inches | ≥ 35 inches |
| Triglycerides | ≥ 150 mg/dL* | ≥ 150 mg/dL |
| HDL cholesterol | ≤ 40 mg/dL | ≤ 50 mg/dL |
| Blood pressure | ≥ 130/85 mm Hg or use of medication for hypertension | ≥ 130/85 mm Hg or use of medication for hypertension |
| Fasting glucose | ≥ 100 mg/dL or use of medication for high blood glucose | ≥ 100 mg/dL or use of medication for high blood glucose |

*Milligrams per deciliter.

Why do the diverse problems that characterize metabolic syndrome tend to show up? The prevailing opinion is that all of them are signs of insulin resistance, which is defined as the diminished ability of a given concentration of insulin to exert its normal biological effect. When insulin resistance develops, it has broad effects on a variety of metabolic pathways that can lead to the specific markers for metabolic syndrome. But not everyone responds to insulin resistance in the same way; moreover, the time frame in which certain signs develop varies. This variability makes defining—and treating—metabolic syndrome tricky.

Treatment of metabolic syndrome is controversial, with nutritional approaches generally downplayed in favor of multiple medications that target the individual components. Conventional recommendations tend to emphasize caloric restriction and reduced fat intake, even though metabolic syndrome can best be described as carbohydrate intolerance. Think of it as the first signs of the metabolic bully leaving marks. Low-carbohydrate diets therefore make intuitive sense as a first-line treatment. Let's take a closer look at how they impact the various features of both metabolic syndrome and heart disease.[5]

## GLUCOSE AND INSULIN

Increased glucose levels are a signal that the body may be having trouble processing dietary carbohydrate. High insulin levels usually go hand in hand with elevated fasting glucose levels. (See "Understanding Blood Sugar Readings" on page 297.) Dietary carbohydrate contributes directly to blood glucose levels and is well accepted as the major stimulator of insulin secretion. Lowering carbohydrate intake is the most direct method to achieve better control of both glucose and insulin levels. Could it really be that simple? Yes, it is. The insulin resistance of metabolic syndrome is characterized by intolerance to carbohydrate. If you have lactose intolerance, you avoid lactose. If you have gluten intolerance, you avoid gluten. You get the idea.

Not surprising, many studies of low-carbohydrate diets have shown that glucose levels improve significantly in subjects following them.[6] Insulin levels also decrease, regardless of glucose tolerance status and even in the absence of weight loss.[7] The reduction in insulin levels throughout the day, even after meals, is crucial to promoting a metabolic environment that favors fat burning. In this way, controlling carbohydrate intake has an important effect on the way the body handles fat, along with profound effects on lipid and cholesterol levels. But before we discuss the research on lipids, a quick tutorial on insulin is in order.

## HOW INSULIN WORKS

The pancreas makes and releases the hormone insulin in response to increases in blood glucose. Its most recognized function is to restore glucose levels to normal by facilitating the transport of blood glucose into (mainly) muscle and fat cells. However, insulin has a multitude of other effects and is generally described as the "storage hormone" because it promotes the storage of protein, fat, and carbohydrate. For example, insulin facilitates the conversion of amino acids into protein and also promotes the conversion of dietary carbohydrate into either glycogen (the storage form of carbohydrate in the body) or fat. While insulin promotes the storage of nutrients, it simultaneously blocks the breakdown of protein, fat, and carbohydrate in the body. Put another way, when insulin is increased, it puts the brakes on burning fat for fuel and at the same time encourages storage of incoming food, mostly as fat. But when you limit your carbohydrate consumption, you stimulate increased fat burning and decreased fat synthesis.

In fact, fat breakdown and fat burning are exquisitely sensitive to changes in the amount of insulin released in response to dietary carbohydrate.[8] Small decreases in insulin can almost immediately increase fat burning severalfold. Insulin also increases glucose uptake and activates key enzymes that transform glucose into fat. Because low-carbohydrate diets significantly blunt insulin levels throughout the day, the Atkins Diet is associated with significant changes in fat metabolism that favor decreased storage and increased breakdown. Translation: you burn more body fat and store less. This is an important adaptation that contributes to a decreased risk for heart disease with better lipid profiles and improvement in all features of metabolic syndrome. This is why dietary fat is your friend and consuming carbohydrate above your tolerance level acts as a metabolic bully.

## CONTROL CARBS TO BURN FAT

Controlling carbohydrate intake and the subsequent decline in insulin levels permits most of the body's cells to use fat almost exclusively for energy, even while an individual is exercising.[9] During Induction and OWL, body fat provides a large share of that energy. During Pre-Maintenance and Lifetime Maintenance, the diet provides most of the needed fuel. Either way, the final effect of the core principle of the Atkins Diet, keeping carb intake at or just below one's individual carb threshold, is the creation of a metabolic state characterized by enhanced mobilization and utilization of both dietary and body fat. Many of the beneficial effects of the Atkins Diet on risk factors for metabolic syndrome and heart disease are extensions of this powerful transformation.

## THE SATURATED FAT PARADOX

Now that you know that you shouldn't avoid dietary fat on a low-carbohydrate diet, you might still have some skepticism about eating saturated fat. After all, just about every health expert would advise you to limit it, and one of the major criticisms of the Atkins Diet is that it contains more saturated fat than is currently recommended. Let us put your mind at rest.

When one nutrient in the diet decreases, usually one or more other nutrients replace it. In fact, researchers have explored the question of what happens when you reduce saturated fat in the diet and replace it with carbohydrate. A recent metastudy made up of eleven American and European cohort studies that followed more than 340,000 subjects for up to ten years came to the conclusion that replacing saturated fat with carbohydrate increases the risk of coronary events.[10] Yes, according to the best scientific evidence, the very recommendation made by most health experts to reduce saturated fat actually *increases* your chances of having heart disease. Yet this is the same dietary pattern adopted by many Americans.[11] The failure of low-fat dietary approaches is partially explained by the lack of understanding that many people consume more carbohydrates when they lower their saturated fat intake. The culprit is not saturated fat per se. If your carbohydrate intake is low, there's little reason to worry about saturated fat in your diet.

However, if your carbohydrate intake is high, increasing the levels of saturated fat in your diet may become problematic. Higher levels of saturated fatty acids in the blood have been shown to occur in individuals with heart disease.[12] As you now know, the Atkins Diet is all about controlling your carbohydrate intake to ensure that fat remains your body's primary fuel. This explains why, on Atkins, saturated fat intake is not associated with harmful effects. Two of the authors of this book explored what happens to saturated fat levels in subjects who were placed on the Atkins Diet.[13] In this experiment, the Atkins subjects consumed three times the levels of saturated fat as did subjects consuming a low-fat diet. Both diets contained the same number of calories, meaning that all the subjects were losing weight.

After twelve weeks, the Atkins group subjects showed consistently greater reductions in the relative proportion of saturated fat in their blood.

This inverse association between dietary intake and blood concentrations of saturated fat prompted further experiments to validate the effect under controlled conditions. The additional study involved weight-stable men who habitually consumed a typical American diet. They followed a low-carbohydrate diet akin to the Lifetime Maintenance Phase, which contained more saturated fat than did their regular diet. All foods were prepared and provided to the subjects during each feeding period. Enough food was provided to maintain their weight. After six weeks on the diet, despite consuming more saturated fat, the men showed a significant reduction in their blood levels of saturated fat. They also improved their triglyceride and HDL cholesterol levels, LDL particle size, and insulin level. This study further supports the conclusion that low dietary carbohydrate is a key stimulus positively impacting the metabolic processing of ingested saturated fat.[14]

These studies clearly show that low-carbohydrate diets high in saturated fat show effects that are very different from results in studies of individuals following a moderate- to high-carbohydrate diet. The likely cause is a combination of less storage and greater burning of saturated fat. This research supports the conclusion that dietary fat, even saturated fat, isn't harmful in the context of a low-carbohydrate diet.[15]

## A LONG HISTORY OF SAFE USE

An equally valid indication of the long-term safety of low carbohydrate diets can be found in the documented experience of Europeans as they explored the North American continent and its established cultures. Very often, the most successful explorers were those who adopted the diet of the indigenous cultures, which in many regions consisted mostly of meat and fat with little carbohydrate. Examples of explorers who documented such experiences include Lewis and Clarke, John Rae,[16] Frederick Schwatka,[17] and even Daniel Boone.

The explorer whose experience living as a hunter was the most carefully documented was the controversial anthropologist Vilhjalmur Stefansson. After spending a decade in the Arctic among the Inuit in the early 1900s, he wrote extensively about their diet around the same time that scientists discovered the existence of vitamins. Challenged to prove that he could remain healthy on a diet of meat and fat, he ate an Inuit diet under close medical observation for a year. The result, published in a prestigious scientific journal,[18] demonstrated that Stefansson remained well and physically capable while consuming a diet of more than 80 percent animal fat and about 15 percent protein.

In addition to recounting some remarkable stories of physical stamina and courage, the reports of these explorers provide valuable insight into the dietary practices of aboriginal hunting societies that lived for millennia on little or no dietary carbohydrate. Of particular importance was the practice of valuing fat over protein, so that the preferred mix of dietary energy was high in fat and moderate in protein. Also of note: Rae, Boone, and Stefansson all lived into their eighties, despite eating mostly meat and fat for years.

Though these historical lessons don't, in and of themselves, prove the long-term safety of low-carbohydrate diets, they constitute strong supporting evidence. When this accumulated history of safe use is combined with our recent research into the effects of carbohydrate restriction on blood lipids and indicators of inflammation, the inescapable conclusion is that a properly formulated low-carbohydrate diet can be safely utilized for months or even years.

## RESEARCH ON SEIZURE CONTROL

In the early 1920s, physicians observed that people subject to epileptic seizures experienced relief when they were placed on a total fast for two weeks. However the benefits of this treatment didn't continue when eating resumed, and a complete fast causes muscle wasting, so this was obviously not a sustainable treatment. But in a series of reports, a Minnesota physician, Mynie Peterman, demonstrated that a very-low-carb diet produced a similar effect in children, reducing or stopping their seizures, and that this diet could be effectively followed for years.[19]

In 1927, Dr. Henry Helmholz reported on more than one hundred cases of childhood seizures treated with Dr. Peterman's ketogenic diet.[20] His results indicated that about one-third of the children were cured of seizures, one-third improved, and one-third didn't respond to the treatment. A ketogenic diet remained the "standard of care" for seizure disorders until effective antiseizure drugs were developed in the 1950s. Between 1922 and 1944, doctors at the Mayo Clinic in Minnesota prescribed the ketogenic diet to 729 seizure patients, with success rates similar to those originally reported by Dr. Peterman.[21] Most of these patients stayed on the diet for a year or two, but some continued it for more than three decades.

The development of antiseizure drugs with similar efficacy rates superseded the ketogenic diet between 1960 and 1980. Although the diet is equally effective, it's far easier for a doctor to write a prescription for a drug than to educate and motivate an individual or family to make a major dietary change. In the 1990s, Dr. John Freeman at Johns Hopkins University revived the ketogenic diet and reported that many children whose seizures didn't respond to drugs did respond to the low-carb diet. With Dr. Eric Kossoff, Dr. Freeman also noted that children experienced fewer side effects from the low-carbohydrate diet than they did from the antiseizure drugs. For example, not surprisingly, their school performance was better when they were off the drugs. These observations have led to a resurgence of interest in low-carbohydrate diets to treat both children and adults suffering from seizures.[22] Today, more than seventy clinics in the United States report the use of this dietary treatment for seizures.

## INDICATORS OF IMPROVEMENT

Now let's take a closer look at some of the most common markers improved by low-carbohydrate diets.

### TRIGLYCERIDES

Much of the fat circulating in your blood, and much of that available to be burned as fuel, is in the form of triglycerides. Increased blood levels of triglycerides are a key feature of metabolic syndrome and have been shown to be an independent risk factor for heart disease. One of the most dramatic and consistent effects of lowering carbohydrate consumption is a reduction in triglyceride levels. In fact, the decline rivals that produced by any current drugs. Most studies focus on fasting levels of triglycerides, but after a meal, fat is packaged into triglycerides within the gastrointestinal tract that are dumped into your blood. The liver can also pump out triglycerides after a meal, especially one high in carbohydrate. People who have an exaggerated and prolonged elevation of blood triglycerides, whether from a high-fat or high-carbohydrate meal, have been shown to be at increased risk for heart disease. The good news is that low-carbohydrate diets consistently decrease triglycerides both in the fasting state *and* in response to meals.[23] Interestingly, this beneficial effect occurs even when weight loss is minimal.[24]

### HDL CHOLESTEROL

The clinical significance of increased HDL levels is well established as an important target for good health.[25] Higher levels are desirable because this lipoprotein offers protection against heart disease. Typical lifestyle changes such as exercise and weight loss are often recommended to increase HDL, but their effects are small compared to those achieved by following a low-carbohydrate diet, which consistently outperform low-fat diets in raising HDL levels.[26] The effects are prominent in men and even more so in women.[27] Dietary saturated fat and cholesterol are actually important nutrients that contribute to an increase in HDL cholesterol levels. Replacing carbohydrate with fat has also been shown to increase HDL.

## KETONES: WHAT ARE THEY, AND WHAT DO THEY DO?

Antiseizure diets are often referred to as ketogenic diets because restricting carbohydrates requires that the body use an alternative to glucose (blood sugar) as the brain's primary fuel. In place of glucose, the liver uses fat molecules to make acetoacetate and hydroxybutyrate, two compounds known as ketones. The body adopts this same fuel strategy during a total fast of more than a few days. Ketones have gotten a bad name because they can rise to very high levels in individuals with uncontrolled type 1 diabetes, a state known as diabetic ketoacidosis. However, there is more than a tenfold difference between the ketone levels seen in ketoacidosis and those achieved with a carbohydrate-restricted diet, which we call nutritional ketosis. Equating the two is comparable to confusing a major flood with a gentle shower. Far from overwhelming the body's acid-base defenses, nutritional ketosis is a completely natural adaptation that is elegantly integrated into the body's energy strategy whenever carbs are restricted and fat becomes its primary fuel.

## LDL CHOLESTEROL

The main aim of low-fat diets and many drugs such as statins is to lower concentrations of LDL cholesterol. On average, low-fat diets are more effective at lowering LDL cholesterol levels than are low-carbohydrate diets. But before you chalk up this marker to low fat, consider that simply lowering LDL cholesterol by restricting dietary fat doesn't reduce your risk of developing heart disease.[28] Why? An obvious reason is that low-fat diets exacerbate other risk factors; they increase triglycerides and reduce HDL cholesterol. But there's another explanation that relates to the LDL particles themselves. Not all forms of LDL particles share the same potential for increasing heart disease. Within the category labeled LDL, there is a continuum of sizes, and research shows that smaller LDL particles contribute more to plaque formation in arteries (atherosclerosis) and are associated with a higher risk for heart disease. Although low-fat diets may decrease total LDL concentration, they tend to *increase* the proportion of small particles,[29] making them more dangerous. However, going in the other direction, numerous studies indicate that replacing carbohydrate with fat or protein leads to increases in LDL size.[30] Therefore, it's clear that carbohydrate intake is strongly and directly related to promoting the forms of LDL that contribute to arterial plaque formation,[31] whereas replacing carbohydrates in the diet with fat, even saturated fat, seems to promote the forms of LDL that are harmless.

## INFLAMMATION

As discussed above, when inflammation stays elevated because of a repeated insult such as a poor diet, it spells bad news. Researchers now appreciate the importance of this ongoing low-grade condition in contributing to many chronic health problems, including diabetes, heart disease, and even cancer. We typically think of inflammation in respect to fighting off bacteria and viruses. However, other substances, including excess carbohydrates and trans fats, can contribute to inflammation. A single high-carbohydrate meal can lead to increased inflammation.[32] Over time, eating a high-carbohydrate diet can lead to increased markers of inflammation.[33]

What about low-carbohydrate diets? Levels of CRP, a cytokine marker for inflammation, have been shown to decrease by approximately one-third on the Atkins Diet.[34] In subjects with higher levels of inflammation, CRP levels decreased more in response to a low-carbohydrate diet than to a fat-restricted diet.[35] A recently published study compared subjects with metabolic syndrome on a low-fat diet to those who were consuming a very-low-carbohydrate diet. The low-carb group showed a greater decrease in eight different circulating inflammatory markers compared to the low-fat group.[36] These data implicate dietary carbohydrate rather than fat as a more significant nutritional factor contributing to inflammation, although the combination of both increased fat and a high carbohydrate intake may be particularly harmful.

The anti-inflammatory effects of the omega-3 fats EPA and DHA have been shown in cell culture and animal studies, as well as in trials using humans.[37] These effects partially explain why these fats appear to have widespread health-promoting effects, especially in reducing the risk of heart disease and diabetes. Several hundred studies have demonstrated the cardioprotective effects of fish oil, and numerous review studies have summarized this body of work.[38] That's why we recommend regular consumption of fatty fish or use of a supplement containing EPA and DHA.

## VASCULAR FUNCTION

An early event in heart disease, vascular dysfunction is now considered part of metabolic syndrome because of its likely origins in insulin resistance in cells that line the interior artery walls.[39] An ultrasound technique that measures the ability of an artery in the arm (the brachial artery) to dilate detects the proper functioning of blood vessels.[40] In previous studies, a high-fat meal has been shown to temporarily impair dilation of the brachial artery.[41] The adverse effects of single meals high in fat, especially saturated fat, on lipid levels after a meal[42] and on vascular and inflammatory functions have been used as evidence to discourage low-carbohydrate diets. The test subject's prior diet history, however, has a fundamentally important effect on the metabolic response to meals. For example, research has repeatedly shown that adaptation to a very-low-carbohydrate diet results in a substantial reduction in the triglyceride response to a high-fat meal.[43] This means that studies that show short-term harmful effects of a high-fat meal on vascular function may show very different results after subjects are adapted to a low-carbohydrate diet.

When the effects of a high-fat meal on vascular function are assessed in subjects with metabolic syndrome who consumed a high-fat, very-low-carb diet,[44] there is a marked decrease in the triglyceride response to the high-fat meal. In contrast, control subjects consuming a low-fat diet showed little change. After twelve weeks on a very-low-carbohydrate diet, subjects showed improved vascular function after a high-fat meal compared to a control group of subjects who consumed a low-fat diet.

## THE ATKINS DIET IS GOOD MEDICINE

A series of low-carbohydrate-diet studies show that improvement in metabolic syndrome is intimately connected with controlling carbohydrate consumption.[45] Although metabolic syndrome can manifest in various ways, the nutritional benefits of a low-carbohydrate diet hold the promise of improving *all* the syndrome's features. Most physicians would treat each symptom individually, with the result that an individual might be taking multiple medications, increasing both the expense and the chance of developing side effects. Because having metabolic syndrome means you're on the fast track to diabetes and heart disease, getting all of its components under control is a unique benefit of the Atkins Diet. In the next chapter, you'll learn that these same dietary modifications can also reduce the likelihood of developing type 2 diabetes or even reverse its course, as evidenced by our final Success Story.

SUCCESS STORY 10

# WHEN PROFESSIONAL AND PERSONAL WORLDS COLLIDE

His self-diagnosis of diabetes launched the Canadian physician Jay Wortman on a personal odyssey of discovery and recovery. It also spurred a professional quest to push the boundaries of diabetes management at a time when the disease is becoming a global health crisis.

## VITAL STATISTICS

Current phase: Lifetime
  Maintenance
Daily Net Carb intake:
  20–30 grams
Age: 59
Height: 5 feet, 9 inches
Before weight: 185 pounds
Current weight: 160 pounds
Weight loss: 25 pounds
Current blood sugar: Under
  6 mmol/Ll (108 mg/dL)
Current HbA1c: 5.5%

Former blood pressure: 150/95
Current blood pressure: 130/80
Current HDL cholesterol:
  91 mg/dL
Current LDL cholesterol:
  161 mg/dL
Current triglycerides: 52.4 mg/dL
Current total cholesterol:
  272 mg/dL
Current C-reactive protein:
  0.3 mg/dL

**What is your background?**
As a physician who has focused on aboriginal health, I was acutely aware of the high rates of diabetes, as well as obesity and metabolic syndrome,

in this population. These epidemics were devastating aboriginal communities and incurring huge costs for health care services. When I traveled to the affected communities, there was almost a feeling that the situation was hopeless. Even in communities with extra resources and research programs, we weren't able to reverse the terrible trend.

**Did you have a family history of diabetes?**
I grew up in a small village in northern Alberta, Canada. Some of my ancestors were settlers in the Hudson Bay area and had intermarried with aboriginal peoples. Both my maternal grandparents developed type 2 diabetes, as did my mother and other close relatives. The aboriginal genetic tendency toward this disease had slowly snaked its way up through my family tree to bite me.

**How did you react to this realization?**
I was stunned. As a physician, you somehow believe that you're going to be immune to the diseases that you diagnose and treat in others. This, coupled with the fact that I had a very young son, made my self-diagnosis doubly shocking. Of all the concerns about serious health problems and a shortened life expectancy, however, the prospect of not seeing my two-year-old son grow into maturity was the thing that disturbed me most.

I had taken extra training in diabetes in my last year of family medicine residency and knew about the diabetic diet and how lifestyle change was supposed to be the cornerstone of diabetes management. I also knew that, for the most part, newly diagnosed type 2 diabetics went on drug therapy immediately because of the ineffectiveness of lifestyle interventions and that, even then, most tended to struggle and fail in their attempts to maintain normal blood glucose values. Further complicating my situation was the fact that I abhorred the use of medication.

**Did the diabetes occur out of the blue?**
Clearly, I'd been in denial. I'd put on some weight and was fatigued all the time. I struggled through bouts of afternoon drowsiness. I got

up at night to urinate, was constantly thirsty, and needed to squint to see the television news. My blood pressure was also rising into the zone that would require treatment. I rationalized all these developing problems as the natural and inevitable effects of aging until it suddenly dawned on me that I had the typical symptoms of diabetes. I tested myself and confirmed that my blood sugar was way too high. In order to buy time while I looked at the recent science and formulated a management plan, I decided not to eat anything that would exacerbate my soaring blood sugar. I immediately stopped eating sugar and starchy foods, but at the time I didn't have a clue about low-carb diets.

**What was the result of your dietary shift?**
Almost immediately, my blood sugar normalized, followed by a dramatic and steady loss of weight—about a pound a day. My other symptoms swiftly vanished, too. I started seeing clearly, the excessive urination and thirst disappeared, my energy level went up, and I began to feel immensely better. I bought an exercise bike and started riding it for thirty minutes every day as I continued to avoid starches and sugars. It was my wife who pointed out that I was on the Atkins Diet. She had struggled to lose weight after the birth of our son and had tried various diets. I recall that when she brought home an Atkins book I was dismissive, suggesting that it was just another of the fad diets and that it probably wouldn't work over the long haul. As I read the book, I realized that I wasn't actually following Dr. Atkins's phased approach to carb restriction, I was simply avoiding all carbs.

**How did your personal situation impact your practice?**
As I began to realize that my simple dietary intervention was rapidly and effectively resolving my own diabetes, I naturally started to look at the broader aboriginal diabetes epidemic through this lens. In my travels to First Nations communities, I started to question people, especially the elders, about their traditional ways of eating. It was common, especially in coastal communities, to consume traditional

foods like salmon, halibut, and shellfish. Inland, one would eat moose, deer, and elk. It was also common to eat modern fare, such as potato and pasta salads with the salmon and moose, cakes and cookies for dessert, all chased with juices and soda pop.

I began to understand that the traditional diet didn't have a significant source of starch or sugar. People ate berries, but the vast majority of calories came in the form of protein and fat. A number of seasonal wild plants, akin to modern greens, were all low in starch and sugar. The traditional diet was looking very much like a modern-day low-carb diet in terms of its macronutrient content.

### How did you test your theory?

Around this time a medical journal published a study in which a group of overweight men were put on the Atkins Diet and followed it for six months. The men lost significant weight and experienced an improvement in their cholesterol levels. I suggested to my two community medicine specialists that we design a similar study for a cohort of First Nations subjects.

I had started speaking to First Nation audiences about my ideas of a link between their changing diet and the epidemics of obesity and diabetes. Ultimately, the Canadian government agreed to fund a trial study to look at the effects of a traditional low-carb diet on obesity and diabetes. I was also able to spend two years on research leave at the University of British Columbia Department of Health Care.

### How is your health today?

For about seven years, I've adhered to the diet and continue to maintain normal blood sugar and blood pressure and a weight loss of about 25 pounds. After the first six months, I had my cholesterol checked. I'd become accustomed to eating lots of fatty foods, including my own wickedly delicious low-carb chocolate ice cream recipe. I have to admit I was afraid. I'd been taught that a diet high in saturated fat would lead to an unhealthy lipid profile. Much to my surprise and relief, I had excellent cholesterol. I was clearly on the right track.

My most recent blood tests continue to demonstrate excellent results. Although my total cholesterol and LDL cholesterol are above normal limits, I know from reading the scientific literature that this is not a concern given that the important markers for cardiovascular risk, HDL and triglycerides, are well within normal limits and my C-reactive protein is exceptionally low. With a pattern like this, although I have not tested for small, dense LDL, I can assume that my LDL is of the healthy variety. I am convinced that my health is better than it has ever been. I have learned an enormous amount in an area of science that physicians, unfortunately, tend to ignore: nutrition.

**Has your research been published yet?**
At this point, we're collecting data. After statistical analysis, we'll write the paper and submit it for publication in a scientific journal. Meanwhile, the study and how it affected the people of the Namgis First Nation and other residents of Alert Bay is the subject of the documentary *My Big Fat Diet*.
(For more information, see www.cbc.ca/thelens/bigfatdiet.)

# Chapter 14

# MANAGING DIABETES, AKA THE BULLY DISEASE

Diabetes now affects more than 18 million people in the United States alone, but because the early stages can be completely silent, as many as 8 million of them are unaware that they have the disease.

The Atkins Diet is more than just a healthy lifestyle. As you've learned in the previous chapter, this way of eating can significantly reduce your chances of developing heart disease and metabolic syndrome. Now you'll learn that the Atkins Diet is also an extremely effective tool to manage diabetes. We've previously pointed out that dietary carbohydrates act like a metabolic bully, demanding that they be burned first and pushing fats to the back of the line, which promotes the buildup of excess fat stores. Just as an individual who has been bullied for years may stop fighting back, some people's bodies eventually give in to the ongoing stress of too much sugar and other refined carbohydrates. The result is type 2 diabetes, which occurs when the body loses its ability to keep blood sugar within a safe range. When this happens, the swings in blood sugar—sometimes too low, but mostly too high—start to do their damage.

## ONE NAME, TWO DISEASES

Though most people know that diabetes has something to do with insulin, they're generally confused about exactly what that means. That's not surprising, considering that two different conditions (type 1 diabetes and type 2 diabetes) share the name. Both types involve insulin, the hormone that facilitates the movement of glucose into cells to be burned or stored. Simply put, type 1 diabetes reflects a problem in insulin production that results in low insulin levels. Type 2, on the other hand, reflects a problem in insulin action (insulin resistance), which results in high insulin levels.

Type 2 occurs mainly in adults and is the much more common form, representing 85 to 90 percent of all cases worldwide. Type 1 is more common in children, but thanks to the rapid increase in obesity among younger people, tragically this age group is also now developing type 2 diabetes.

If you've already been diagnosed with type 2 diabetes and have been testing your blood sugar after meals—or you live with someone who does—you've probably noticed that foods rich in carbohydrates drive blood sugar higher than those composed mostly of proteins and fats. If so, this chapter will confirm your suspicions that a healthful diet should limit carbohydrates to an amount that doesn't elevate blood sugar to the level that can inflict damage. And for the rest of us who don't (yet) have diabetes, it will soon become apparent that the best way to prevent this illness is by reducing dietary carbs to the point where they no longer function as a metabolic bully.

## A "SILENT" DISEASE ... BUT AN ENORMOUS EPIDEMIC

About one-third of people with type 2 diabetes in the United States are unaware that they have this disease. Fortunately, diagnosing diabetes is as simple as checking a small amount of your blood for its blood sugar (glucose) level or your blood level of hemoglobin A1c (HbA1c), which indicates your blood glucose level over the last several months. Your health care provider can perform either of these tests at a routine checkup, and many employers provide workplace screening (see the sidebar "Understanding Blood Sugar Readings" for more on testing). Because diabetes is so common and checking for it is so easy, if you don't know if you have diabetes, there's no reason not to find out as soon as possible.

Understanding the role of carbohydrate restriction in the prevention and treatment of diabetes is especially important because of the enormous scope of the diabetes epidemic. Despite the best efforts of the traditional medical approach, which is based upon aggressive use of drugs, the tide of this disease continues to rise. According to the American Diabetes Association, the disease now affects 18.2 million people in the United States, but because the early stages of diabetes can be completely silent, 8 million of them are unaware that they have the disease. Nor are the numbers likely to improve soon. As other nations adopt a diet high in sugar and processed carbohydrates, the epidemic has escalated to involve 246 million people worldwide, with projections of 380 million by 2025.

## UNDERSTANDING BLOOD SUGAR READINGS

The amount of glucose (sugar) in your blood changes throughout the day and night. Your levels vary depending upon when, what, and how much you have eaten and whether or not you've exercised. The American Diabetes Association (ADA) categories for normal blood sugar levels follow, based on how your glucose levels are tested.

*Fasting blood glucose.* This test is performed after you have consumed no food or liquids (other than water) for at least eight hours. A normal fasting blood glucose level is between 60 and 110 mg/dL (milligrams per deciliter). A reading of 126 mg/dL or higher indicates a diagnosis of diabetes. (In 1997, the ADA changed it from 140 mg/dL or higher.) A blood glucose reading of 100 indicates that you have 100 mg/dL.

*"Random" blood glucose.* This test may be taken at any time, with a normal blood glucose range in the low to midhundreds. A diagnosis of diabetes is made if your blood glucose reading is 200 mg/dL or higher and you have such symptoms of the disease as fatigue, excessive urination, excessive thirst, or unplanned weight loss.

*Oral glucose tolerance.* After fasting overnight, you'll be asked to drink a sugar-water solution. Your blood glucose levels will then be tested over several hours. In a person without diabetes, glucose levels rise and then fall quickly after drinking the solution. If a person has diabetes, blood glucose levels rise higher than normal and don't fall as quickly. A normal blood glucose reading two hours after drinking the solution is less than 140 mg/dL, and all readings in the first two hours must be less than 200 mg/dL for the test to be considered normal. Blood glucose levels of 200 mg/dL or higher at any time indicate a diagnosis of diabetes.

*Hemoglobin A1c (HbA1c).* This is a substance that goes up as a result of high blood glucose levels, and, once elevated, it stays up for a couple of months. Because blood glucose levels bounce around a lot depending on diet and exercise, the HbA1c test offers the advantage of smoothing out a lot of this variability. A level below 5.5 is considered good; a level above 6.5 indicates a diagnosis of diabetes.

As of this writing, the American Diabetes Association is intending to adopt the HbA1c test as a diagnosis for diabetes.

# DIABETES AND INFLAMMATION: A CHICKEN-AND-EGG SITUATION?

The underlying cause of type 2 diabetes is a controversial topic. In general, diabetes is a disorder of carbohydrate metabolism caused by a combination of hereditary and environmental factors. The latter includes the composition of the diet, obesity, and inactivity. However, many people eat a poor diet and are sedentary but never develop obesity or diabetes. Similarly, some obese, sedentary people have normal blood sugar levels. Nonetheless, overall, obesity and inactivity increase an individual's risk of developing diabetes, but some individuals seem more protected than others. This indicates that genetics play an important role in the development of the disorder. Another important factor is age: your body may tolerate bad behavior at age 30 but not necessarily at 60.

Your body uses the hormone insulin to trigger the movement of blood sugar into the cells, but, as you learned in the previous chapter, at high levels insulin also promotes metabolic syndrome, including excess fat storage, inflammation, and the formation of plaque in your arteries. Inflammation has increasingly become a topic of interest because people with type 2 diabetes typically have increased blood levels of inflammation biomarkers such as C-reactive protein (CRP), and this biomarker in turn accurately predicts who will later develop such complications of type 2 diabetes as heart disease, stroke, and kidney failure.[1]

More important, however, when large populations of adults without diabetes are screened for CRP levels and then followed for five to ten years, the quarter of the population with the highest levels has two to four times the likelihood of subsequently developing diabetes.[2] What this means is that inflammation comes before the overt signs of diabetes develop. In other words, inflammation looks less like an effect of diabetes and more like an (if not the) underlying cause. Coming back to our analogy of carbohydrate as a bully, it's simple but appealing to think that dietary carbohydrates repeatedly "bruise" the body. Further, it would seem that some people respond to this bruising by becoming inflamed, and this inflammation eventually results in damage that causes cells to become insulin-resistant and organs to eventually fail.

So how does this simple analogy help us understand something as complex as the underlying cause of type 2 diabetes? Well, take away the bully, and the bruising stops. Right? In the previous chapter we gave you strong evidence that carbohydrate restriction in people with metabolic syndrome (aka prediabetes) results in a sharp reduction in the biomarkers of inflammation. Now we'll show you that type 2 diabetics consuming a low-carb diet experience improvements in blood sugar, blood lipids, and body weight—sometimes dramatically so.

# A LOOK AT THE RESEARCH

There are several different types of studies used to understand the effect of eating different foods on human health. In previous decades, scientists tended to rely on observational studies of what people ate and how that affected their long-term health (nutritional epidemiology), but prospective clinical trials are considered more accurate. Studies on individuals in an "inpatient" clinical research ward provide tight control over what people eat, but they tend to be limited to a week or two, during which research subjects remain hospitalized, with a few notable exceptions.

In other studies, researchers give subjects food to take home to eat. However, there's no assurance that people won't eat other food in addition to the supplied meals. Finally, another type of research involves instructing people to buy and eat certain foods and return for instruction and support—often over a period of several years. These "outpatient" or "free-living" studies tell us a lot about whether a certain diet is sustainable in the "real-world" setting. But the interpretation of such studies is limited because people don't necessarily follow the dietary instructions. Here are some examples of studies that have shown that the Atkins Diet is a safe and effective treatment for type 2 diabetes.

## INPATIENT STUDIES

In a pioneering study done thirty years ago, seven obese type 2 diabetics were placed on a very-low-calorie ketogenic diet, first as inpatients and later as outpatients.[3] Initially, these subjects had fair-to-poor blood glucose control despite the fact that they were already taking 30 to 100 units of insulin per day. Within twenty days of starting the low-carbohydrate diet, all the subjects were able to discontinue their insulin injections. Nonetheless, their blood glucose control improved, as did their blood lipid profiles. The authors noted that blood glucose control improved much more rapidly than did the rate at which they lost weight, indicating that carbohydrate intake was the primary determinant of glucose control and insulin requirement rather than obesity itself.

In a 2005 inpatient study ten obese people with type 2 diabetes were fed their usual diet for seven days, followed by a low-carbohydrate diet (the Induction phase of Atkins) of 20 grams of carbs a day for fourteen days.[4] In both cases, subjects were allowed to choose how much they ate, so the only change after the first week was eliminating most carbohydrate foods. Because this study took place in a research ward, the researchers were able to document the subjects' total food intake. They found that when subjects followed the low-carb diet, they continued to eat about the same amount of protein and fat as before, even after two weeks of carb restriction and although they could have eaten more protein and/or fat to make up for the missing carbohydrate calories if they desired. This means that they naturally ate fewer calories when carbs were restricted. In addition to losing weight, the subjects also showed improvements in their blood glucose and insulin levels. Many were able to eliminate their medications, and their insulin sensitivity improved by 75 percent on average, similar to the observations of the 1976 study cited above. More important, this recent study showed that instructing people to limit their grams of carbohydrate (without restricting calories or portion size) resulted in their eating less food and rapidly improving their insulin sensitivity.

## OUTPATIENT STUDIES

A recent outpatient study compared a low-carbohydrate diet to a portion-controlled, low-fat diet in seventy-nine patients over a three-month period.[5] After three months, subjects in the low-carb group were reportedly consuming 110 grams of carbohydrate per day (the upper range of the Atkins Lifetime Maintenance phase). Compared to the low-fat group, the low-carb group had improvements in glucose control, weight, cholesterol, triglycerides and blood pressure. In addition, more people in the low-carb group were able to reduce medications than those in the low-fat group.

Another, very recent outpatient study compared the Induction phase of Atkins (20 grams of carbohydrate daily) to a reduced-calorie diet (500 calories a day below their previous intake level, low in fat and sugar but high in complex carbs) over a six-month period.[6] They found greater improvements in blood sugar levels and greater weight loss in the Atkins Induction group. What was especially exciting, however, was that individuals who were taking insulin often found the beneficial effects of the low-carb diet quite powerful. Subjects taking from 40 to 90 units of insulin before participating in the study were able to eliminate insulin altogether, while also improving glycemic control. These results were similar to the inpatient studies described above.

And finally, the Kuwaiti low-carb study cited in chapter 1 included thirty-five subjects whose blood glucose was elevated at the start of the study. The average value for this group returned into the normal range within eight weeks of following the low-carb diet, and at fifty-six weeks, this group's average fasting blood glucose had been reduced by 44 percent.

In summary, these five studies, in a variety of settings, all showed dramatic improvements in blood glucose control and blood lipids in type 2 diabetics consuming a low-carb diet. When these studies included a low-fat, high-carb comparison group, the low-carb diet consistently showed superior effects on blood glucose control, medication reduction, blood lipids, and weight loss. Weight loss is particularly important because treatment goals for patients with type 2 diabetes always emphasize weight loss if the individual is overweight, yet the drugs used to treat diabetics almost all cause weight gain. So let's look at this briefly, as the ability to deliver improved blood sugar control *and* weight loss distinguishes a low-carb approach from all other nonsurgical treatments for type 2 diabetes.

## WEIGHING THE OPTIONS: COMMON SIDE EFFECTS OF MEDICATION

On its surface, the management of type 2 diabetes seems pretty easy: just get your blood glucose back down into the normal range. But insulin resistance characterizes this form of diabetes; put simply, the glucose level "doesn't want to go down." This means that the body is less responsive to the most powerful drug used to treat it: insulin. So the dose of insulin that most type 2 diabetics are prescribed is very high. Moreover, because insulin not only drives glucose into muscle cells but also accelerates fat synthesis and storage, weight gain is usually one side effect of aggressive insulin therapy.[7] Other pills and injected medications have been developed to reduce this effect, but on average, the harder one tries to control blood glucose, the greater the tendency to gain weight.[8] The other major side effect of attempting to gain tight control of blood sugar is driving it too low, causing hypoglycemia, which causes weakness, shakiness, confusion, and even coma. If these symptoms appear, the advice is to immediately eat a lot of sugar to stop the symptoms, which jump-starts the blood sugar roller coaster all over again. Interestingly, once type 2 diabetics complete the first few weeks of the Atkins program, they rarely experience hypoglycemia. That's because of the body's adaptation to burning fat for most of its fuel during carb restriction, in concert with the ability to reduce or stop most diabetic medications (including insulin) within a few days or weeks of starting the Atkins Diet.

So why isn't it good enough just to cut back on one's calories without cutting back on carbs? It's true that going on a diet and losing weight typically improve diabetes control. Well, first of all, dieting won't necessarily result in weight loss, and any weight loss may not be sustained. Second, even weight loss is usually not enough to significantly reduce medication dosage. Finally, since diabetic drugs still produce side effects and appetite stimulation, losing weight on a standard diet is a difficult tightrope for a diabetic to walk.

Once you understand this tightrope of weight loss during drug treatment—some would call it a Catch-22—it's easier to appreciate the advantage of using the Atkins Diet to manage type 2 diabetes. When you remove added sugar, significantly reduce carb intake overall, and confine your consumption primarily to the foundation vegetables allowed in Induction, your insulin resistance rapidly improves, and blood glucose control improves—usually dramatically. Additionally, most people find that they can stop or substantially reduce their diabetes medications. As a result, the path to meaningful weight loss changes from a tightrope to a wide road. As long as you stay within your carb tolerance range, you should be able to navigate your way to health.

## IF AND WHEN TO EXERCISE

You might be familiar with many of the potential health benefits of exercise, but you probably don't know that exercise has insulinlike effects. This is relevant for type 2 diabetics with insulin resistance, because performing just a single bout of exercise improves insulin resistance for several hours. A number of studies have shown that regular exercise improves blood sugar control, even if it doesn't significantly improve weight loss.[9] Because weight loss is so difficult for people with type 2 diabetes and because doctors have little else to offer (other than drugs) in the way of effective remedies, exercise is always near the top of the list of official guidelines.

Given this information, simple logic dictates that we should tell everyone with diabetes to get out and exercise. But not so fast. First, exercise holds an exalted position in diabetic treatment because the usual diets almost always fail. We need to consider what role exercise should play if the tables are turned and you have access to a diet like Atkins that almost always "works" and that simultaneously causes insulin resistance and blood sugar control to improve significantly. Unfortunately, we don't yet have the perfect answer. Yes, we've proved that once people adapt to the Atkins

Diet, they're capable of lots of exercise. But no one has done a study of diabetics on Atkins in which some of them exercise and some of them don't, to prove that adding exercise to an already successful diet improves blood sugar control or increases weight loss enough to justify the added effort.

Second, if you're diabetic, you're at increased risk for heart attack, and most people with type 2 diabetes are overweight (at least, before they start Atkins). So if you were offered the choice of either starting the program and exercising at the same time, or alternatively starting Atkins first, getting your blood sugar under control, reducing or stopping medications you might be taking for diabetes, and getting some weight off your ankles, knees, hips, and lower back, which would you choose?

Clearly, the key question is not really *if* but *when*. The Atkins Diet opens the door for you to exercise, and exercise has a lot of benefits other than weight loss (and may even improve your blood sugar control). As we've said previously, if you're already physically active, keep it up, being careful not to overdo it while you're adapting to fat burning in the first few weeks. But if it's been a while since you did much of anything vigorous, consider giving yourself a few weeks or months to unburden your heart and joints before taking on a 10K run or trying to burn out the treadmill or pump iron at the gym.

## THE CURRENT OFFICIAL GUIDELINES

Okay, we've explained how Atkins offers unique benefits to someone with type 2 diabetes. So why isn't everyone with the disorder doing it? The answer is that the low-fat-diet fad of the last forty years, backed by the food industry and government-sanctioned committees, has taken a long time to run its course. Only with the recent research we've cited in the last few chapters has the mainstream medical community begun to be receptive to the value of low-carbohydrate diets. Standard treatment guidelines are beginning to reflect this change. This is where we stand today.

The goal of medical nutrition therapy for type 2 diabetes is to attain and maintain optimal metabolic outcomes, including:

- Blood glucose levels in the normal range or as close to normal as is safely possible to prevent or reduce the risk for complications of diabetes
- Lipid and lipoprotein profiles that reduce the risk for blood vessel disease (i.e., blockage of blood flow to your heart, brain, kidneys, and legs)
- Blood pressure levels that reduce the risk of developing vascular disease

The American Diabetes Association (ADA) has acknowledged the use of a low-carbohydrate diet in achieving these goals in its 2008 guidelines, which include:[10]

- Modest weight loss has been shown to improve insulin resistance in overweight and obese insulin-resistant individuals.
- Weight loss is recommended for all overweight individuals who have or are at risk for the disease.
- Either low-carbohydrate or low-fat calorie-restricted diets may be effective for weight loss in the short term (up to one year).
- Patients on low-carbohydrate diets should have their lipid profiles, kidney function, and protein intake (for those with kidney damage) monitored regularly.
- To avoid hypoglycemia, patients following a low-carb diet who are taking blood sugar–lowering medications need to have them monitored and adjusted, as needed.

## PRACTICAL POINTERS

How can those of you who are diabetic translate all of this information into action to transform your health? Here are three practical considerations:

1. The focus of this chapter has been on type 2 diabetes because it's usually associated with being overweight, and also because most type 2 diabetics probably won't need insulin injections if they can find and comply with their threshold for carbohydrate tolerance (CLL or ACE). Type 1 diabetics will always need some insulin, making its management much more technical on a carb-restricted diet. Though some doctors are now using the Atkins Diet for selected type 1 diabetics, instructions on how to do this safely are beyond the scope of this book. If you've been diagnosed with type 1 diabetes, or if you've ever been diagnosed with diabetic ketoacidosis, you should not try the Atkins Diet on your own. And if you do try it under medical supervision, be sure that you're being instructed and closely monitored by a doctor familiar with Atkins.

2. Second, if you're taking medications to control blood sugar (diabetic drugs) or drugs for high blood pressure, be sure to work closely with your doctor, particularly in the first weeks and months of the diet. It's during this time that diabetes and blood pressure improve rapidly, which usually requires

reducing or stopping the medications used to treat these problems. This should always be done with your doctor's knowledge and consent.

3. Be consistent about sticking with the program. While we advise this for everyone following a low-carb diet—whether your problem is weight, diabetes, high blood lipids, or high blood pressure—consistency is of the greatest importance if you start out with diabetes. This is because type 2 diabetes represents the highest level of insulin resistance, so if you break the diet, your body's return to carbohydrate intolerance will be rapid and the swings in blood sugar wide. If you've gotten off of most of your diabetes or high-blood-pressure drugs in the first two weeks of the diet and celebrate this victory by three days of eating everything in Vegas, the metabolic bully will beat you up and you'll return home with these problems once again out of control. (In this case, what happened in Vegas won't stay in Vegas!) Yes, as you lose weight, your underlying tendency to be insulin-resistant often improves. But most diabetics still remain somewhat insulin-resistant even after substantial weight loss, so staying at or under your carbohydrate threshold has greater importance for you in order to avoid the long-term medical problems caused by poorly controlled diabetes.

## A CHALLENGE THAT'S WORTH THE EFFORT

Using the Atkins Diet to manage type 2 diabetes is probably the most potent use of this powerful tool, but it's also the most demanding. Make sure that you (and your doctor) are ready to apply the time and energy necessary to be successful—both in the near term and for years to come. To that end, we have provided a combination of scientific and practical information in this chapter so that both you and your physician can be assured that this use of the Atkins Diet can be safe and effective.

# Acknowledgments

We are like dwarfs on the shoulders of giants, so that we can see
more than they, and things at a greater distance, not by virtue of
any sharpness of sight on our part, or any physical distinction, but
because we are carried high and raised up by their giant size.
                                              —*Bernard of Chartres, 1159*

For a quarter century, as an academic physician doing research on low-carbohydrate metabolism, my life ran parallel to that of Robert C. Atkins. Sadly, our paths never crossed. About a decade ago, however, two leaders of a new generation of medical scientists contacted me. Building a bridge between the heretofore separate realms of academic research and the clinical brilliance of Dr. Atkins, Dr. Eric Westman and Dr. Jeff Volek have forged the scientific foundation of the New Atkins. As a result of their efforts and the support of the Atkins Foundation, there has been a resurgence of scientific interest in the Atkins Diet. It has been my very great pleasure to collaborate with them, first on current research studies and now on the creation of this book.

I also wish to thank Drs. Ethan Sims, Edward Horton, Bruce Bistrian, and George Blackburn for teaching me to subject standard dietary practices to scientific scrutiny. Their guidance helped to shape my life and my career. I also owe a debt of gratitude to my many patients and research subjects for opening my eyes to unanticipated results. And, most important, thanks to my lovely family—Huong, Lauren, and Eric—for their unquestioning support and their tolerance of my cooking.
                                              —*Stephen D. Phinney*

I must first thank those people who have shaped my scientific thinking and specifically contributed to a line of research on carbohydrate restriction. Dr. William J. Kraemer initially sparked my interest in science and has offered unwavering support for almost twenty years as we have continued to collaborate on research and become best friends. I'm not sure if he qualifies for MENSA, but my coauthor Dr. Stephen Phinney is a bona fide nutritional genius. In 1994, I first read his enlightening papers on experiments he conducted in the early 1980s on metabolic adaptations to very-low-carbohydrate diets. A decade later I'm fortunate to consider him a close friend and colleague. Several other colleagues have significantly influenced my views of nutrition and positively impacted my research. Drs. Maria Luz Fernandez, Richard Feinman, and Richard Bruno are all brilliant collaborators on past and current research projects whose relationships I treasure. I have also been privileged to work with several tireless and talented graduate students over the years, all of whom dedicated countless hours to conducting more than a dozen experiments aimed at better understanding how low-carbohydrate diets improve health.

It's been a pleasure working with Eric Westman and Stephen Phinney. It is also necessary to acknowledge Dr. Robert C. Atkins, who had a remarkable and permanent impact on my life. His recognition of the importance of science to validate his dietary approach and his generous philanthropy has been a major reason I was able to conduct cutting-edge research on low-carbohydrate diets over the last decade.

I am forever grateful to my selfless mother, Nina, and my father, Jerry, for their unconditional love and support, and all the sacrifices they have made in order to make my life better. My two cherished boys, high-spirited Preston, who recently turned two, and Reese, who was born during the writing of this book, give me a deep sense of purpose and perspective. Coming home to them is the perfect antidote to a stressful day of work. Most important, thanks to my beloved wife, Ana, who keeps me balanced and makes life infinitely more fun.

—*Jeff S. Volek*

I acknowledge first the enthusiastic love and support of my wife, Gretchen, and our children, Laura, Megan, and Clay. I learned to tilt at windmills from my parents, Jack C. and Nancy K. Westman, and brothers, John C. Westman and D. Paul Westman. Innumerable friends, colleagues, and data-driven academic environments enabled this book—and the science behind it—to materialize.

Thanks to Dr. Robert C. Atkins and Jackie Eberstein for having the openness to invite me to visit their clinical practice. Thanks to Veronica Atkins and Dr. Abby Bloch of the Robert C. Atkins Foundation for continuing his legacy. Thanks also to the doctors and researchers who allowed me to visit their practices or collaborate on research studies with them: Mary C. Vernon, Richard K. Bernstein, Joseph T. Hickey, Ron Rosedale, members of the American Society of Bariatric Physicians, William S. Yancy, Jr., James A. Wortman, Jeff S. Volek, Richard D. Feinman, Donald Layman, Manny Noakes, and Stephen D. Phinney.

—*Eric C. Westman*

As a team, we wish to acknowledge the Herculean effort expended in bringing together all the components of this book by project editor Olivia Bell Buehl and Atkins nutritionist Colette Heimowitz. Dietician Brittanie Volk developed the meal plans. Thanks also to Monty Sharma and Chip Bellamy of Atkins Nutritionals, Inc., for their insight on the importance of publishing this book and their patience as it took on a life of its own.

# Glossary

**ACE:** See *Atkins Carbohydrate Equilibrium*.

**Aerobic exercise:** Sustained rhythmic exercise that increases your heart rate; also referred to as cardio.

**Amino acids:** The building blocks of protein.

**Antioxidants:** Substances that neutralize harmful free radicals in the body.

**Atherosclerosis:** Clogging, narrowing, and hardening of blood vessels by plaque deposits.

**Atkins Carbohydrate Equilibrium (ACE):** The number of grams of Net Carbs that a person can consume daily without gaining or losing weight.

**Atkins Edge:** A beneficial state of fat-burning metabolism, caused by carbohydrate restriction, that makes it possible to lose weight and maintain weight loss without extreme hunger or cravings; a metabolic edge.

**Beta cells:** Specialized cells in the pancreas that produce insulin.

**Blood lipids:** The factors of total cholesterol, triglycerides, and HDL and LDL cholesterol in your blood.

**Blood pressure:** The pressure your blood exerts against the walls of your arteries during a heartbeat.

**Blood sugar:** The amount of glucose in your bloodstream; also called blood glucose.

**BMI:** See *Body mass index*.

**Body mass index (BMI):** An estimate of body fatness that takes into account body weight and height.

**Carbohydrate:** A macronutrient from plants and some other foods broken down by digestion into simple sugars such as glucose to provide a source of energy.

**Cholesterol:** A lipid; a waxy substance essential for many of the body's functions, including manufacturing hormones and making cell membranes.

**C-reactive protein (CRP):** A chemical in blood that serves as a marker for inflammation.

**Diabetes:** See *Type 1 diabetes* and *Type 2 diabetes*.

**Diuretic:** Anything that removes fluid from the body by increasing urination.

**Essential fatty acids (EFAs):** Two classes of essential dietary fats that your body cannot make on its own and that must be obtained from food or supplements.

**Fat:** One of the three macronutrients; an organic compound that dissolves in other oils but not in water. A source of energy and building blocks of cells.

**Fatty acids:** The scientific term for fats, which are part of a group of substances called lipids.

**Fiber:** Parts of plant foods that are indigestible or very slowly digested, with little effect on blood glucose and insulin levels; sometimes called roughage.

**Foundation vegetables:** Leafy greens and other low-carbohydrate, nonstarchy vegetables suitable for Phase 1, Induction, and the basis upon which later carb intake builds.

**Free radicals:** Harmful molecules in the environment and naturally produced by our bodies. Excess free radicals can damage cells and cause oxidation.

**Glucose:** A simple sugar. Also see *Blood sugar*.

**Glycogen:** The storage form of carbohydrate in the body.

**HDL cholesterol:** High-density lipoprotein; the "good" type of cholesterol.

**Hydrogenated oils:** Vegetable oils processed to make them solid and improve their shelf life. See *Trans fats*.

**Hypertension:** High blood pressure.

**Inflammation:** Part of the body's delicately balanced natural defense system against potentially damaging substances. Excessive inflammation is associated with increased risk of heart attack, stroke, diabetes, and some forms of cancer.

**Insulin:** A hormone produced by the pancreas that signals cells to remove glucose and amino acids from the bloodstream and stop the release of fat from fat cells.

**Ketoacidosis:** The uncontrolled overproduction of ketones characteristic of untreated type 1 diabetes, typically five to ten times higher than nutritional ketosis.

**Ketones:** Substances produced by the liver from fat during accelerated fat breakdown that serve as a valuable energy source for cells throughout the body.

**Ketosis:** A moderate and controlled level of ketones in the bloodstream that allows the body to function well with little dietary carbohydrate; also called nutritional ketosis.

**LDL cholesterol:** Low-density lipoprotein. Commonly referred to as the "bad" type of cholesterol, but not all LDL cholesterol is "bad."

**Lean body mass:** Body mass minus fat tissue; includes muscle, bone, organs, and connective tissue.

**Legumes:** Most members of the bean and pea families, including lentils, chickpeas, soybeans, peas, and numerous others.

**Lipids:** Fats, including triglycerides, and cholesterol in the body.

**Macronutrients:** Fat, protein, and carbohydrate, the dietary sources of calories and nutrients.

**Metabolic syndrome:** A group of conditions, including hypertension, high triglycerides, low HDL cholesterol, higher-than-normal blood sugar and insulin levels, and weight carried in the middle of the body. Also known as syndrome X or insulin resistance syndrome, it predisposes you to heart disease and type 2 diabetes.

**Metabolism:** The complex chemical processes that convert food into energy or the body's building blocks, which in turn become part of organs, tissues, and cells.

**Monounsaturated fat:** Dietary fat typically found in foods such as olive oil, canola oil, nuts, and avocados.

**Net Carbs:** The carbohydrates in a food that impact your blood sugar, calculated by subtracting fiber grams in the food from total grams. In a low-carb product, sugar alcohols, including glycerin, are also subtracted.

**Omega-3 fatty acids:** A group of essential polyunsaturated fats found in green algae, cold-water fish, fish oil, flaxseed oil, and some other nut and vegetable oils.

**Omega-6 fatty acids:** A group of essential polyunsaturated fats found in many vegetable oils and also in meats from animals fed corn, soybeans, and certain other vegetable products.

**Partially hydrogenated oils:** See *Trans fats.*

**Plaque:** A buildup in the arteries of cholesterol, fat, calcium, and other substances that can block blood flow and result in a heart attack or stroke.

**Polyunsaturated fats:** Fats with a chemical structure that keeps them liquid in the cold; oils from corn, soybean, sunflower, safflower, cottonseed, grape seed, flaxseed, sesame seed, some nuts, and fatty fish are typically high in polyunsaturated fat.

**Prediabetes:** Blood sugar levels that are higher than normal but fall short of full-blown diabetes.

**Protein:** One of the three macronutrients found in food, used for energy and building blocks of cells; chains of amino acids.

**Resistance exercise:** Any exercise that builds muscle strength; also called weight-bearing or anaerobic exercise.

**Satiety:** A pleasurable sense of fullness.

**Saturated fats:** Fats that are solid at room temperature; the majority of fat in butter, lard, suet, palm and coconut oil.

**Statin drugs:** Pharmaceuticals used to lower total and LDL cholesterol.

**Sucrose:** Table sugar, composed of glucose and fructose.

**Sugar alcohols:** Sweeteners such as glycerin, mannitol, erythritol, sorbitol, and xylitol that have little or no impact on most people's blood sugar and are therefore used in some low-carb products.

**Trans fats:** Fats found in partially hydrogenated or hydrogenated vegetable oil; typically used in fried foods, baked goods, and other products. A high intake of trans fats is associated with increased heart attack risk.

**Triglycerides:** The major form of fat that circulates in the bloodstream and is stored as body fat.

**Type 1 diabetes:** A condition in which the pancreas makes so little insulin that the body can't use blood glucose as energy, producing chronically high blood sugar levels and overproduction of ketones.

**Type 2 diabetes:** The more common form of diabetes; high blood sugar levels caused by insulin resistance, an inability to use insulin properly.

**Unsaturated fat:** Monounsaturated and polyunsaturated fats.

# Notes

## Chapter 1: Know Thyself

1. C. D. Gardner, A. Kiazand, S. Alhassan, S. Kim, R. S. Stafford, R. R. Balise, et al., "Comparison of the Atkins, Zone, Ornish, and LEARN Diets for Change in Weight and Related Risk Factors among Overweight Premenopausal Women: The A TO Z Weight Loss Study: A Randomized Trial," *The Journal of the American Medical Association* 297 (2007), 969–977; I. Shai, D. Schwarzfuchs, Y. Henkin, D. R. Shahar, S. Witkow, I. Greenberg, et al., "Weight Loss with a Low-Carbohydrate, Mediterranean, or Low-Fat Diet," *The New England Journal of Medicine* 359 (2008), 229–241; J. S. Volek, M. L. Fernandez, R. D. Feinman, and S. D. Phinney, "Dietary Carbohydrate Restriction Induces a Unique Metabolic State Positively Affecting Atherogenic Dyslipidemia, Fatty Acid Partitioning, and Metabolic Syndrome," *Progress in Lipid Research* 47 (2008), 307–318.

2. Shai et al., "Weight Loss with a Low-Carbohydrate, Mediterranean, or Low-Fat Diet"; A. J. Nordmann, A. Nordmann, M. Briel, U. Keller, W. S. Yancy, Jr., B. J. Brehm, et al., "Effects of Low-Carbohydrate vs Low-Fat Diets on Weight Loss and Cardiovascular Risk Factors: A Meta-analysis of Randomized Controlled Trials," *Archives of Internal Medicine* 166 (2006), 285–293.

3. C. D. Gardner et al., "Comparison of the Atkins, Zone, Ornish, and LEARN Diets for Change in Weight and Related Risk Factors among Overweight Premenopausal Women."

4. G. Boden, K. Sargrad, C. Homko, M. Mozzoli, and T. P. Stein, "Effect of a Low-Carbohydrate Diet on Appetite, Blood Glucose Levels, and Insulin Resistance in Obese Patients with type 2 Diabetes," *Annals of Internal Medicine* 142 (2005), 403–411; E. C. Westman, W. S. Yancy, Jr., J. C. Mavropoulos, M. Marquart, and J. R. McDuffie, "The Effect of a Low-Carbohydrate, Ketogenic Diet Versus a Low-Glycemic Index Diet on Glycemic Control in type 2 Diabetes Mellitus," *Nutrition & Metabolism* (London) 5 (2008), 36.

5. E. H. Kossoff, and J. M. Rho, "Ketogenic Diets: Evidence for Short- and Long-Term Efficacy," *Neurotherapeutics* 6 (2009), 406–414; J. M. Freeman, J. B. Freeman, and M. T. Kelly, *The Ketogenic Diet: A Treatment for Epilepsy*, 3rd ed. (New York: Demos Health, 2000).

6. T. A. Wadden, J. A. Sternberg, K. A. Letizia, A. J. Stunkard, and G. D. Foster, "Treatment of Obesity by Very Low Calorie Diet, Behavior Therapy, and Their Combination: A Five-Year Perspective," *International Journal of Obesity* 13 suppl. 2 (1989), 39–46.

7. Gardner et al., "Comparison of the Atkins, Zone, Ornish, and LEARN Diets for Change in Weight and Related Risk Factors among Overweight Premenopausal Women: The A TO Z Weight Loss Study: A Randomized Trial"; I. Shai et al., "Weight Loss with a Low-Carbohydrate, Mediterranean, or Low-Fat Diet."

8.  G. Boden et al., "Effect of a Low-Carbohydrate Diet on Appetite, Blood Glucose Levels, and Insulin Resistance in Obese Patients with type 2 Diabetes"; J. S. Volek, M. J. Sharman, A. L. Gomez, D. A. Judelson, M. R. Rubin, G. Watson, et al., "Comparison of Energy-Restricted Very Low-Carbohydrate and Low-Fat Diets on Weight Loss and Body Composition in Overweight Men and Women," *Nutrition & Metabolism* (London) 1 (2004), 13.

9.  E. A. Sims, E. Danforth, Jr., E. S. Horton, G. A. Bray, J. A. Glennon, and L. B. Salans, "Endocrine and Metabolic Effects of Experimental Obesity in Man," *Recent Progress in Hormonal Research* 29 (1973), 457–496; C. Bouchard, A. Tremblay, J. P. Despres, G. Theriault, A. Nadeau, P. J. Lupien, et al., "The Response to Exercise with Constant Energy Intake in Identical Twins," *Obesity Research* 2 (1994), 400–410.

10.  Gardner et al., "Comparison of the Atkins, Zone, Ornish, and LEARN Diets for Change in Weight and Related Risk Factors among Overweight Premenopausal Women: The A TO Z Weight Loss Study: A Randomized Trial"; I. Shai et al., "Weight Loss with a Low-Carbohydrate, Mediterranean, or Low-Fat Diet"; B. J. Brehm, R. J. Seeley, S. R. Daniels, and D. A. D'Alessio, "A Randomized Trial Comparing a Very Low Carbohydrate Diet and a Calorie-Restricted Low Fat Diet on Body Weight and Cardiovascular Risk Factors in Healthy Women," *Journal of Clinical Endocrinology & Metabolism* 88 (2003), 1617–1623; M. L. Dansinger, J. A. Gleason, J. L. Griffith, H. P. Selker, and E. J. Schaefer, "Comparison of the Atkins, Ornish, Weight Watchers, and Zone Diets for Weight Loss and Heart Disease Risk Reduction: A Randomized Trial," *The Journal of the American Medical Association* 293 (2005), 43–53; G. D. Foster, H. R. Wyatt, J. O. Hill, B. G. McGuckin, C. Brill, B. S. Mohammed, et al., "A Randomized Trial of a Low-Carbohydrate Diet for Obesity," *The New England Journal of Medicine* 348 (2003), 2082–2090; L. Stern, N. Iqbal, P. Seshadri, K. L. Chicano, D. A. Daily, J. McGrory, et al., "The Effects of Low-Carbohydrate Versus Conventional Weight Loss Diets in Severely Obese Adults: One-Year Follow-up of a Randomized Trial," *Annals of Internal Medicine* 140 (2004), 778–785; W. S. Yancy, Jr., M. K. Olsen, J. R. Guyton, R. P. Bakst, and E. C. Westman, "A Low-Carbohydrate, Ketogenic Diet versus a Low-Fat Diet to Treat Obesity and Hyperlipidemia: A Randomized, Controlled Trial," *Annals of Internal Medicine* 140 (2004), 769–777.

11.  H. M. Dashti, N. S. Al-Zaid, T. C. Mathew, M. Al-Mousawi, H. Talib, S. K. Asfar, et al., "Long Term Effects of Ketogenic Diet in Obese Subjects with High Cholesterol Level," *Molecular and Cellular Biochemistry* 286 (2006), 1–9.

## Chapter 2: The Road Ahead

1.  J. S. Volek, M. J. Sharman, A. L. Gomez, D. A. Judelson, M. R. Rubin, G. Watson, et al., "Comparison of Energy-Restricted Very Low-Carbohydrate and Low-Fat Diets on Weight Loss and Body Composition in Overweight Men and Women," *Nutrition & Metabolism* (London) 1 (2004), 13; J. S. Volek, S. D. Phinney, C. E. Forsythe, E. E. Quann, R. J. Wood, M. J. Puglisi, et al., "Carbohydrate Restriction Has a More Favorable Impact on the Metabolic Syndrome than a Low Fat Diet," *Lipids* 44 (2008), 297–309.

2.  C. D. Gardner, A. Kiazand, S. Alhassan, S. Kim, R. S. Stafford, R. R. Balise, et al., "Comparison of the Atkins, Zone, Ornish, and LEARN Diets for Change in Weight and Related Risk Factors among Overweight Premenopausal Women: The A TO Z Weight Loss Study: A Randomized Trial," *The Journal of the American Medical Association* 297 (2007), 969–977; I. Shai, D. Schwarzfuchs, Y. Henkin, D. R. Shahar, S. Witkow, I. Greenberg, et al., "Weight Loss with a Low-Carbohydrate, Mediterranean, or Low-Fat Diet," *The New England Journal of Medicine* 359 (2008), 229–241; J. S. Volek et al., "Carbohydrate Restriction Has a More Favorable Impact on the Metabolic Syndrome than a Low Fat Diet."

## Chapter 3: The Right Carbs in the Right Amounts

1. See www.ers.usda.gov/publications/sb965/sb965h.pdf for more information.
2. S. S. Elliott, N. L. Keim, J. S. Stern, K. Teff, and P. J. Havel. "Fructose, Weight Gain, and the Insulin Resistance Syndrome," *American Journal of Clinical Nutrition* 76 (2002), 911–922; G. A. Bray, S. J. Nielsen, and B. M. Popkin, "Consumption of High-Fructose Corn Syrup in Beverages May Play a Role in the Epidemic of Obesity," *American Journal of Clinical Nutrition* 79 (2004), 537–543.
3. Bray, Nielsen, and B. M. Popkin, "Consumption of High-Fructose Corn Syrup in Beverages May Play a Role in the Epidemic of Obesity."
4. www.cspinet.org/new/pdf/final_soda_petition.pdf.
5. K. L. Teff, J. Grudziak, R. R. Townsend, T. N. Dunn, R. W. Grant, S. H. Adams, et al., "Endocrine and Metabolic Effects of Consuming Fructose- and Glucose-Sweetened Beverages with Meals in Obese Men and Women: Influence of Insulin Resistance on Plasma Triglyceride Responses," *Journal of Clinical Endocrinology & Metabolism* 94 (2009), 1562–1569.
6. C. Bouchard, A. Tremblay, J. P. Despres, A. Nadeau, P. J. Lupien, G. Theriault, et al., "The Response to Long-Term Overfeeding in Identical Twins," *The New England Journal of Medicine* 322 (1990), 1477–1482.
7. C. Bouchard, A. Tremblay, J. P. Despres, G. Theriault, A. Nadeau, P. J. Lupien, et al., "The Response to Exercise with Constant Energy Intake in Identical Twins," *Obesity Research* 2 (1994), 400–410.

## Chapter 4: The Power of Protein

1. G. H. Anderson, and S. E. Moore, "Dietary Proteins in the Regulation of Food Intake and Body Weight in Humans," *The Journal of Nutrition* 134 (2004), 974S–979S.
2. E. Jequier, "Pathways to Obesity," *International Journal of Obesity and Related Metabolic Disorders* 26 suppl. 2 (2002), S12–S17.
3. F. Q. Nuttall, K. Schweim, H. Hoover, and M. C. Gannon, "Metabolic Effect of a LoBAG30 Diet in Men with type 2 Diabetes," *American Journal of Physiology—Endocrinology and Metabolism* 291 (2006), E786–E791; D. K. Layman, P. Clifton, M. C. Gannon, R. M. Krauss, and F. Q. Nuttall, "Protein in Optimal Health: Heart Disease and type 2 Diabetes," *American Journal of Clinical Nutrition* 87 (2008), 1571S–1575S.
4. J. W. Krieger, H. S. Sitren, M. J. Daniels, and B. Langkamp-Henken, "Effects of Variation in Protein and Carbohydrate Intake on Body Mass and Composition during Energy Restriction: A Meta-regression," *American Journal of Clinical Nutrition* 83 (2006), 260–274.
5. L. J. Hoffer, B. R. Bistrian, V. R. Young, G. L. Blackburn, and D. E. Matthews, "Metabolic Effects of Very Low Calorie Weight Reduction Diets," *The Journal of Clinical Investigation* 73 (1984), 750–758; P. G. Davis, and S. D. Phinney, "Differential Effects of Two Very Low Calorie Diets on Aerobic and Anaerobic Performance," *International Journal of Obesity* 14 (1990), 779–787.
6. R. P. Heaney and D. K. Layman, "Amount and Type of Protein Influences Bone Health," *American Journal of Clinical Nutrition* 87 (2008), 1567S–1570S.
7. Ibid.

## Chapter 5: Meet Your New Friend: Fat

1. "Trends in Intake of Energy and Macronutrients—United States, 1971–2000," *Morbidity and Mortality Weekly Report (MMWR)* 53 (2004), 80–82.
2. S. Klein, and R. R. Wolfe, "Carbohydrate Restriction Regulates the Adaptive Response to Fasting," *American Journal of Physiology* 262 (1992), E631–E636.

3. D. Mozaffarian, E. B. Rimm, and D. M. Herrington, "Dietary Fats, Carbohydrate, and Progression of Coronary Atherosclerosis in Postmenopausal Women," *American Journal of Clinical Nutrition* 80 (2004), 1175–1184.

4. J. S. Volek, M. J. Sharman, and C. E. Forsythe, "Modification of Lipoproteins by Very Low-Carbohydrate Diets," *The Journal of Nutrition* 135 (2005), 1339–1342.

5. Ibid.; R. M. Krauss, "Dietary and Genetic Probes of Atherogenic Dyslipidemia," *Arteriosclerosis, Thrombosis, and Vascular Biology* 25 (2005), 2265–2272; R. M. Krauss, P. J. Blanche, R. S. Rawlings, H. S. Fernstrom, and P. T. Williams, "Separate Effects of Reduced Carbohydrate Intake and Weight Loss on Atherogenic Dyslipidemia," *American Journal of Clinical Nutrition* 83 (2006), 1025–1031.

6. C. E. Forsythe, S. D. Phinney, M. L. Fernandez, E. E. Quann, R. J. Wood, D. M. Bibus, et al., "Comparison of Low Fat and Low Carbohydrate Diets on Circulating Fatty Acid Composition and Markers of Inflammation," *Lipids* 43 (2008), 65–77.

7. R. Micha and D. Mozaffarian, "Trans Fatty Acids: Effects on Cardiometabolic Health and Implications for Policy," *Prostaglandins, Leukotrienes and Essential Fatty Acids* 79 (2008), 147–152.

8. D. Mozaffarian, A. Aro, and W. C. Willett, "Health Effects of Trans-Fatty Acids: Experimental and Observational Evidence," *European Journal of Clinical Nutrition* 63 suppl. 2 (2009), S5–S21.

9. W. S. Harris, D. Mozaffarian, E. Rimm, P. Kris-Etherton, L. L. Rudel, L. J. Appel, et al., "Omega-6 Fatty Acids and Risk for Cardiovascular Disease: A Science Advisory from the American Heart Association Nutrition Subcommittee of the Council on Nutrition, Physical Activity, and Metabolism; Council on Cardiovascular Nursing; and Council on Epidemiology and Prevention," *Circulation* 119 (2009), 902–907.

10. S. D. Phinney, A. B. Tang, S. B. Johnson, and R. T. Holman, "Reduced Adipose 18:3 Omega-3 with Weight Loss by Very Low Calorie Dieting," *Lipids* 25 (1990), 798–806.

11. C. E. Forsythe, S. D. Phinney, M. L. Fernandez, E. E. Quann, R. J. Wood, D. M. Bibus, et al., "Comparison of Low Fat and Low Carbohydrate Diets on Circulating Fatty Acid Composition and Markers of Inflammation," *Lipids* 43 (2008), 65–77.

## Chapter 6: Atkins for You: Make It Personal

1. L. E. Armstrong, D. J. Casa, C. M. Maresh, and M. S. Ganio, "Caffeine, Fluid-Electrolyte Balance, Temperature Regulation, and Exercise-Heat Tolerance," *Exercise and Sport Sciences Reviews* 35 (2007), 135–140.

2. D. L. Costill, G. P. Dalsky, and W. J. Fink, "Effects of Caffeine Ingestion on Metabolism and Exercise Performance," *Medicine & Science in Sports & Exercise* 10 (1978), 155–158.

3. S. D. Phinney, B. R. Bistrian, W. J. Evans, E. Gervino, and G. L. Blackburn, "The Human Metabolic Response to Chronic Ketosis without Caloric Restriction: Preservation of Submaximal Exercise Capability with Reduced Carbohydrate Oxidation," *Metabolism* 32 (1983), 769–776; S. D. Phinney, B. R. Bistrian, R. R. Wolfe, and G. L. Blackburn, "The Human Metabolic Response to Chronic Ketosis without Caloric Restriction: Physical and Biochemical Adaptation," *Metabolism* 32 (1983), 757–768.

4. E. E. Quann, T. P. Scheett, K. D. Ballard, M. J. Puglusi, C. E. Forsythe, B. M. Volk et al., "Carbohydrate Restriction and Resistance Training Have Additive Effects on Body Composition during Weight Loss in Men," *Journal of the American Dietetic Association* (abstract), 107(8) (April 2007), A14.

5. C. Bouchard, A. Tremblay, J. P. Despres, G. Theriault, A. Nadeau, P. J. Lupien, et al., "The Response to Exercise with Constant Energy Intake in Identical Twins," *Obesity Research* 2 (1994), 400–410.

## Chapter 7: Welcome to Phase 1, Induction

1. E. Lopez-Garcia, R. M. van Dam, S. Rajpathak, W. C. Willett, J. E. Manson, and F. B. Hu, "Changes in Caffeine Intake and Long-Term Weight Change in Men and Women," *American Journal of Clinical Nutrition* 83(2006):674–80.

2. A. G. Dulloo, C. A. Geissler, T. Horton, A. Collins, and D. S. Miller. "Normal Caffeine Consumption: Influence on Thermogenesis and Daily Energy Expenditure in Lean and Postobese Human Volunteers," *American Journal of Clinical Nutrition* 49 (1989):44–50; K. J. Acheson, B. Zahorska-Markiewicz, P. Pittet, K. Anantharaman, and E. Jéquier, "Caffeine and Coffee: Their Influence on Metabolic Rate and Substrate Utilization in Normal Weight and Obese Individuals," *American Journal of Clinical Nutrition* 33 (1980):989–997; K. J. Acheson, G. Gremaud, L. Meirim, F. Montigon, Y. Krebs, L. B. Fay, L. J. Gay, P. Schneiter, C. Schindler, and L. Tappy. "Metabolic Effects of Caffeine in Humans: Lipid Oxidation or Futile Cycling?" *American Journal of Clinical Nutrition* 79 (2004):40–46.

3. A. I. Qureshi, F. K. Suri, S. Ahmed, A. Nasar, A. A. Divani, and J. F. Kirmani, "Regular Egg Consumption Does Not Increase the Risk of Stroke and Cardiovascular Diseases," *Medical Science Monitor* 13 (2007), CR1–CR8.

4. J. S. Vander Wal, A. Gupta, P. Khosla, and N. V. Dhurandhar, "Egg Breakfast Enhances Weight Loss," *International Journal of Obesity* (London) 32 (2008), 1545–1551.

5. J. S. Vander Wal, J. M. Marth, P. Khosla, K. L. Jen, and N. V. Dhurandhar, "Short-Term Effect of Eggs on Satiety in Overweight and Obese Subjects," *Journal of the American College of Nutrition* 24 (2005), 510–515.

6. G. Mutungi, J. Ratliff, M. Puglisi, M. Torres-Gonzalez, U. Vaishnav, J. O. Leite, et al., "Dietary Cholesterol from Eggs Increases Plasma HDL Cholesterol in Overweight Men Consuming a Carbohydrate-Restricted Diet," *The Journal of Nutrition* 138 (2008), 272–276.

## Chapter 10: Keeping It Off: Lifetime Maintenance

1. J. O. Hill, and H. R. Wyatt, "Role of Physical Activity in Preventing and Treating Obesity," *Journal of Applied Physiology* 99 (2005), 765–770.

## Chapter 13: Metabolic Syndrome and Cardiovascular Health

1. B. V. Howard, J. E. Manson, M. L. Stefanick, S. A. Beresford, G. Frank, B. Jones, et al., "Low-Fat Dietary Pattern and Weight Change over 7 Years: The Women's Health Initiative Dietary Modification Trial," *The Journal of the American Medical Association* 295 (2006), 39–49; L. F. Tinker, D. E. Bonds, K. L. Margolis, J. E. Manson, B. V. Howard, J. Larson, et al., "Low-Fat Dietary Pattern and Risk of Treated Diabetes Mellitus in Postmenopausal Women: The Women's Health Initiative Randomized Controlled Dietary Modification Trial," *Archives of Internal Medicine* 168 (2008), 1500–1511; S. A. Beresford, K. C. Johnson, C. Ritenbaugh, N. L. Lasser, L. G. Snetselaar, H. R. Black, et al., "Low-Fat Dietary Pattern and Risk of Colorectal Cancer: The Women's Health Initiative Randomized Controlled Dietary Modification Trial," *The Journal of the American Medical Association* 295 (2006), 643–654; R. L. Prentice, C. A. Thomson, B. Caan, F. A. Hubbell, G. L. Anderson, S. A. Beresford, et al., "Low-Fat Dietary Pattern and Cancer Incidence in the Women's Health Initiative Dietary Modification Randomized Controlled Trial," *Journal of the National Cancer Institute* 99 (2007), 1534–1543.

2. E. S. Ford, W. H. Giles, and W. H. Dietz, "Prevalence of the Metabolic Syndrome among US Adults: Findings from the Third National Health and Nutrition Examination Survey," *The Journal of the American Medical Association* 287 (2002), 356–359.

3. G. M. Reaven, "Banting Lecture 1988: Role of Insulin Resistance in Human Disease," *Diabetes* 37 (1988), 1595–1607.

4.  S. M. Grundy, H. B. Brewer, Jr., J. I. Cleeman, S. C. Smith, Jr., and C. Lenfant, "Defini-
    tion of Metabolic Syndrome: Report of the National Heart, Lung, and Blood Institute/
    American Heart Association Conference on Scientific Issues Related to Definition,"
    *Circulation* 109 (2004), 433–438.

5.  J. S. Volek, M. J. Sharman, and C. E. Forsythe, "Modification of Lipoproteins by Very
    Low-Carbohydrate Diets," *The Journal of Nutrition* 135 (2005), 1339–1342; J. S. Volek
    and R. D. Feinman, "Carbohydrate Restriction Improves the Features of Metabolic
    Syndrome. Metabolic Syndrome May Be Defined by the Response to Carbohydrate
    Restriction," *Nutrition & Metabolism* (London) 2 (2005), 31.

6.  G. Boden, K. Sargrad, C. Homko, M. Mozzoli, and T. P. Stein, "Effect of a Low-
    Carbohydrate Diet on Appetite, Blood Glucose Levels, and Insulin Resistance in Obese
    Patients with type 2 Diabetes," *Annals of Internal Medicine* 142 (2005), 403–411.

7.  J. S. Volek, M. J. Sharman, D. M. Love, N. G. Avery, A. L. Gomez, T. P. Scheett, et
    al., "Body Composition and Hormonal Responses to a Carbohydrate-Restricted Diet,"
    *Metabolism* 51 (2002), 864–870.

8.  M. D. Jensen, M. Caruso, V. Heiling, and J. M. Miles, "Insulin Regulation of Lipolysis
    in Nondiabetic and IDDM Subjects," *Diabetes* 38 (1989), 1595–1601.

9.  S. D. Phinney, B. R. Bistrian, R. R. Wolfe, and G. L. Blackburn, "The Human Meta-
    bolic Response to Chronic Ketosis without Caloric Restriction: Physical and Biochem-
    ical Adaptation," *Metabolism* 32 (1983), 757–768.

10. M. U. Jakobsen, E. J. O'Reilly, B. L. Heitmann, M. A. Pereira, K. Balter, G. E. Fraser,
    et al., "Major Types of Dietary Fat and Risk of Coronary Heart Disease: A Pooled
    Analysis of 11 Cohort Studies," *American Journal of Clinical Nutrition* 89 (2009),
    1425–1432.

11. "Trends in Intake of Energy and Macronutrients—United States, 1971–2000," *Morbid-
    ity and Mortality Weekly Report (MMWR)* 53 (2004), 80–82.

12. L. Wang, A. R. Folsom, Z. J. Zheng, J. S. Pankow, and J. H. Eckfeldt, "Plasma Fatty
    Acid Composition and Incidence of Diabetes in Middle-Aged Adults: The Atheroscle-
    rosis Risk in Communities (ARIC) Study," *American Journal of Clinical Nutrition* 78
    (2003), 91–98; E. Warensjo, U. Riserus, and B. Vessby, "Fatty Acid Composition of
    Serum Lipids Predicts the Development of the Metabolic Syndrome in Men," *Diabeto-
    logia* 48 (2005), 1999–2005.

13. C. E. Forsythe, S. D. Phinney, M. L. Fernandez, E. E. Quann, R. J. Wood, D. M. Bibus,
    et al., "Comparison of Low Fat and Low Carbohydrate Diets on Circulating Fatty Acid
    Composition and Markers of Inflammation," *Lipids* 43 (2008), 65–77.

14. J. S. Volek, M. L. Fernandez, R. D. Feinman, and S. D. Phinney, "Dietary Carbohy-
    drate Restriction Induces a Unique Metabolic State Positively Affecting Atherogenic
    Dyslipidemia, Fatty Acid Partitioning, and Metabolic Syndrome," *Progress in Lipid Re-
    search* 47 (2008), 307–318.

15. S. K. Raatz, D. Bibus, W. Thomas, and P. Kris-Etherton, "Total Fat Intake Modifies
    Plasma Fatty Acid Composition in Humans," *The Journal of Nutrition* 131 (2001),
    231–234; I. B. King, R. N. Lemaitre, and M. Kestin, "Effect of a Low-Fat Diet on Fatty
    Acid Composition in Red Cells, Plasma Phospholipids, and Cholesterol Esters: Inves-
    tigation of a Biomarker of Total Fat Intake," *American Journal of Clinical Nutrition* 83
    (2006), 227–236.

16. John Rae, *John Rae's Correspondence with Hudson's Bay Company on the Arctic Explora-
    tion, 1844–1855* (London: Hudson's Bay Record Society, 1953).

17. E. A. Stackpole, *The Long Arctic Search: The Narrative of Lt. Frederick Schwatka* (Mys-
    tic, Connecticut: Marine Historical Association, 1965).

18. E. F. Dubois and W. S. McClellan, "Clinical Calorimetry. XLV: Prolonged Meat Di-
    ets with a Study of Kidney Function and Ketosis," *The Journal of Biological Chemistry*
    87 (1930), 651–668; V. R. Rupp, M. C. McClellan, and V. Toscani, "Clinical Calo-

rimetry. XLVI: Prolonged Meat Diets with a Study of the Metabolism of Nitrogen, Calcium, and Phosphorus," *The Journal of Biological Chemistry* 87 (1930), 669–680.

19. M. G. Peterman, "The Ketogenic Diet in Epilepsy," *The Journal of the American Medical Association* 84 (1925), 1979–1983.

20. H. F. Helmholz, "The Treatment of Epilepsy in Childhood: Five Years' Experience with the Ketogenic Diet," *The Journal of the American Medical Association* 88 (1927), 2028–2032.

21. H. M. Keith, *Convulsive Disorders in Children* (Boston: Little, Brown, 1963), 167–172.

22. E. H. Kossoff, and J. M. Rho, "Ketogenic Diets: Evidence for Short- and Long-Term Efficacy," *Neurotherapeutics* 6 (2009), 406–414.

23. M. J. Sharman, A. L. Gomez, W. J. Kraemer, and J. S. Volek, "Very Low-Carbohydrate and Low-Fat Diets Affect Fasting Lipids and Postprandial Lipemia Differently in Overweight Men," *The Journal of Nutrition* 134 (2004), 880–885.

24. M. J. Sharman, W. J. Kraemer, D. M. Love, N. G. Avery, A. L. Gomez, T. P. Scheett, et al., "A Ketogenic Diet Favorably Affects Serum Biomarkers for Cardiovascular Disease in Normal-Weight Men," *The Journal of Nutrition* 132 (2002), 1879–1885; J. S. Volek, M. J. Sharman, A. L. Gomez, T. P. Scheett, and W. J. Kraemer, "An Isoenergetic Very Low Carbohydrate Diet Improves Serum HDL Cholesterol and Triacylglycerol Concentrations, the Total Cholesterol to HDL Cholesterol Ratio and Postprandial Pipemic Responses Compared with a Low Fat Diet in Normal Weight, Normolipidemic Women," *The Journal of Nutrition* 133 (2003), 2756–2761.

25. P. P. Toth, "High-Density Lipoprotein as a Therapeutic Target: Clinical Evidence and Treatment Strategies," *American Journal of Cardiology* 96 (2005), 50K–58K; discussion at 34K–35K.

26. J. S. Volek, M. J. Sharman, and C. E. Forsythe, "Modification of Lipoproteins by Very Low-Carbohydrate Diets," *The Journal of Nutrition* 135 (2005), 1339–1342.

27. J. S. Volek et al., "An Isoenergetic Very Low Carbohydrate Diet Improves Serum HDL Cholesterol and Triacylglycerol Concentrations, the Total Cholesterol to HDL Cholesterol Ratio and Postprandial Pipemic Responses Compared with a Low Fat Diet in Normal Weight, Normolipidemic Women."

28. B. V. Howard, L. Van Horn, J. Hsia, J. E. Manson, M. L. Stefanick, S. Wassertheil-Smoller, et al., "Low-Fat Dietary Pattern and Risk of Cardiovascular Disease: The Women's Health Initiative Randomized Controlled Dietary Modification Trial," *The Journal of the American Medical Association* 295 (2006), 655–666.

29. D. M. Dreon, H. A. Fernstrom, B. Miller, and R. M. Krauss, "Low-Density Lipoprotein Subclass Patterns and Lipoprotein Response to a Reduced-Fat Diet in Men," *The FASEB Journal* 8 (1994), 121–126; D. M. Dreon, H. A. Fernstrom, P. T. Williams, and R. M. Krauss, "A Very Low-Fat Diet Is Not Associated with Improved Lipoprotein Profiles in Men with a Predominance of Large, Low-Density Lipoproteins," *American Journal of Clinical Nutrition* 69 (1999), 411–418.

30. Volek, Sharman, and Forsythe, "Modification of Lipoproteins by Very Low-Carbohydrate Diets"; R. M. Krauss, "Dietary and Genetic Probes of Atherogenic Dyslipidemia," *Arteriosclerosis, Thrombosis, and Vascular Biology* 25 (2005), 2265–2272.

31. Krauss, "Dietary and Genetic Probes of Atherogenic Dyslipidemia."

32. A. Aljada, J. Friedman, H. Ghanim, P. Mohanty, D. Hofmeyer, A. Chaudhuri, et al., "Glucose Ingestion Induces an Increase in Intranuclear Nuclear Factor κb, a Fall in Cellular Inhibitor κb, and an Increase in Tumor Necrosis Factor Alpha Messenger RNA by Mononuclear Cells in Healthy Human Subjects," *Metabolism* 55 (2006), 1177–1185; P. Mohanty, W. Hamouda, R. Garg, A. Aljada, H. Ghanim, and P. Dandona, "Glucose Challenge Stimulates Reactive Oxygen Species (ROS) Generation by Leucocytes," *Journal of Clinical Endocrinology & Metabolism* 85 (2000), 2970–2973.

33. S. E. Kasim-Karakas, A. Tsodikov, U. Singh, and I. Jialal., "Responses of Inflammatory Markers to a Low-Fat, High-Carbohydrate Diet: Effects of Energy Intake," *American Journal of Clinical Nutrition* 83 (2006), 774–779; S. Liu, J. E. Manson, J. E. Buring, M. J. Stampfer, W. C. Willett, and P. M. Ridker, "Relation between a Diet with a High Glycemic Load and Plasma Concentrations of High-Sensitivity C-reactive Protein in Middle-Aged Women," *American Journal of Clinical Nutrition* 75 (2002), 492–498.

34. M. L. Dansinger, J. A. Gleason, J. L. Griffith, H. P. Selker, and E. J. Schaefer, "Comparison of the Atkins, Ornish, Weight Watchers, and Zone Diets for Weight Loss and Heart Disease Risk Reduction: A Randomized Trial," *The Journal of the American Medical Association* 293 (2005), 43–53; K. A. McAuley, C. M. Hopkins, K. J. Smith, R. T. McLay, S. M. Williams, R. W. Taylor, et al., "Comparison of High-Fat and High-Protein Diets with a High-Carbohydrate Diet in Insulin-Resistant Obese Women," *Diabetologia* 48 (2005), 8–16.

35. P. Seshadri, N. Iqbal, L. Stern, M. Williams, K. L. Chicano, D. A. Daily, et al., "A Randomized Study Comparing the Effects of a Low-Carbohydrate Diet and a Conventional Diet on Lipoprotein Subfractions and C-reactive Protein Levels in Patients with Severe Obesity," *The American Journal of Medicine* 117 (2004), 398–405.

36. C. E. Forsythe, S. D. Phinney, M. L. Fernandez, E. E. Quann, R. J. Wood, D. M. Bibus, et al., "Comparison of Low Fat and Low Carbohydrate Diets on Circulating Fatty Acid Composition and Markers of Inflammation," *Lipids* 43 (2008), 65–77.

37. P. C. Calder, "Polyunsaturated Fatty Acids and Inflammation," *Prostaglandins, Leukotrienes and Essential Fatty Acids* 75 (2006), 197–202.

38. T. A. Jacobson, "Secondary Prevention of Coronary Artery Disease with Omega-3 Fatty Acids," *American Journal of Cardiology* 98 (2006), 61i–70i.

39. H. O. Steinberg, H. Chaker, R. Leaming, A. Johnson, G. Brechtel, and A. D. Baron, "Obesity/Insulin Resistance Is Associated with Endothelial Dysfunction. Implications for the Syndrome of Insulin Resistance," *The Journal of Clinical Investigation* 97 (1996), 2601–2610.

40. M. C. Corretti, T. J. Anderson, E. J. Benjamin, D. Celermajer, F. Charbonneau, M. A. Creager, et al., "Guidelines for the Ultrasound Assessment of Endothelial-Dependent Flow-Mediated Vasodilation of the Brachial Artery: A Report of the International Brachial Artery Reactivity Task Force," *Journal of the American College of Cardiology* 39 (2002), 257–265.

41. A. Ceriello, C. Taboga, L. Tonutti, L. Quagliaro, L. Piconi, B. Bais, et al., "Evidence for an Independent and Cumulative Effect of Postprandial Hypertriglyceridemia and Hyperglycemia on Endothelial Dysfunction and Oxidative Stress Generation: Effects of Short- and Long-Term Simvastatin Treatment," *Circulation* 106 (2002), 1211–1218; M. J. Williams, W. H. Sutherland, M. P. McCormick, S. A. De Jong, R. J. Walker, and G. T. Wilkins, "Impaired Endothelial Function Following a Meal Rich in Used Cooking Fat," *Journal of the American College of Cardiology* 33 (1999), 1050–1055; M. C. Blendea, M. Bard, J. R. Sowers, and N. Winer, "High-Fat Meal Impairs Vascular Compliance in a Subgroup of Young Healthy Subjects," *Metabolism* 54 (2005), 1337–1344.

42. Ibid.

43. M. J. Sharman, A. L. Gomez, W. J. Kraemer, and J. S. Volek, "Very Low-Carbohydrate and Low-Fat Diets Affect Fasting Lipids and Postprandial Lipemia Differently in Overweight Men," *The Journal of Nutrition* 134 (2004), 880–885; J. S. Volek, M. J. Sharman, A. L. Gomez, T. P. Scheett, and W. J. Kraemer, "An Isoenergetic Very Low Carbohydrate Diet Improves Serum HDL Cholesterol and Triacylglycerol Concentrations, the Total Cholesterol to HDL Cholesterol Ratio and Postprandial Pipemic Responses Compared with a Low Fat Diet in Normal Weight, Normolipidemic Women," *The Journal of Nutrition* 133 (2003), 2756–2761.

44. J. S. Volek, K. D. Ballard, R. Silvestre, D. A. Judelson, E. E. Quann, C. E. Forsythe, et al., "Effects of Dietary Carbohydrate Restriction versus Low-Fat Diet on Flow-Mediated Dilation," *Metabolism* 58 (2009), 1769–1777.

45. J. S. Volek and R. D. Feinman, "Carbohydrate Restriction Improves the Features of Metabolic Syndrome. Metabolic Syndrome May Be Defined by the Response to Carbohydrate Restriction," *Nutrition & Metabolism* (London) 2 (2005), 31; J. S. Volek, M. L. Fernandez, R. D. Feinman, and S. D. Phinney, "Dietary Carbohydrate Restriction Induces a Unique Metabolic State Positively Affecting Atherogenic Dyslipidemia, Fatty Acid Partitioning, and Metabolic Syndrome," *Progress in Lipid Research* 47 (2008), 307–318.

## Chapter 14: Managing Diabetes, aka the Bully Disease

1. S. D. De Ferranti, and N. Rifai, "C-reactive Protein: A Nontraditional Serum Marker of Cardiovascular Risk," *Cardiovascular Pathology* 16 (2007), 14–21; P. M. Ridker, "Inflammatory Biomarkers and Risks of Myocardial Infarction, Stroke, Diabetes, and Total Mortality: Implications for Longevity," *Nutrition Reviews* 65 (2007), S253–S259.

2. A. D. Pradhan, J. E. Manson, N. Rifai, J. E. Buring, and P. M. Ridker, "C-reactive Protein, Interleukin 6, and Risk of Developing type 2 Diabetes Mellitus," *The Journal of the American Medical Association* 286 (2001), 327–334; J. I. Barzilay, L. Abraham, S. R. Heckbert, M. Cushman, L. H. Kuller, H. E. Resnick, et al., "The Relation of Markers of Inflammation to the Development of Glucose Disorders in the Elderly: The Cardiovascular Health Study," *Diabetes* 50 (2001), 2384–2389; G. Hu, P. Jousilahti, J. Tuomilehto, R. Antikainen, J. Sundvall, and V. Salomaa, "Association of Serum C-Reactive Protein Level with Sex-Specific type 2 Diabetes Risk: A Prospective Finnish Study," *Journal of Clinical Endocrinology & Metabolism* 94 (2009), 2099–2105.

3. B. R. Bistrian, G. L. Blackburn, J. P. Flatt, J. Sizer, N. S. Scrimshaw, and M. Sherman, "Nitrogen Metabolism and Insulin Requirements in Obese Diabetic Adults on a Protein-Sparing Modified Fast," *Diabetes* 25 (1976), 494–504.

4. G. Boden, K. Sargrad, C. Homko, M. Mozzoli, and T. P. Stein, "Effect of a Low-Carbohydrate Diet on Appetite, Blood Glucose Levels, and Insulin Resistance in Obese Patients with type 2 Diabetes," *Annals of Internal Medicine* 142 (2005), 403–411.

5. M. E. Daly, R. Paisey, R. Paisey, B. A. Millward, C. Eccles, K. Williams, et al., "Short-Term Effects of Severe Dietary Carbohydrate-Restriction Advice in type 2 Diabetes—A Randomized Controlled Trial," *Diabetic Medicine* 23 (2006), 15–20.

6. E. C. Westman, W. S. Yancy, Jr., J. C. Mavropoulos, M. Marquart, and J. R. McDuffie, "The Effect of a Low-Carbohydrate, Ketogenic Diet Versus a Low-Glycemic Index Diet on Glycemic Control in type 2 Diabetes Mellitus," *Nutrition & Metabolism* (London) 5 (2008), 36.

7. A. Daly, "Use of Insulin and Weight Gain: Optimizing Diabetes Nutrition Therapy," *Journal of the American Dietetic Association* 107 (2007), 1386–1393.

8. H. C. Gerstein, M. E. Miller, R. P. Byington, D. C. Goff, Jr., J. T. Bigger, J. B. Buse, et al., "Effects of Intensive Glucose Lowering in type 2 Diabetes," *The New England Journal of Medicine* 358 (2008), 2545–2559.

9. N. G. Boule, E. Haddad, G. P. Kenny, G. A. Wells, and R. J. Sigal., "Effects of Exercise on Glycemic Control and Body Mass in type 2 Diabetes Mellitus: A Meta-analysis of Controlled Clinical Trials," *The Journal of the American Medical Association* 286 (2001), 1218–1227.

10. J. P. Bantle, J. Wylie-Rosett, A. L. Albright, C. M. Apovian, N. G. Clark, M. J. Franz, et al., "Nutrition Recommendations and Interventions for Diabetes: A Position Statement of the American Diabetes Association," *Diabetes Care* 31 suppl. 1 (2008), S61–S78.

# Index

# About the Authors

**DR. STEPHEN D. PHINNEY** has spent thirty years studying diet, exercise, essential fatty acids, and inflammation. He has held positions at the University of Vermont, the University of Minnesota, and the University of California at Davis. Following early retirement from U.C. Davis as professor of medicine, he has worked at the leadership level and later as a consultant in nutrition biotechnology. Dr. Phinney has published more than seventy papers in the peer-reviewed literature and has several patents. His medical degree is from Stanford University and his Ph.D. in nutritional biochemistry is from MIT. He also did postgraduate training at the University of Vermont and Harvard University.

**DR. JEFF S. VOLEK** is currently an associate professor and exercise and nutrition researcher in the Department of Kinesiology at the University of Connecticut. In the last decade, he has published more than two hundred peer-reviewed studies, including seminal work on low-carbohydrate diets that points to the Atkins Diet as a powerful tool to lose weight and improve metabolic health. He has provided some of the most convincing evidence that dietary fat, even saturated fat, can be healthy when consumed in the context of a lower-carbohydrate diet.

**DR. ERIC C. WESTMAN** is an associate professor of medicine at the Duke University Health System and director of the Duke Lifestyle Medicine Clinic. He combines clinical research and clinical care in lifestyle treatments for obesity, diabetes, and tobacco dependence. He is an internationally known researcher for his work on low-carbohydrate nutrition. He is currently the vice president of the American Society of Bariatric Physicians and a fellow of the Obesity Society and the Society of General Internal Medicine.

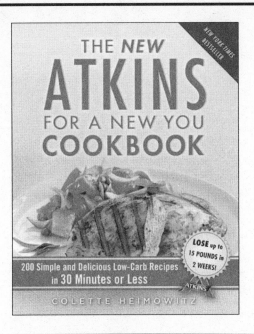
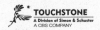